Supportive Cancer Care with Chinese Medicine

William C.S. Cho
Editor

Supportive Cancer Care with Chinese Medicine

Springer

Editor
Dr. William Chi-Shing Cho
Department Clinical Oncology
Queen Elizabeth Hospital
13/F Block R 30 Gascoigne Road
Kowloon
Hong Kong SAR
chocs@ha.org.hk

ISBN 978-90-481-3554-7 e-ISBN 978-90-481-3555-4
DOI 10.1007/978-90-481-3555-4
Springer Dordrecht Heidelberg London New York

Library of Congress Control Number: 2009942718

Printed on acid-free paper

Springer is part of Springer Science+Business Media (www.springer.com)

Preface

Cancer is a chronic disease. There are increasing cancer survivors after curative cancer treatment and this makes supportive cancer care an important area that more attention is needed. Chinese medicine has a long history of practice; it has aroused much interest from both Oriental and Western countries. A number of laboratory evidences and clinical trials demonstrated the effectiveness and efficacies of Chinese medicine for supportive cancer care. This book attempts to take a comprehensive approach to overview the different areas of Chinese medicine for supportive cancer care.

This book not only serves as an introduction to novices to the area and a useful reference for those already involved, but also serves as a stimulus to these and others to employ alternative approaches to current cancer care.

Hong Kong
December 2009

William C.S. Cho

Contents

Contributors

Ting Bao Marlene and Stewart Greenebaum Cancer Center; School of Medicine, Center for Integrative Medicine, University of Maryland, Baltimore, MD, USA, tingbao@gmail.com

Aditya Bardia School of Medicine, The Sidney Kimmel Comprehensive Cancer Center, Johns Hopkins University, Baltimore, MD, USA, adityabardia@gmail.com

Huijuan Cao Centre for Evidence Based Chinese Medicine, Beijing University of Chinese Medicine, Beijing, China, huijuancao327@hotmail.com

Dennis HT Chang College of Health and Science, Centre for Complementary Medicine Research, Penrith South DC, NSW, Australia, D.Chang@uws.edu.au

Yi-Hung Chen Graduate Institute of Acupuncture Science, China Medical University, Taichung, Taiwan, yihungchen@mail.cmu.edu.tw

Kevin W. Chen Center for Integrative Medicine, University of Maryland School of Medicine, Baltimore, MD, USA, chenke@umdnj.edu

Yung-Chi Cheng Pharmacology Department, School of Medicine, Yale University, New Haven, CT, USA, yccheng@yale.edu

Delia Chiaramonte Center for Integrative Medicine, School of Medicine, University of Maryland, Baltimore, MD, USA, dc@insightmedicalconsultants.com

Peter Dorsher Mayo Clinic, Rochester, MN, USA, dorsher.peter@mayo.edu

Thomas Efferth German Cancer Research Centre (DKFZ), Pharmaceutical Biology (C015), Heidelberg, Germany, t.efferth@dkfz.de

Edzard Ernst Complementary Medicine, Peninsula Medical School, Universities of Exeter and Plymouth, Exeter, UK, eernst@pms.ac.uk

Lixing Lao School of Medicine, Center for Integrative Medicine, University of Maryland, Baltimore, MD, USA, llao@compmed.umm.edu

Myeong S. Lee Division of Standard Research, Korea Institute of Oriental Medicine, Daejeon, South Korea; Complementary Medicine, Peninsula Medical School, Universities of Exeter and Plymouth, Exeter, UK, drmslee@gmail.com mslee@kiom.re.kr

Xun Li Centre for Evidence Based Chinese Medicine, Beijing University of Chinese Medicine, Beijing, China, tina000341@163.com

Henry LM Liang College of Health and Science, Centre for Complementary Medicine Research, University of Western Sydney, Penrith South DC, NSW, Australia, h.liang@uws.edu.au

Jaung-Geng Lin Graduate Institute of Chinese Medical Science, China Medical University, Taichung, Taiwan, jglin@mail.cmu.edu.tw.

Shwu-Huey Liu Phyto Ceutica Inc, New Haven, CT, USA, shliu@phytoceutica.com

Jianping Liu Centre for Evidence Based Chinese Medicine, Beijing University of Chinese Medicine, Beijing, China, jpliutcm@yahoo.co.uk

Zengfu Peng Mayo Clinic, Rochester, MN, USA, peng.zengfu@gmail.com

Peter K Plinkert Department of Otorhinolaryngology, Head and Neck Surgery, University Heidelberg, Heidelberg, Germany, peter.plinkert@med.uni-heidelberg.de

Stephen M. Sagar Radiation Oncology, Juravinski Cancer Centre, Hamilton, ON, Canada, stephen.sagar@jcc.hhsc.ca

Muhammad W. Saif Pharmacology Department; Department of Medicine, School of Medicine, Yale Cancer Center, Yale University, New Haven, CT, USA, wasif.saif@yale.edu

Francis Seow-Choen Seow-Choen Colorectal Centre, 3 Mt Elizabeth Medical Centre, Singapore, seowchoen@gmail.com

Serkan Sertel Department of Otorhinolaryngology, Head and Neck Surgery, University Heidelberg; German Cancer Research Centre (DKFZ), Pharmaceutical Biology (C015), Heidelberg, Germany, s.sertel@gmx.net

Zhou Shu-feng Discipline of Chinese Medicine, School of Health Sciences, RMIT University, Bundoora, VIC, Australia, shufeng.zhou@rmit.edu.au

Torkel Snellingen Centre for International Health, University of Tromsø, Tromsø, Norway, torkel.snellingen@gmail.com

Kok-Yang Tan Department of Surgery, Colorectal Service, Alexandra Hospital, Singapore, kokyangtan@gmail.com

Raimond K. Wong Department of Medicine, Juravinski Cancer Centre, McMaster University, Hamilton, ON, Canada, raimond.wong@jcc.hhsc.ca

Xiaoxiu Wu Beijing Ton-Ren-Tang Science Arts (Singapore) Co. Pte. Ltd, Singapore, sarahwu@singnet.com.sg

Ruixin Zhang School of Medicine, Center for Integrative Medicine, University of Maryland, Baltimore, MD, USA, Rzhan001@umaryland.edu

Chapter 1
Supportive Cancer Care Using Chinese Medicine

Raimond Wong and Stephen M. Sagar

Abstract Complementary and alternative medicine (CAM) has been increasingly utilized by cancer patients in developed countries. Among the various forms of CAM, traditional Chinese medicine (TCM) is one of the few that has a well constructed theoretical framework and established treatment approaches for diseases including cancer. Recent research has revealed growing evidence suggesting that TCM is effective in the supportive care of cancer patients during and after major conventional cancer treatments (surgery, chemotherapy and radiotherapy). This effectiveness seems to mediate mainly through three approaches: (1) Improvement of tumour response and reduction of adverse treatment effects; (2) Immunity modulation and (3) Enhancement of symptom control. This chapter reviewed the concepts behind which TCM treatment approaches in supportive care of cancer patients are formulated and the published laboratory and clinical evidence supporting the usage of various TCM treatment strategies including herbal medicine, acupuncture, dietary modifications and qigong energy therapy.

1.1 Introduction

Up to 80% of cancer patients in the Western countries have utilized some forms of complementary and alternative medicine (CAM) to support their conventional cancer therapies (Ernst and Cassileth 1998; Boon et al. 1999). Among the various forms of CAM, traditional Chinese medicine (TCM) is one of the few that has a well constructed theoretical framework and established treatment approaches for diseases including cancer. In its country of origin, TCM has been used for thousands of years for treating cancers and continuous to be a well accepted form of treatment modality for effective cancer management, particularly when used in combination with other major conventional therapies such as surgery, radiotherapy and chemotherapy.

R. Wong (✉)
Juravinski Cancer Centre, Hamilton, ON, L8V 5C2, Canada
e-mail: raimond.wong@jcc.hhsc.ca

W.C.S. Cho (ed.), *Supportive Cancer Care with Chinese Medicine*,
DOI 10.1007/978-90-481-3555-4_1, © Springer Science+Business Media B.V. 2010

The acceptance of TCM as an effective supportive treatment for cancer in China is likely rooted from deep cultural influence, as well as recent emerging evidence from clinical and laboratory research supports the potential effectiveness of TCM in cancer therapies. This chapter aimed to review the concepts behind which TCM treatment approaches in supportive care of cancer patients are formulated and the published laboratory and clinical evidence supporting the usage of various TCM treatment strategies including herbal medicine, acupuncture, dietary modifications and energy exercise (qigong) energy therapy.

1.2 Cancer: Traditional Chinese Medicine and Conventional Perspective

Traditional Chinese medicine recognizes the human body functions as a body-mind system that are connected not only by physical anatomical structures but also by theoretical communication channels, collectively known as meridian network, in which vital energy (qi) and informational signals (blood) travel to adjust and coordinate bodily functions (Ikemi and Ikemi 1986). This complex dynamic body-mind system constantly seeks to achieve homeostasis, a balanced and harmonic state, the healthy state. The system is also autopoietic that it can recreate itself and evolve through adaptation to changing environments with which the human body interacts. External and internal pathological factors can disturb this system resulting in a transient or permanent imbalance unhealthy state. The presence of an imbalance system can be detected through observable patterns of signs and symptoms, syndrome patterns, presented by the person affected. Similar imbalance of the system presenting with similar syndrome patterns can be caused by very different disease processes. For example, a syndrome pattern with fatigue, shortness of breath and back discomfort can be presented in a patient with a primarily untreated lung cancer or a treated colon cancer on adjuvant cancer treatment. Traditional Chinese medicine practitioners learned the skill of identifying and differentiating different syndrome patterns. Once a syndrome pattern is identified, treatment with various approaches including, dietary adjustment, qigong, massage (tuina), acupuncture and herbal treatment, that have been recorded to be effective in TCM literature, can be utilized to correct the syndrome patterns and rebalance the body-mind system. However, the process of healing of the body-mind system is also dynamic that syndrome patterns can change over time and a number of different treatment approaches for various patterns may need to be used to achieve system balance.

In conventional Western medicine, cancer is considered a development in which the transformed cells acquire the ability to disregard the constraints of its environment and the body normal control mechanisms. The main conventional treatment strategies are aimed to remove or destroy these cancer cells with aggressive approaches such as radical surgery, radiotherapy and chemotherapy that inevitably lead to treatment complications (Macek 1984; Wong et al. 2001). In TCM, however, cancer is a systemic disease from the start, and the terrain is considered to be as important as the tumour itself (Schipper et al. 1995). The development of cancer is interpreted as a result of disturbance of the balance in the body-mind system by external and/or internal pathological (emotional) factors (Macek 1984). This disturbance affects the normal flow of vital energy and informational signals through the system resulting in unchecked, prolonged stagnation of these elements that in turn, transform normal healthy tissues in the stagnated area to morbid tissues and eventually cancerous growth. Vital energy may be viewed as a model for intra- and inter-cellular information and potential energy transfer. This would correlate with the known abnormalities of signal transduction, cell contact and electrophysiology of cancer cells (Coffey 1998; Cuzick et al. 1998; Kang et al. 2000). It has also been shown that there is increased fluid content and a stagnant blood supply in malignant tumours (Baxter and Jain 1989; Sagar et al. 1993; Milosevic et al. 1998). The emphasis of internal or emotional pathological factors in TCM is intriguing. Experiments in rats show that chronic restraint stress promotes lymphocyte apoptosis through modulating *CD95* gene expression via a pathway that involves opioid receptors (Yin et al. 2000). In other words, stress can influence both the function and structure of the nervous system that, in turn, may modulate lymphocyte gene expression, thereby influencing immunity and resistance to cancer (Yin et al. 2000). It is interesting that there is correspondence with the TCM model of cancer predisposition being associated with rising qi or liver fire (representing anger), and the scientific evidence that repressed anger both suppresses the immune system and may increase the risk of breast cancer in the so-called Type C personality (Amkraut and Solomon 1972; Temoshok 1985; Temoshok and Dreher 1992). The presence of cancerous growth then further generates more disturbance in the body-mind system through additional blockage of energy and signal flow and the secretion of factors, referred as a form of toxin that critically damage healthy organ functions. This continuous system disturbance leads to diminishing healthy qi that, in conventional medicine, is related to the body nutritional, hormonal and immune status. Throughout this process, a variety of syndrome patterns can appear depending on the types of imbalance present.

It is believed that if one can strengthen and rebalance the body-mind network, the normal pattern will be restored and this will help to resolve the cancer. Traditional Chinese medicine treatments for cancer aim to assist the cancer patient to reacheive body-mind system balance and treatment approaches are individualized with constant adjustment according to the pathological patterns present and the constitutional status of the patients. Consequently, approaches include reduction of stagnation of qi and blood, information signals; elimination of toxin and enhancement of healthy qi are commonly utilized. Success of treatment is reflected with elimination of syndrome patterns; improvement in patient's symptoms and overall being. In combination with major conventional Western medicine cancer treatment strategies, these TCM approaches have been shown to support cancer patients through their treatment with improved symptoms control, enhanced cancer treatment response and improved survival.

1.3 Traditional Chinese Medicine and Surgery

Surgery is the commonest strategy in managing cancer. In early stage where cancers are confined to an anatomical location, most cancers, for example, breast, lung, prostate and colorectal cancers, can be effectively managed or even cured with radical surgery. However, surgical procedures usually involve analgesia and destruction of normal anatomical structures. From a TCM perspective, any major surgery weakens the body, the healthy qi, causing a reduction in the immune function and generating imbalance of the body-mind network. Thus it is important to maintain normal functioning of the body-mind network through surgery to allow the system imbalance to readjust and the healthy qi to recover.

1.3.1 Herbal

1.3.1.1 Preoperative Nutritional and General Status Improvement

A number of strategies have been advocated in TCM practice to prepare patients for their up-coming surgery. The use of TCM formulas such as Shiquan Dabao Decoction (Decoction of Ten Powerful Tonics), containing herbs: *Panax ginseng* (ginseng), *Angelica sinensis* (Chinese angelica root), *Paeonia lactiflora* (white peony root), *Atractylodes macrocephala* (bighead atractylodes rhizome), *Poria cocos* (tuckahoe), *Cinnamomum cassia* (cinnamom twig), *Astragalus membranaceus* (astragalus root), *Ligusticum chuanxiong* (chuanxiong rhizome), *Glycyrrhiza uarlensis* (licorice root) and *Rheum palumatum* (rhubarb), that traditionally used to improve the healthy qi of the body has been suggested in most TCM practice. There is however, no published clinical trial to examine its usage in preoperative settings in cancer patients. In an in vivo study, this formula has been shown to enhance T-cell immunity, through intestinal Peyer's patches stimulation, and this function correlates with the description of enhancing healthy qi and exert anti-tumour and anti-metastatic effects (Ohnishi et al. 1998; Dai et al. 2001). Moreover, surgery always causes some loss in blood and usage of TCM formulas, such as the Decoction of Ten Powerful Tonics, which also possesses hematopoietic effects, is also practiced preoperatively (Ohnishi et al. 1990).

Traditional Chinese medicine also recognizes the importance of the ability to absorb nutrition. Without this ability, even with the provision of rich nutritional food, normal bodily functions will not be sustainable and will result in a decline of the general status and poor disease prognosis. In patients with suboptimal nutritional status due to systemic effects of cancer where poor appetite is one of the main symptoms, TCM practice has engaged herbal treatments to improve patients' nutritional and overall performance status for enhancing their tolerance to invasive surgical procedures such as radical cancer surgery. Commonly used TCM formulas including the popular Buzhong Yiqi Decoction (Decoction for Reinforcing Middle-energizer and Replenishing Qi) containing *Codonopsis pilosula* (dangshen), tuckahoe, bighead atractylodes rhizome, Chinese angelica root, stir-fried *Setaria italica* (millet sprout) and stir-fried *Hordeum vulgre* (malt), astragalus root, *Cimicifuga heracleifolia* (buybane rhizome), *Bupleurum chinense* (thorowax root), *Amomum villosum* (villous amomum fruit) and licorice root. The potential usefulness of this formula in preoperative intervention has not been evaluated clinically, but in a randomized controlled study of patients suffering from cancer related anorexia-cachexia, patients randomized to this formula showed greater improvement of body weight, increased food intake and better quality of life when compared to controlled group. Its effect is comparable to a third group randomized to medroxyprogesterone, a hormone that has been a standard conventional treatment for cancer-related anorexia. The formula however had not induced any side effects while medroxyprogesterone usage was associated with fluid retention, vaginal bleeding and hypertension resulting in cessation of therapy in a few patients (Cai 2003). This preoperative intervention approach is thus worth further research for its potential in improving patient's tolerance to surgery.

Cautions have been raised regarding the use of herbs in the perioperative period, particularly for the fear of adverse events caused by the interactions between herbs with anaesthesia and with blood coagulation mechanisms. For example, herbs including bighead atractylodes rhizome, *Salvia miltiorrhiza* (red sage root) and chuanxiong rhizome have been found to have anticoagulation effects, while herbs like Chinese angelica root, *Carthamus tinctorius* (safflower), *Curcuma longa* (common turmeric) and *Leonurus heterophyllus* (motherwort herb) affect thrombus formation. *Pueraria lobata* (pueraria root), *Cornus officinalis* (Asian cornelian cherry fruit), *Corydalis turtschaninovii* (corydalis tuber), *Ginkgo biloba* (ginkgo seed) and *Epimedium grandiflorum* (epimedium) inhibit platelets aggregation. Thus, it is generally recommended to stop herbal consumption for at least 2 weeks before the surgery (Zhu 1998; Ang-Lee et al. 2001).

1.3.2 Acupuncture and Other Approaches

1.3.2.1 Reduction of Acute Postoperative Nausea and Pain

Unlike herbal treatment, a variety of acupuncture and related techniques have been evaluated for its effectiveness in the perioperative period for reduction of postoperative nausea and pain.

Postoperative nausea and vomiting is common among cancer patients following anaesthesia and surgery. Acupuncture treatment at acupoint PC6 has been shown to increase the anti-emetic effect of drugs for peri-operative and chemotherapy-induced nausea and vomiting (Dundee et al. 1986, 1989). Innovative randomized single-blind controlled trials have since confirmed these results (Al-Sadi et al. 1997; Schlager et al. 1998; Lee and Done 1999) and led to the NIH (US) consensus statement that, "acupuncture is a proven effective treatment modality for nausea and vomiting" (NIH Consensus Development Panel on Acupuncture 1998). Stimulation of PC6 may be done more conveniently with a small transcutaneous nerve stimulation (TENS) device, such as the Reliefband, which is worn like a wrist watch. In a recent Cochrane database systematic review of randomized trials examine stimulation of PC6 using invasive or non-invasive techniques was showed to be effective in preventing postoperative nausea and vomiting. Side effects of PC6 stimulation were minor and there was no significant difference between the effectiveness of PC6 stimulation compared to antiemetic drug treatments (Lee and Fan 2009).

1.3.2.2 Reduction of Analgesia Requirement

Acupuncture was first known to the conventional medicine world by its demonstrated analgesic property. Subsequent studies have suggested possible mechanisms through induced endorphin secretion and modification of thalamus and cortical activities in functional MRI studies (Lin and Chen 2008; Luo and Wang 2008). Intraoperative use of acupuncture and related techniques has been examined in a few randomized trials. In one trial, patients undergoing hip arthroplasty were randomized to auricular acupuncture and sham control. The treatment group was treated with indwelling needles to lung, shenman, forehead and hip points while the control group received needles to four non-acupuncture points on the helix. The results showed a reduction of 21% of fentanyl during surgery in the treatment group (Usichenko et al. 2006). Several other randomized studies also support the effect of auricular acupuncture on anaesthetic requirements (Greif et al. 2002; Taguchi et al. 2002). However, acupuncture on a few selected body acupuncture points was not shown to be effective in reducing anaesthetic requirement (Morioka et al. 2002).

1.3.2.3 Acute Postoperative Pain Control

Acute postoperative pain control after cancer surgery has been a common subject of recent acupuncture studies. In a controlled trial of breast cancer patients after breast cancer surgery and axillary lymph node resection, acupuncture was found to significant improve pain control and range of shoulder movement compared to a controlled group without acupuncture. The importance of individualized selected acupuncture points in the successful management of patients was emphasized (He et al. 1999).

Post thoracotomy pain is another pain condition that the analgesic effect of acupuncture has been examined in randomized controlled trials. In one trial, body acupuncture points including LI4, GB34, TE8 and GB36 on the same side of the thoracotomy. These points were chosen for its recognized influence on the chest wall, upper body and pain control. Treatments were given with electrical stimulation on the first 7 postoperative days. A sham group using non-piercing needles was used as control. Analgesic usage on postoperative day 2 was found to be significantly lowered than controlled group and there was a trend of lower pain score in the treatment group from day 3 to 6 but it was not significant statistically (Wong et al. 2006). In another trial, a more invasive approach was used. Two groups of patients were treated with implanted intradermal needles or sham needles prior to thoracotomy. The needles were left for 4 weeks postoperatively. The study result was a negative outcome but was criticized for not a common TCM acupuncture practice (Deng et al. 2008b).

Evaluation of acupuncture effect in acute postoperative pain control continuous to be hampered by problems of appropriate sham control, placebo effects and multiple confounding variables. With the increase in evidence from randomized trials demonstrating the effectiveness of acupuncture and related techniques in postoperative pain control, acupuncture will likely be continuously used and examined as a component of acute pain control strategies after cancer surgery (Sun et al. 2008). The types of acupuncture techniques to be utilized should be carefully chosen to balance the ease of delivery and expected effectiveness based on TCM principles and practice.

1.3.2.4 Improvement of Postoperative Urinary Dysfunction

Apart from pain control, other symptoms arising in the acute post operative period has also been treated with acupuncture techniques. Patients underwent pelvic surgery commonly experience temporary urinary dysfunction that may lengthen hospital stay. In a couple of reported studies, acupuncture treatments using electrical stimulation, on body acupuncture points including ST36, SP6, TE5, ST28 and ST29, have been shown to improve urinary flow rate, lower residual bladder volume and shorten post operative hospital stay compared to controls (Shi et al. 2008; Yi et al. 2008). Another report on patients with urinary retention after rectal cancer surgery, acupuncture using various body points aimed to strengthen the flow of qi through Bladder meridian and improve water flow, was shown to be effective in relieving urinary retention in over 90% of patients (Dong et al. 2003). However, all studies still involved small number of patients and had suboptimal study design.

1.4 Traditional Chinese Medicine and Radiotherapy

Radiotherapy is one of main conventional treatment modalities for cancer. Upward to 50% or more of cancer patients undergo radiotherapy through the course of their diseases. For radiotherapy to be effective, the availability of optimal oxygen level among the treated cells is important since cancer cells that survive in a low oxygen tension environment are found to be more resistant to radiotherapy and some types of chemotherapy (Brizel et al. 1997; Fyles et al. 1998). However, it has been shown that there is increased fluid content and a stagnant blood supply in malignant tumours (Sagar et al. 1993; Milosevic et al. 1998; Baxter and Jain 1989). The microcirculation within a tumour is also very abnormal in functions and in anatomical distribution, as a result, there are regions within the tumour where the blood flow is sluggish. The impaired blood circulation leads to areas of poor oxygenation in the tumour and can induce radio-resistance. In TCM, stagnation of blood and vital energy is classically considered to be associated with tumours and conceptually describes the similar phenomena observed in recent scientific research.

Radiotherapy treatment typically creates a sense of warmth, dryness and ultimate atrophy of the irradiated volume of tissue. This leads to TCM interpretation that therapeutic radiation is a form of external heat factor that can drive away stagnated cold blood seen in tumour and has the effect of drying up the fluid accumulated in tumour causing a regression in its size. However, these effects can also affect irradiated normal tissue resulting in complications that characterized by dryness and shrinkage similar to what is observed in fibrotic tissue. Thus therapeutic radiation is also viewed as a form of heat toxin that can consume body fluid and blood. If excessively delivered to a particular area of the body, can affect the person not only locally but also systemically presenting with general sense of warmth, dryness, red tongue, irritability, fatigue and ultimately a reduction in the healthy qi. These observations are supported by the recent finding of radiation-induced endothelial cells damage resulting in initial vessel dilatation, leakage with tissue edema and eventual vessel collapse and consequent ischemic necrosis of tissue (Girinsky 2000). Several studies also reported the suppressive effect of the body immune system by therapeutic local radiotherapy also support the concept that radiation heat toxin can gradually consume the healthy qi of the person treated (Thomas et al. 1971; Hoppe et al. 1977; Uh et al. 1994).

Traditional Chinese medicine treatment strategies in combination with radiotherapy thus focus on the reduction in stagnation of blood and vital energy accumulated in the tumour and in facilitating the elimination of accumulated heat toxin in the normal tissue.

1.4.1 Herbal

1.4.1.1 Enhancement of Radiotherapy Response

Destagnation or detoxification herbs are used to promote the movement of blood and vital energy that has accumulated in pathological tissue, such as malignant tumors. Interestingly, the use of anticoagulants, such as heparin and coumadin (warfarin), as an adjunctive treatment to chemotherapy, has been shown to prevent the development of blood-borne metastases in animal laboratory studies, and to improve the survival of cancer patients in clinical studies (Lebeau et al. 1994; Hejna et al. 1999).

Traditional Chinese medicinal herbs have been extensively investigated in the laboratory and are known to have multiple pharmacological effects (Wang et al. 1992; Tode et al. 1993; Lau et al. 1994; Boik 1996a, b; Shoemaker et al. 2005; Yance and Sagar 2006). Many of these herbs are also proving to be anti-angiogenic agents that may improve tumour blood flow and oxygenation status (Yance and Sagar 2006). There are plenty of examples of TCM herbs that have destagnation properties and process multiple anticancer therapeutic properties. Ginseng has anti-tumour activity, inhibits platelet aggregation, and inhibits chemotherapy-induced immunosuppression. Licorice root acid has anti-tumour activity, is anti-inflammatory through increasing serum cortisol, and also increases natural killer (NK) cell activity against cancer cells. Astragalus root is a powerful stimulator of the immune system, has anti-tumour activity and inhibits platelet aggregation. Chinese angelica root stimulates the immune system, has anti-tumour activity, inhibits platelet aggregation, and inhibits vascular permeability. Bighead atractylodes rhizome has anti-tumour activity, and is an anti-thrombotic and fibrinolytic agent. Ginkgo seed has multiple effects including inhibition of platelet activation factor (PAF), stimulation of the immune system, fibrinolysis and anti-thrombosis, scavenging of free radicals, and dilation of blood vessels to increase perfusion. The effects on the haemostatic coagulation system are intriguing as more evidence emerges suggesting the existence of an interactive roles of the bone marrow, hemopoietic system, and angiogenesis in the progression of cancer (Yance and Sagar 2006).

The possible usefulness of destagnation herbs was demonstrated in a randomized controlled clinical trial evaluating the combined modality treatment of Chinese herbal destagnation formula and radiotherapy in patients with nasopharyngeal carcinoma (Xu et al. 1989). In this trial, 90 patients received combined herbal and radiotherapy compared to 98 patients who were randomized to receive radiotherapy alone. The ingredients of the herbal formula included astragalus root, *Paeonia veitchii* (red peony root), chuanxiong rhizome, Chinese angelica root, *Prunus persica* (peach seed), safflower, *Spatholobus suberectus* (suberect stem), pueraria root, *Citrus reticulata* (green tangerine orange peel) and dangshen. The combined treatment group showed a statistically significant increase in local tumour control and overall 5-year survival as compared with the group treated with radiotherapy alone. The rate of local recurrence in the intervention group was halved from 29% in those receiving radiotherapy alone, to 14% in the group receiving destagnation herbs as well. The 5-year disease free survival was increased from 37% in the control group to 53% in the group receiving destagnation herbs. It is postulated that this herbal destagnation formula may have improved tumour microcirculation and increased tumour blood flow leading to an improvement in the oxygen tension inside the tumour. The oxygen tension increases the radiosensitivity of the tumour. In other words, the destagnation formula has acted as a radiation sensitizer. Results from several other randomized controlled studies using similar TCM destagnation and blood invigorating herbs in combination with radiotherapy supported the effectiveness of this strategy (Li et al. 2002; Liu et al. 2002).

In animal experiments, ginkgo seed has also been shown to increase perfusion and radiosensitivity (Kleijnen and Knipschild 1992; Ha et al. 1996). Chinese herbs, such as red sage root, which inhibit tumour oedema caused by free radicals, may also increase tumour perfusion, oxygenation and response to radiotherapy (Sagar et al. 1995; Kuang et al. 1996). Other herbs may directly sensitize neoplastic cells to radiotherapy (Sun et al. 1994). Some herbs may protect normal tissues from radiotherapy. For example, ginseng and *Panax quinquefolium* (American ginseng) water extract (Rh2 ginsenoside) radioprotect through mechanisms involving antioxidative and immunomodulating properties (Lee et al. 2005a). The presence of a variety of chemicals in a single herb; the common usage of multiple herbs for therapy and the multiple pharmacological actions of a single herb may explain the observed multiple benefits of herbal treatment, in terms of radiosensitization of tumour; improved treatment tolerance and reduction of treatment side effects. The subtle balance between anticancer effects and protection of normal tissue, is however still unknown.

1.4.1.2 Improvement of Symptoms in Radiation Enteritis

Apart from radiation sensitization for cancer treatment, TCM herbal treatments have also been reported to successfully treat radiation-induced side effects. Radiation-induced enteritis is a common side effect in patient received radiotherapy for abdominal or pelvic cancers presenting with symptoms of abdominal cramps, diarrhoea, feacal incontinence and tenesmus. When chronic, ischemic changes and adhesions of intestine can occur and can severely affect patients' quality of life. Treatment of radiation enteritis has been mainly for symptomatic relief with dietary adjustments and medications. A TCM formula, known in Kampo medicine practice in Japan, called Daikenchuto that consists of three herbs: dry *Zingiber officinale* (ginger), ginseng and *Zanthoxylum bungeanum* (peppertree pricklyash seed) traditionally used for treating abdominal pain and distension has been reported to be effective in alleviating this condition (Takeda et al. 2008). This report illustrated a practical approach in the choice of herbal formulas for treatment. The herbal formula should best be founded on traditional TCM reported experience. This should be further supported by evidence of its effectiveness in related conditions and the presence of possible underlying mechanisms by which the herbal ingredients may exert their effects.

Ginger has been shown to increase intestinal blood flow and enhance bowel motility. Ginseng possesses anti-inflammatory effects and may reduce radiation-induced bowel inflammation and peppertree pricklyash seed induces intestinal neural acetylcholine release promoting intestinal motility (Satoh et al. 2001; Murata et al. 2002; Hofseth and Wargovich 2007).

Traditional Chinese medicine enemas have also been reported to be helpful in managing radiation bowel injury. A solution prepared mainly with astragalus root, bighead atractylodes rhizome, dangshen and *Coptis chinensis* (coptis root) has been shown to induce symptom improvement in over 90% of patients (Ding et al. 2004). Possible mechanism may involve the suppression of nitric oxide production resulting in less inflammation of the bowel mucosa. Experiments using this herbal solution on irradiated rat bowel mucosa showed a significant increase in the number and height of bowel villi suggesting mucosal cells regeneration was promoted (Ding et al. 2003).

1.4.1.3 Prevention and Treatment of Radiation Pneumonitis

Despite the advance in radiotherapy techniques for locally advanced lung cancer, radiation pneumonitis remains the most serious and often dose-limiting complication. Traditional Chinese herbal treatment may be able to prevent or treat radiation pneumonitis. A proprietary TCM herbal infusion preparation, Shenqi Fuzheng Injection, with dangshen and astragalus root as the main components was evaluated in a randomized study. Fifty-eight lung cancer patients were randomized to a control group treated with radiotherapy alone and a treatment group with herbal infusion given on day 3 after radiotherapy initiation to 1 week after radiotherapy completion. Radiation pneumonitis of grade 2 or greater, according to RTOG criteria, was significantly less than the control group. Plasma level of TNF-alpha and ratio of IL-10/TNF-alpha was also significantly lower in the treatment group compared to that of control suggesting the herbal injection may be able to down regulate cytokines and thus effective in preventing and treating radiation pneumonitis (Liu et al. 2007). In another randomized study in patients with established radiation pneumonitis, Shenqi Fuzheng Injection combining with antibiotics and hormone therapy has been shown to shorten pneumonitis and enhance immune function in patients compared to controls (Zheng et al. 2007). Similar effectiveness in treating radiation pneumonitis was also reported using a different an oral TCM preparation, Qingjin Runfei Decoction. This preparation was formulated, according to TCM herbal properties, to literally clear the lung dryness and smooth lung function (Zhang et al. 2007b).

1.4.1.4 Other Symptoms

Other radiation-induced symptoms that TCM herbal treatment has been shown to be effective include radiation-induced oral mucositis, visual pathway damage, dermatitis and symptom patterns developed during radiotherapy for nasopharyngeal cancer (Xu et al. 2003; Ma et al. 2007; Song et al. 2007; Wu et al. 2007). The successful results of these studies again emphasized the importance in choosing TCM herbal formulas based on observed herbal properties and the symptom pattern differentiation to be treated. However, studies involving proprietary herbal combinations reporting without the herbal ingredients listed continue to be a significant problem in scientifically evaluation and the acceptance of study results, and represent one of the road blocks in understanding and advancing the science of TCM herbal treatments.

1.4.2 Acupuncture and Other Related Techniques

Although acupuncture has been shown in studies to be a useful modality for a variety of symptoms in cancer patients, along with other interventions, clinical studies focused in acupuncture for radiation-induced symptoms are scarce (Thompson and Filshie 1998). The fewer reports may be due to the relatively under utilization of acupuncture by patients undergoing radiotherapy. A recent study showed that there was only 1.9% of surveyed cancer patients used acupuncture (Swarup et al. 2006). Direct radiotherapy induced symptoms that have been reported to benefit from acupuncture include xerostomia, post irradiation masseter muscle contracture and radiation proctitis. Among these reports, radiation-induced xerostomia has been the most studied.

1.4.2.1 Reduction of Symptoms in Radiation-induced Xerostomia

Radiation-induced xerostomia is one of the distressing late side effects seen in patients who received radiotherapy that involved the parotid glands. Patients with this condition suffer loss of taste and difficulty in speaking and swallowing. Recently, acupuncture treatment has been found to increase blood flow to the parotid glands and may stimulate tissue regeneration in parotid glands damaged by radiotherapy (Talal et al. 1992; Blom et al. 1992, 1993; Rydholm and Strang 1999). A randomized controlled trial of 38 patients with radiation xerostomia was reported from the Karolinska Institute (Sweden) (Blom et al. 1996). Subjects were randomized to either deep acupuncture treatment or superficial acupuncture treatment. The latter group was used as the control, despite previous evidence that superficial acupuncture treatment can have a certain degree of effectiveness and should not be used as a control in acupuncture treatment trials. In this study it was found that in both groups, there was more than a 20% increase in saliva flow rate in more than 50% of patients. In the deep acupuncture group, 68% of patients demonstrated an increase in salivary flow rate. Changes in the control group were smaller and appeared after a longer latency phase. Moreover, patients in the treatment group reported less dryness, less hoarseness and improved taste. In another study, 70 patients with xerostomia due to either Sjögren's syndrome or irradiation were treated with acupuncture (Blom and Lundeberg 2000). A statistically significant increase in unstimulated and stimulated salivary flow rates (SFR) was found in all patients immediately after acupuncture treatment, and up to 6 months follow-up. After a review at 3 years, those patients who chose to be treated with additional acupuncture demonstrated a consistently higher median SFR, compared to those not having additional acupuncture. Despite, some limitations in the study's design, both studies provide evidence suggesting acupuncture can be effective in treating radiation-induced xerostomia, with minimal side effects. In a prospective single cohort, visual analogue assessed study of acupuncture in palliative care patients with xerostomia, there was a highly significant alleviation of subjective xerostomia (Rydholm and Strang 1999). Other studies are confirming the clinical use of acupuncture for relief of radiation-induced xerostomia (Johnstone et al. 2001; Braga et al. 2008; Cho et al. 2008).

At the Juravinski Cancer Centre (Canada), a phase I and II study of acupuncture like (AL)-TENS in the treatment of radiation-induced xerostomia has been completed (Wong et al. 2003). Forty five patients were randomized into three treatment groups with AL-TENS stimulation using the Codetron to three different sets of acupuncture points (Group A: CV24, ST36, SP6, LI4; Group B: CV24, ST36, SP6, PC6; and Group C, CV24, ST5, ST6, SP6, PC6). The goal of this study was to determine the optimum pattern of stimulation (based on TCM theory) prior to designing a placebo-controlled study. AL-TENS treatment was administered twice a week for a total of 12 weeks. Unstimulated and stimulated salivary flow rates before, during and after treatment were measured, and a survey of the patients' quality of life was assessed during a follow up of 1 year. There was an improvement in xerostomia symptoms with a mean increase in the visual analogue score at 3 and 6 months after treatment completion. All patients demonstrated a significant increase in the mean basal and citric-acid primed saliva production. The results suggest that AL-TENS treatment improves saliva production and related symptoms in patients suffering from radiation-induced xerostomia. Treatment effects are sustained at least 6 months after completion of treatment. Built on the results of this phase I/II study, a randomized phase III trials is currently underway by the Radiation Therapy Oncology Group, comparing AL-TENS with oral pilocarpine in established radiation-induced xerostomia patients. A recent fMRI study showed activation of the insula region of the brain, the location associated with gustatory function suggesting one of the possible mechanisms of acupuncture effectiveness in xerostomia is the stimulation of the central nervous system that may be followed by a cascade of physiological effects (Deng et al. 2008a).

1.4.2.2 Reduction of Radiation Proctitis Symptoms

Only one reported study examined the use of acupuncture in radiation proctitis. In this study varies acupuncture points were used to treat acute radiation proctitis in cervix cancer patients undergoing radiotherapy and reported 73% complete response rate (Zhang 1987). At the Juravinski Cancer Centre (Canada), acupuncture has been used for patients who suffered from tenesmus, pressure sensation and increased mucous secretion per rectum during preoperative combined chemradiotherapy for locally advanced rectal cancer. In 15 symptomatic rectal cancer patients treated using only the acupuncture point GV20 weekly during the third to fifth week of radiotherapy, all patients reported marked improvement of their symptoms after one or two treatments (unpublished data). GV20 is classically used to treat organs prolapsed and to limit leakage symptoms. It is commonly indicated in treating bleeding haemorrhoid.

1.5 Traditional Chinese Medicine and Chemotherapy and/or Biological Modifiers

Chemotherapy and biological modifiers have been one of the main treatment modalities for many types of cancers. Increasingly, multiagents are being used and are found to be more effective than single agent therapy. However, the severity of side effects almost always positively correlates with the number of agents used and is often dose limiting. Minimizing chemotherapy and biological modifier treatment side effects can improve dose tolerance and may translate to better treatment outcome and better patients' quality of life. Traditional Chinese medicine treatments have been shown to potentially improve not only treatment side effects but also act synergistically with chemotherapy and other agents against cancer cells.

1.5.1 Herbal

1.5.1.1 Synergistic Actions Against Cancer Cells

Many TCM herbs contain a variety of chemicals that may act synergistically to increase tumour cell death (apoptosis), inhibit tumour cell division, increase the proportion of immune cells within the tumour, and increase blood flow through the tumour (Motoo and Sawabu 1994; Yano et al. 1994; So et al. 1997; Ikemoto et al. 2000; Liu et al. 2000). These observable changes were found to be associated with changes in the balance of cytokines and other communicating peptides released by immune cells, resulting in a reduction in the proliferation of tumour cells and an increase in tumour cell death, whilst minimizing many side effects for normal tissues. This synergy appears to be secondary to inducing apoptosis, anti-angiogenesis, antagonism of the viral genome, and induction of an immune response. In addition, some herbs can reverse multidrug resistance (Zhou and Liu 2005).

Extracts of multiple Chinese herbs traditionally used for anti-cancer therapy, such as *Anemarrhena asphodeloides* (wind-weed rhizome), *Artemisia argyi* (argyi wormwood leaf), *Commiphora molmol* (myrrh), *Potentilla indica* (mock strawberry), *Gleditsia sinensis* (Chinese honeylocust spine), *Ligustrum lucidum* (glossy privet fruit), rhubarb, *Rubia cordifolia* (India madder root), *Salvia chinensis* (Chinese sage), *Scutellaria barbata* (barbat skullcap), *Uncaria rhynchophylla* (uncaria stem with hooks), *Vaccaria segelalis* (cow-fat seed), demonstrate growth inhibitory activity against various cancer cell lines, but limited inhibitory activity against normal cell proliferation (Shoemaker et al. 2005). Coptis root induces cell growth arrest and apoptosis by up regulating interferon-beta and TNF-alpha in human breast cancer cells (Kang et al. 2005). Recent meta-analyses confirm the utility for Chinese herbs to both enhance the control of particular cancers (particularly viral-induced cancers such as hepatocellular carcinoma and nasopharyngeal carcinoma) and reduce side effects of chemotherapy (Shu et al. 2005; Taixiang et al. 2005; Meng et al. 2008; Cho and Chen 2009a, b). Laboratory studies suggest that some herbs increase the effectiveness of conventional chemotherapy. For example, red ginseng acidic polysaccharide (RGAP) increases the cytotoxicity of paclitaxel (Shin et al. 2004) and *Phellinus linteus* (sanghuang) enhances the cytotoxicity of doxorubicin (Collins et al. 2006). A meta-analysis of Astragalus-based Chinese herbs and platinum-based chemotherapy for advanced non-small-cell lung cancer indicates a promising therapeutic gain (McCulloch et al. 2006). Occasionally herbs alone are associated with tumour regression. In one report, a 51-year old lady with pathological proven squamous cell carcinoma of the lung attained complete regression with sole treatment using a combination of herbs "*Hedyotis diffusa* (spreading hedyotis herb), *Ophiopogon japonicus* (dwarf lilyturf tuber root), *Taraxacum mongolicum* (dandelion herb), *Panax notoginseng* (notoginseng), *Cremastra variabilis* (bulb of Chinese tulip), American ginseng, *Houttuynin cordata* (heartleaf houttuynia herb), *Fritillaria cirrhosa* (fritillary bulb), *Pinellia ternata* (pinellia tuber)" (Liang et al. 2004). This reported anecdote is unusual, but deserves further exploration. More clinical trials need to be done to further evaluate this promising role of herbs in potentially improving the therapeutic gain.

1.5.1.2 Reduction of Chemotherapy Side Effects

Cancer patients receiving chemotherapy develop common side effects including gastrointestinal upset with nausea, vomiting, oral mucositis and diarrhoea; myelosuppression with lowered blood counts resulting in anaemia, bleeding and increased risk of infection; skin toxicities with hair loss and dermatitis; poor appetite with weight loss and general fatigue and poor quality of life. From TCM perspective, most chemotherapies are causing disturbance in the balance of the body-mind network, affecting mainly the vital energy of the spleen and kidney system resulting in syndrome patterns such as deficient spleen qi that manifests as diarrhoea; heart fire manifests as stomatitis; disturbed spleen and stomach qi with nausea and vomiting and physically as damage to the stomach and intestinal lining (Rosenberg 1997). With weakening of the whole body-mind network, a reduction in the healthy qi is resulted with suppression of the immune system and a deterioration of the general status of patients.

1.5.1.3 Prevention and Reduction of Myelosuppression

Traditional Chinese medicine associates the depressed immunity and susceptibility to infection and cancer progression with the weakening of the body healthy qi. Treatment approaches using herbs are focused on the qi strengthening potential either by the herbs alone or by the ability of the herbs to strengthen the spleen function to improve nutrients absorption and transformation and to strengthen the kidney function that facilitate the formation of blood elements. This may be viewed as correcting the basic imbalance of the body-mind communication network and is reflected by an enhancement in immunity. This is called reinforce the healthy qi (Fuzheng) treatment and is mediated by specific group of TCM herbs collectively called Fuzheng herbs. Examples of these herbs include ginseng, *Ganoderma lucidum* (lucid ganoderma), astragalus root, Chinese angelica root, *Cordyceps sinensis* (cordyceps) and *Lycium barbarum* (wolfberry fruit), have been shown to enhance the body's defence mechanisms. Clinical studies, including two randomized trials, have found that cell counts of NK cells and CD4 (Th) lymphocytes were increased with the use of Fuzheng herbs (Ning et al. 1988; Ling et al. 1989; Chen 1990; Yu et al. 1990; Hou et al. 1991; Rao et al. 1991; Li 1992; Yu et al. 1993; Cao et al. 1994; Cheng 1994; Horie et al. 1994; Lin et al. 1995). These immunocytes are known to attack cancer cells. Many of these herbs are associated with an increase in cytokines, such as interferon and interleukin (Kawakita et al. 1990; Jin et al. 1994; Feng et al. 1995). In a study of gastric cancer patients, increased survival was found in the combined treatment group (receiving both Fuzheng herbs and chemotherapy) as compared with the chemotherapy-alone group (Wang 1990).

Single herb, particularly medicinal mushrooms, such as lucid ganoderma, cordyceps and *Lentinus edodes* (Shiitake mushroom), rather than a formula, have been used clinically in cancer patients for its immune enhancement and anti-cancer properties. Data from controlled clinical trials suggest that medicinal mushrooms may be beneficial as adjunctive anticancer therapies (Lin 2005; Matsui et al. 2002). A randomized controlled trial in colorectal cancer patients receiving curative resection compared adjuvant chemotherapy alone to chemotherapy plus an extract (PSK) from the fungus *Coriolus versicolor* (multicolored polypore). Both disease-free and overall survival was significantly higher in the group that received PSK (Mitomi et al. 1992). Medicinal mushrooms contain a class of polysaccharides known as β-glucans that promote antitumour immunity. They may act synergistically with some of the new therapeutic antibodies and chemotherapy agents and protect normal marrow (Cheung et al. 2002; Lin et al. 2004). However, in most clinical trials involving cancer patients, the effect on immune functions rather than the blood profile of cancer patients were examined. For instance, in one randomized trial in which lucid ganoderma extract capsules were used on 68 lung cancer patients. Significant increases of total T-cells and NK cells and a slight increase of CD4/CD8 ratios were found in the treatment group compared with the placebo group. The quality of life, in terms of Karnofsky scores, was improved in ~65% of the patients (Gao et al. 2003). Extracts of various medicinal mushrooms can be easily obtained over-the-counter and it is predictable that many patients may use these extracts during their cancer treatments despite the lack of well controlled clinical trials. Although, medicinal mushrooms have been regarded as safe in most TCM practice, recent data has emerged that cautions are needed in using such extracts. In one study, lucid ganoderma extracts were found to be toxic to some human peripheral blood mononuclear cells and this may be significant in patients receiving chemotherapy (Gill and Rieder 2008).

A number of clinical trials, some with randomized controlled design, have been conducted to evaluate the benefits of TCM herbal formulas in patients having chemotherapy. Results of these studies have shown that TCM herbal treatments can reduce the severity of myelosuppression, improve gastrointestinal side effects and increase the patient's appetite. Most importantly, TCM can also increase the probability of patients completing the scheduled chemotherapy that may improve the overall treatment outcome.

One randomized trial recruited 669 patients with late-stage gastric cancer (Yu et al. 1993). One group of patients was treated with herbs that support the spleen and kidney function (Jianpi Yishen Prescription) twice daily for 4–6 weeks with concurrent chemotherapy, while another group was treated with the same type of chemotherapy alone. The combined treatment group showed significantly higher leukocyte and platelet counts with less general and gastrointestinal side effects. The percentage of patients completing the scheduled chemotherapy was 95% in the combined treatment group versus 74% in the chemotherapy alone group ($P < 0.01$).

Zhang (2004) described 47 patients undergoing chemotherapy with a Fuzheng Peiben herbal formula consisted of astragalus root, *Atractylodes lancea* (atractylodes rhizome), *Dioscorea opposita* (Chinese yam), dangshen, Chinese angelica root, white peony root, *Citrus reticulata* (tangerine peel), *Coix lacryma-jobi* (coix seed) and *Bambusa tuldoides* (bamboo shavings). Thirty of the 47 patients (63.8%) managed to maintain normal white cell counts, haemoglobin and platelets counts. There were only 10 patients reported mild symptoms related to chemotherapy. All patients did not experience fatigue and had normal appetite.

It is interested to know that, in another recent double-blind randomized trial where 120 breast and colorectal cancer patients underwent adjuvant chemotherapy were randomized. The treatment group received TCM herbal treatments prescribed by dedicated TCM practitioners according to individualized conditions. The control group received placebo made with similar taste and appearance of common herbal decoction. The study design was intended to have a reasonable representation of real-life community situation where patients seek their own TCM practitioners to initiate the combined treatment. There was a wide variety of herbal formulas prescribed. All herbs came from a central herbal pharmacy stock where quality assurance was maintained. Results of this study showed no significant difference between the two groups in regards to the chemotherapy associated myelosuppression. Both groups were associated with a moderate incidence of severe (CTC-V2 grades 3 and 4) neutropenia, 52.7% in the TCM group versus 44.7% in control ($P = 0.63$) and leukopenia, 47.3% in the treatment group versus 32.2% in control ($P = 0.37$). Severe anemia and thrombocytopenia were infrequent and the incidence in the two groups was similar. However, there was significant difference in nausea control (Mok et al. 2007).

A Cochrane systematic review of Chinese medicinal herbs for chemotherapy side effects in colorectal cancer patients found some merit in the concoction termed astragalus root compounds (Taixiang et al. 2005). Another Cochrane systematic review of Chinese medicinal herbs to treat the side effects of chemotherapy in breast cancer patients provides limited evidence, even though there was a suggestion of benefit in bone marrow improvement and quality of life (Zhang et al. 2007a).

There were no reported adverse effects since these are rarely documented in Chinese studies that most data have been generated. There are potential detrimental interactions and idiosyncratic toxicity when Chinese herbs and conventional Western pharmaceuticals are used together. Well designed randomized trials, preferably with study endpoints including haematological toxicity parameters and rate of chemotherapy completion, will be necessary to provide the evidence of TCM in decreasing the severity of chemotherapy-induced myelosuppression.

1.5.1.4 Nausea and Vomiting Control and Better Quality of Life

There were a lot of trials with TCM herbal treatments to examine the effects of nausea control during chemotherapy. However, most trials were not randomized and involved small number of patients (Zhang and Fei 2001; Wang and Guan 2004; Jing and Zhang 2005; Mao and Huang 2005).

Mao and Huang (2005) treated 46 patients during chemotherapy with Liujunzi Decoction (Decoction of Six Noble Drugs), a decoction which consists of dangshen, astragalus root, atractylodes rhizome, tuckahoe, pinellia tuber, Chinese angelica root, tangerine peel, *Platycodon grandiflorum* (platycodon root), *Scutellria barbata* (barbat skullcap) and *Paris polyphylla* (herb Paris). Compared with 33 patients who underwent chemotherapy alone, there were only 26% of patients in the TCM group suffered from nausea and vomiting compared with 45% in the control group. Patients in the treatment group also had better sleep and appetite compared to the control group. In another small randomized trial study on 30 patients undergoing chemotherapy for advanced stage colorectal cancer. The treatment group received Da An Pill, which consists of bighead atractylodes rhizome, *Crataegus cuneata* (hawthorn fruit), tangerine peel, *Raphanus sativus* (radish root), *Forsthia suspensa* (weeping forsythia fruit) and other ingredients. Study results showed significant reduction in gastrointestinal discomfort such as nausea and vomiting in the treatment group compared with control (Jing and Zhang 2005).

1.5.1.5 Vasomotor Symptoms Reduction

Vasomotor symptoms with hot flashes and sweating are frequent complications by hormonal manipulative therapies for breast and prostate cancer. Frequent hot flashes with the associated insomnia, fatigue and irritability, were shown to profoundly affect quality of life (Oldenhave et al. 1993). Management of vasomotor symptoms usually involves hormonal replacement therapy with agents like progesterone, megestrol acetate and estrogen or centrally active non-hormonal therapy with agents like gabapentin, antidepressant and venalfaxine (Bordeleau et al. 2007). Chinese herbal treatments may provide an alternative in managing this condition. In TCM perspective, vasomotor symptoms are viewed as kidney deficiencies, blood deficiencies and overactive heart and liver conditions. Correction of these syndrome patterns can result in a reduction of symptoms. Effectiveness of TCM in cancer patients who suffer from vasomotor symptoms has not been studied extensively. Data from non-cancer patients can be extrapolated to study the potential of TCM in treating this condition. However, randomized studies that were reported suffered from poor study design with single herb for the treatment arm. Single herb is rarely used in TCM practice and thus the conclusion from these studies may not be applicable (Hirata et al. 1997; Wiklund et al. 1999).

103 symptomatic women were randomized into treatment and a placebo group in a recently reported randomized study. A TCM herbal formula, Danggui Buxue Decoction (Chinese Angelica Decoction for Replenishing Blood), consisted of a combination of Chinese angelica root and astragalus root was given to the treatment group. Rationale in the choice of this formula was that Chinese angelica root is commonly indicated in treatment menopausal symptoms in TCM and that astragalus root can correct blood and qi deficiencies. Self reported vasomotor symptoms diary and the vasomotor domain of the Menopausal Specific Quality of Life were used to assess outcome for a period of 6 months. Results of this study showed no overall significant difference between the two groups but Chinese Angelica Decoction for Replenishing Blood was found to be effective in treating mild hot flash symptoms compared with the placebo group. The authors suggested that a syndrome patterns diagnosis conducted by TCM practitioners and appropriate herbal treatments may be important than a protocol therapy (Haines et al. 2008).

Keishi-bukuryo-gan (KBG) is a Japanese herbal formula based upon a traditional Chinese medicine formula of the Han Dynasty. This formula is also known as Guizhi Fuling Pill (Pill of Cinnamom Twig and Poria) in Chinese and consists of five herbs: cinnamom twig, tuckahoe, white peony root, *Paeonia suffruticasa* (moutan bark) and peach seed mixed in equal proportion by weight. In Japan, KBG is being widely used as an herbal remedy for hot flashes in post-menopausal women and also in women suffering from hypermenorrhea and dysmenorrea. In vitro studies have shown that KBG has no estrogenic activity. Plasma levels of luteinizing hormone, follicular stimulating hormone and prolactin have not found to be increased by KBG in animal and human studies (Sakamoto 1998; Lerner 2001).

In a recent Japanese pilot trial in 16 prostate cancer patients with hot flushes caused by LHRH agonist, KBG was shown to improve symptoms in 68.8 % (11 out of 16 subjects) of patients after 4 weeks of treatment. A reduction in the average frequency of hot flash attacks from 5.1 to 3 times per day was observed after KBG treatment. Average duration of flash attack was also reduced from 9.1 to 7.3 min. There was no adverse effect observed in all study subjects (Akihiro et al. 2006). A larger randomized placebo trial is pending to open at the Juravinski Cancer Centre (Canada).

1.5.1.6 Potential for Chemotherapy Cognitive Dysfunction

Chinese herbal therapies may have a role in improving cognitive dysfunction due to chemotherapy. Many patients complain about changes in cognitive function during and after chemotherapy. This phenomenon has been particularly studied in breast cancer patients (Ahles et al. 2003; Tannock et al. 2004). At least 18% of cancer patients who have received standard-dose chemotherapy manifest cognitive deficits on post-treatment neuropsychological testing, and this may be sustained 2 years after treatment (Fan et al. 2005). The patients typically complain of a foggy brain. The impairments have an impact on tests that require sustained attention and speed of information processing. Fatigue and depression are associated disorders. Whether the initial cause of dysfunction is due to loss of neuronal integrity or secondary to metabolic pathology is, as yet, unknown. There may be a genetic component, such as the e4 allele of apolipoprotein (Wefel et al. 2004a). Cytokines, such as interleukin-1 and interferons may play a role, according to some animal experiments (Wefel et al. 2004b). Chemotherapy may damage the endothelium of blood vessels, resulting in thromboses and micro-infarcts in the CNS. Currently, the changes that occur in cerebral tissue after anti-cancer treatments are poorly understood and there are no proven interventions.

Interventions that could ameliorate such disabilities would be of great benefit to the patients and their caregivers. Effects of ginkgo seed extracts have been postulated to include improvement of memory, increased blood circulation, as well as beneficial effects to sufferers of Alzheimer's disease. The most unique components of the extracts are the terpene trilactones, that is, ginkgolides and bilobalide. These structurally complex molecules have been attractive targets for total synthesis. Terpene trilactones are believed to be partly responsible for the neuromodulatory properties of ginkgo seed extracts, and several biological effects of the terpene trilactones have been discovered in recent years. Ginkgolides A, B, C, J, K, L and M and bilobalide are rare terpene trilactones that have been isolated from leaves and root bark of the Chinese ginkgo tree. The compounds were found to be potent and selective antagonists of platelet activating factor (PAF), responsible for their effect on increasing bleeding time. Radioactive isotope studies show cerebral availability, particularly in the hippocampus, striatum and hypothalamus (DeFeudis 2002; DeFeudis et al. 2003; Menku et al. 2003). Lipid peroxidation and brain edema are important factors that produce tissue damage in head injury. An investigation of the effect of mexiletine and ginkgo seed extract (EGb 761) on head trauma of rats showed the usefulness of mexiletine and its combination with EGb 761 as a cerebroprotective agent (Ahlemeyer and Krieglstein 2003). Bilobalide has multiple mechanisms of action that may be associated with neuroprotection, including its preservation of mitochondrial ATP synthesis, its inhibition of apoptotic damage induced by staurosporine or by serum-free medium, its suppression of hypoxia-induced membrane deterioration in the brain, and its actions of increasing the expression of the mitochondrial DNA-encoded COX III subunit of cytochrome c oxidase and the ND1 subunit of NADH dehydrogenase. As multiple modes of action may apply to bilobalide, it could be useful in developing therapy for disorders involving cerebral ischemia and neurodegeneration (Santo et al. 2003; Bressler 2005). A Cochrane review concludes that it is promising for treating cognitive dysfunction (Kurz and Van Baelen 2004). However, other randomized controlled trials have not confirmed its effectiveness (Dodge et al. 2008). Potential usefulness of ginseng extracts, ginsenosides has also been examined. The ginsenosides can inhibit NMDA receptor-mediated signals (Bao et al. 2005). A combination of ginseng and ginkgo seed was shown to improve cognitive function in normal volunteers (Kennedy et al. 2001). However, further clinical studies on patients with chemotherapy-induced cognitive dysfunction and laboratory studies will be important to explore the potential usefulness of ginkgo seed and ginseng extracts in managing this significant side effects of chemotherapy.

1.5.2 Acupuncture and Related Techniques

1.5.2.1 Reduction of Vasomotor Symptoms

Acupuncture may be able to reduce the vasomotor symptoms associated with anti-cancer hormone therapy. Many different acupuncture approaches have been tested in non-randomized clinical trials showing a positive reduction in vasomotor symptoms in breast and prostate cancer patients (Hammar et al. 1999; Tukmachi 2000; Cumins and Brunt 2001; Porzio et al. 2002; Filshie et al. 2005; Harding et al. 2009). In one study, 60 prostate cancer patients on luteinizing hormone releasing hormone agonist treatment, were treated with auricular acupuncture using external ear points: autonomic, kidney, shenmen, liver and lung corresponding to the National Acupuncture Detoxification Association protocol for auricular acupuncture. Treatments were given weekly for 10 weeks. 95% of patients reported reduced severity of vasomotor symptoms with a decrease in symptom scores from 5 to 2.1 and $P < 0.01$ (Harding et al. 2009). In another study for 194 breast and prostate cancer patients, an innovative approach of acupuncture treatments given weekly by practitioners to LI4, TE5, LR3 and SP6 and two upper sternal points, but avoiding limbs with lymphoedema or prone to developing it. Patients with no contraindication were instructed to give self acupuncture to SP6 with either semi-permanent needles or conventional needles. Long-term relief of vasomotor symptoms was obtained with 79% of patients gained 50% or greater reduction in hot flushes and 21% with less than 50% reduction (Filshie et al. 2005). These studies suggested acupuncture is a feasible and self approach in managing vasomotor symptoms in cancer patients. In recent years, several randomized trials were reported. These trials compared various acupuncture approaches with or without other interventions versus placebo or self care in cancer and non-cancer patients with vasomotor symptoms (Zaborowska et al. 2007; Frisk et al. 2008; Borud et al. 2009). However, two systematic reviews on the randomized trials of acupuncture for vasomotor symptoms concluded that there is no strong evidence to support the effectiveness of acupuncture (Cho and Whang 2009; Lee et al. 2009). This confusing conclusion is probably due to the absence of rigorous randomized controlled trial with larger enough patients number and the lack of suitable placebo. Further research with robust study design is required to adequately examine the usefulness of acupuncture in vasomotor symptoms.

1.5.2.2 Chemotherapy-induced Peripheral Neuropathy

Besides bone marrow suppression, bowel and renal toxicities, neurotoxicity is often a dose limiting side effect that leads to necessary reduction of chemotherapy dose or even termination of therapy. Chemotherapy-induced peripheral neuropathy (CIPN) appears to occur in 10–20% of patients (Forman 1990). The frequency of this often debilitating toxicity is increasing because of the ability to dose-escalate chemotherapy through improvements in supportive care. Many chemotherapy agencies including platinum compounds, vinca alkaloids, taxols and suramin can cause neurotoxicity. Different components of the peripheral nervous system can be affected resulting in neuropathy. CIPN is most frequently associated with axonal degeneration and a dying-back type of neuropathy. Commonly this occurs weeks to months after exposure to the drug and may continue despite withdrawal of the drug (Kaplan and Wiernik 1982). Symptoms of neurotoxicity can appear immediately during or after the course of chemotherapy and its severity depends on the type and the accumulative dose of chemotherapy used. Sensory or sensory-motor peripheral neuropathy is the predominant presenting symptom while autonomic nervous system dysfunction can occasionally be seen. Patients usually present with continuous or intermittent pain that is described in terms of burning, shooting or electric, and most patients describe more than one pain. Patients may report abnormal pain to normally painful or non-painful stimuli, and may report sensations such as itching, numbness, pins and needles, and tingling. Impaired vibration and joint position sense, ataxia, myalgia and muscle weakness may occur depends on the types of nerve fibre affected. Although damages to the peripheral nerve may recover in most patients, the recovery is incomplete resulting in persistent symptoms (Martin and Hagen 1997). Unrelieved pain can impact patients' functional abilities and severely affecting patient's quality of life.

Current treatments of CIPN are aimed for symptomatic relief of paraesthesia and pain. Tricyclic antidepressant, ion channel blockers: carbamazepine and gabapentin have been shown to be moderately effective, but side effects associate with these medications including sedation, postural hypotension, dry mouth and cardiac problems make their usage limited and may not be acceptable to patients. Moreover, symptoms reappear after these medications are discontinued (Sindrup and Jensen 1999; Quasthoff and Hartung 2002). Thus, better treatments for this debilitating chemotherapy induced peripheral neuropathy are continuously being explored.

Treatment for patients with symptoms consisted of paraesthesia, hyperalgia, pain, pin and needles presenting in both feet and hands have been described in TCM Classics (Flaws 1999). In TCM model, symptoms presented in CIPN are considered to be a state of deficiency in qi and blood and the body's failure in directing these components to the four limbs leading to sensory symptoms and impaired limbs function. Successful treatment with acupuncture has been described based on an approach by improving body qi and blood and directing flow to the extremities. In recent published clinical trials, acupuncture treatment has been shown to induce significant symptom improvement in patients with peripheral neuropathy due to HIV or diabetes mellitus (Phillips et al. 2004; Abuaisha et al. 1998). At Juravinski Cancer Center, a pilot trial was conducted using an acupuncture protocol for patients with CIPN caused by combined taxol and platinum treatments for gynaecological cancers (Wong and Sagar 2006). In this trial, 5 consecutive patients (60–71 years old) with greater than WHO grade II CIPN symptoms were recruited. All received carboplatinum and taxol chemotherapy. Duration of symptoms before acupuncture treatment ranged from 6 to 38 months (median 18 months). 3 patients had Grade II and 2 had Grade III symptoms. Pain, numbness and tingling of fingers and toes were the chief symptoms in all patients. Imbalance in gait was seen in 3 patients. Average pain score was 7.8/10 (range from 6 to 9). At the end of the two courses of acupuncture treatment using a structured protocol, all 5 patients reported improvement of pain, numbness and tingling. Average pain score was 3/10 (range 1–5). Symptoms improvement was seen after first treatment for the patient with 6-month history of CIPN symptoms. All patients had a reduction in analgesic dosage. Gait imbalanced was significantly improved in all 3 patients. At 6 months follow-up, symptoms improvement persisted in 4 patients. One patient with history of diabetes and multiple sclerosis reported symptoms improvement for 1 month only. Although the number of patients studied was small, the results suggest potential usefulness of acupuncture treatment in CIPN and further trials of larger number of patients with more formal assessment is needed. An ongoing Phase II trial using the same acupuncture protocol for CIPN is currently underway at the Juravinski Cancer Centre (Canada).

1.5.2.3 Reduction of Chemotherapy-induced Nausea and Vomiting

Usefulness of acupuncture for nausea and vomiting has been established based on positive results from trials discussed in previous sections. A Cochrane Database systematic review specifically on acupuncture point stimulation using all methods for chemotherapy-induced nausea or vomiting was conducted recently. The conclusion of the review suggested that electroacupuncture is effective and that acupressure can reduce acute nausea but non-invasive electrostimulation is not beneficial. However, the clinical relevance of acupuncture for this condition remains questionable since there is no well conducted study examining the additional benefit of a combination of electroacupuncture with state-of-the-art antiemetics. The management of patients with refractory symptoms is also important to be examined (Ezzo et al. 2006).

1.5.2.4 Chemotherapy-induced Cognitive Dysfunction

The role of acupuncture for cognitive impairment caused by chemotherapy is unclear. An intriguing study in rats showed that it improved cognitive impairment caused by multi-infarcts (Yu et al. 2005). A recent review concluded that there is some limited evidence that acupuncture can be effectively used to manage a range of psychoneurological issues, some of which are similar to those experienced by patients with chemotherapy-associated cognitive dysfunction (Johnston et al. 2007).

1.6 Miscellaneous Symptoms

1.6.1 Pain

Pain is a common symptom in cancer patient. Causes of pain can be due to the cancer or its treatment. Pain relief in cancer patients often aid radical cancer treatments and improve quality of life. Acupuncture has been shown to be effective in managing pain and other symptoms in cancer patients, along with other interventions (Thompson and Filshie 1998). In a retrospective study from the Royal Marsden Hospital (London, UK), 183 cancer patients with malignant pain, iatrogenic pain and radiation-induced chronic ulcers were treated with acupuncture (Filshie 1984; Filshie and Redman 1985). There was an improvement in 82% of the patients, but effectiveness only lasted for more than 3 days in half of the patients. Iatrogenic pain (e.g. pain due to radiation fibrosis or skin ulceration) and pain due to secondary muscle spasm responded better than malignant pain. Furthermore, increased blood flow with improved healing of skin ulcers was demonstrated after treatment with acupuncture. A randomized controlled trial using ear acupuncture showed a profound effect on cancer pain (Alimi et al. 2003). At Juravinski Cancer Centre (Canada), acupuncture is advocated as a useful treatment modality that may best be combined with other treatments to improve pain control and to reduce doses of pharmaceutical analgesics. This has the benefit of reducing the incidence and degree of drug-induced side effects. A systematic review could not support the effectiveness of acupuncture as an adjunctive analgesic method for cancer patients (Lee et al. 2005). However, it included only one randomized controlled trial (Alimi et al. 2003) and all the other studies were generally of poor scientific quality. The intensity of stimulation, especially electrostimulation, may be important (Barlas et al. 2006).

For some patients, TENS has the advantage of easy administration by patients or staff with minimal basic training. AL-TENS devices have been developed to mimic the treatment of acupuncture using low-frequency (e.g. 4 Hz), high-intensity stimulation (Pomeranz and Niznik 1987). The goal is to stimulate the high threshold type III afferent nerve fibers that are potent releasers of endorphins. Recent meta-analyses (including a Cochrane Database systematic review) have shown that AL-TENS is more effective than placebo, and improves function more than standard TENS, when treating chronic pain (Patel et al. 1989; Gadsby and Flowerdew 2000). AL-TENS devices are very simple machines that patients can learn to operate in less than an hour's training. An acupoint prescription may then be given to the patient who can administer the appropriate treatments with AL-TENS at home. Unpublished retrospective audit at the Juravinski Cancer Centre (Canada) in the use of AL-TENS (with a random electrode stimulation set up for reducing habituation of brain) and individualised acupoint prescription for patients with cancer pain not controlled by optimal analgesics, showed positive benefit for AL-TENS as an adjunctive treatment for cancer pain control.

1.6.2 Anxiety, Depression, Cognitive Impairment

Acupuncture has also been reported to be useful in other symptoms experienced by cancer patients. Anxiety is a common reaction in cancer patients. The presence of anxiety can decrease pain threshold, causes insomnia, worsen quality of life and may affect treatment outcome (Jones 2001). Relief of anxiety by acupuncture is associated with an increase in the pain threshold (Widerstrom-Noga et al. 1998).

Depression is another common problem that cancer patients may encounter (Jones 2001). Recent laboratory evidence has demonstrated that tumour alone may be sufficient to induce depression-like behaviour by stimulating cytokine production in the behavior related brain regions and by altering the regulation of the hypothalamic-pituitary-axis (Pyter et al. 2009). The treatment of depression is an important intervention in the management of cancer patients. Conventionally, clinical depression is treated with oral medication, such as amitriptyline or the newer serotonin reuptake inhibitor drugs. Studies indicate that acupuncture treatment may be an equally effective alternative treatment modality to drugs in patients suffering from mild depression. In one study, the profile of side effect associated with acupuncture treatment was shown to be better than amitriptyline (Han 1986). In a single-blind placebo-controlled study of the antidepressant, mianserin, supplementary acupuncture improved the course of depression more than pharmacological treatment with the drug alone (Roschke et al. 2000). A Cochrane review concludes that there is insufficient evidence to determine the efficacy of acupuncture compared to medication, or to wait list control, or sham acupuncture, in the management of depression (Smith and Hay 2005). However, since pharmaceutical antidepressants are not usually effective until 2 weeks after starting therapy, their combination with acupuncture may enable more rapid results with reduced side effects.

1.6.3 Fatigue

Acupuncture can also play a role in the treatment of fatigue through the modulation of cytokines and hormones (Lissoni et al. 1996; Campbell and Murphy 1998; Glaus 1998; Stone et al. 1998). A phase II study of acupuncture for postchemotherapy fatigue (average of 2 years) showed a mean improvement of 30% on the Brief Fatigue Inventory (Vickers et al. 2004). In a recent randomized controlled trial, 47 patients with moderate to severe fatigue were randomized to an acupuncture group, an acupressure group and a sham acupressure group. Results demonstrated significant improvement of the severity of fatigue measured by Multidimensional Fatigue Inventory in both the acupuncture and acupressure group compared to the control group. These findings prompt the feasibility of a larger randomized trial of acupuncture or acupressure versus control in cancer related fatigue management (Molassiotis et al. 2007).

1.6.4 Hiccups and Yawning

Persistent hiccups and yawning are rarely encountered in cancer patients. Underlying causes are still not cleared by can be related to direct tumour irritation or other factors that affect the hiccup reflex arc. One case report has suggested the involvement of brain tumour and effect of radiotherapy on the brain stem. The presence of these symptoms can be distressing for patients. Acupuncture using TCM techniques have been shown to effectively treat these conditions (Yan 1988; Wong and Sagar 2000; Lin 2006; Chang et al. 2008).

1.7 Qigong Exercise

One of the strategies in TCM is to engage patients to motivate their own healing power to improve health. From TCM perspective, this is a manoeuvre by which the vital energy of the body can be supplemented or moved through the body to achieve smooth flow and eventual balance of the body-mind network (Sancier 1996). Qigong can be broadly divided into external and internal qigong. Internal qigong is self-directed and often involve the mind directing body vital energy to move through body meridians or pathways in an orderly fashion with particular attention to body movements or breathing techniques at the same time. There are many forms of internal qigong practice, among which tai chi exercise and Guolin qigong exercise are most popular. External qigong involves qigong practitioners who direct the energy treatment.

Although the scientific basis of qigong is still unclear, results from few clinical trials involving cancer patients have suggested beneficial effects (Oh et al. 2008). According to a recent systematic review, four randomized controlled trials were conducted to examine the effects of qigong on cancer patients. Improvement of chemotherapy related nausea and vomiting, fatigue, immune enhancement, quality of life and even survival has been reported. However, the methodological quality of the trials was poor and there was no large-scale randomized trial reported. It was also not clear how the qigong practice in those trials was conducted and thus a firm conclusion of the benefit of qigong as claimed by some studies cannot be established (Lee et al. 2007a).

As a form of internal qigong, tai chi exercise has been most studied. This exercise is characterized by the meditated like slow physical movements and associated regulated breathing techniques (National Center for Alternative and Complementary

Medicine 2006). This has also been demonstrated to physiological processes, including electromagnetic changes that may represent the flow of qi (Tiller and Pecci 1997; Syldona and Rein 1999). Moderate physical activities also have been shown to improve survival in colorectal and breast cancer patients (Demark-Wahnefried 2006). In another study significant increase in regulatory T-cells and mediators TGFβ and IL10 under varicella zoster virus stimulation and increased helper to suppressor T-cell ratio were found after regular tai chi exercise (Yeh et al. 2006). These techniques encourage a personal sense of control, improve mood, reduce side effects of treatment, increase immunity, and may be associated with an improved outcome from cancer treatment (Meares 1978; Young et al. 1999). There are current few clinical trials that tested tai chi exercise as an adjunct to conventional cancer treatment. A recent systematic review of the currently available 3 randomized trials, there were insufficient evidence to support the effects of tai chi are significantly different from those of conventional forms of exercise (Lee et al. 2007b). Further well designed research is necessary to establish evidence for the usefulness of qigong in cancer patients especially during the treatment period. Innovative research designs will be necessary and multiple disciplines, including qigong practitioners, oncologists and cancer researchers, should be involved in the design of this type of study.

1.8 Nutritional Therapy

Maintenance of good nutrition and adjustment of nutrition for reducing symptoms in cancer patients continue to be an important issue in conventional cancer care (Eldridge and Hamilton 2004). Nutritional therapy for cancer patients is also a main part in TCM cancer treatment. While nutritional therapy in conventional medicine largely involve the improvement and maintenance of patient optimal nutritional status, TCM nutritional therapy aim to individualize recommendation according to patients' presenting syndrome patterns. Traditional Chinese medicine has extensive experience and systematic records regarding the properties of different types of food and their usage in particular syndrome patterns. In TCM, different type of food, like different type of herbal medicine, has different medicinal properties (Kastner and Moje 2004). Food can be classified according to their medicinal properties into five main classes: sweet affects spleen; pungent affects lung; salty affects kidney; sour affects liver, and bitter affects heart. For examples, barley is considered to be sweet, papaya is sour, and crab is salty. Food in each class also has other properties, including warm or cold nature; supportive or dispersive nature, and others. Nutritional therapeutic recommendations are given according to the observed syndrome patterns. For instance, a patient presented with syndrome pattern that suggests spleen and stomach deficiency and cold, with symptoms including reduction in appetite, tasteless sense, nausea, mental and physically fatigue and avoidance of cold temperature; warm food, like red dates, logan, beef or mutton, should be recommended while cold food like watermelon, rabbit meat, duck and soy, should be avoided. Sweet food, but not sugary food, for example, grains like barley or root vegetables should be consumed to support the deficient spleen and stomach. This nutritional therapy of TCM is intriguing, but to date, published evidence to support the effectiveness of such practice is still lacking.

1.9 Chinese Massage Therapy, Tuina

Chinese massage therapy, called tuina, is also one of the main modalities in TCM that is recommended as part of the care for cancer patients. In tuina, massage techniques utilized are very similar to many other styles of massage, for example Swedish massage with similar techniques like gliding, kneading, percussion, shaking, pulling, rotation, rocking and friction. The main difference between tuina and other conventional styles of massage is the emphasis on applying pressure to acupuncture points or other physical manipulation that are indicated in particular clinical situations and thus, individualized treatments are applied to patients. Shiatsu, a Japanese style of massage is more closely related to tuina with special massage techniques tailored to the presenting symptoms of the patients. To date there is just a few published clinical research that examined the benefit of tuina in cancer patients. However, research studies of massage therapy in general for cancer patients has suggested benefit, in terms of reduction in chemotherapy and radiation therapy side effects, improvement of immune function, reduction in stress and anxiety, reduction in pain and better quality of life (Kutner et al. 2008; Myers et al. 2008; Billhult et al. 2009; Sturgeon et al. 2009). Massage therapy appears to be safe in cancer patients even in those with bone metastasis (Jane et al. 2009).

1.10 Conclusion

Traditional Chinese medicine is one of the few that has a well constructed theoretical framework and established treatment approaches for diseases including cancer. There is increasing evidence that TCM can be an effective adjunctive treatment to support cancer patients through their major conventional cancer therapies. Future research will continue to provide the underlying mechanism and optimal clinical indications of TCM in cancer care. Innovative research designs are needed to generate high quality research of TCM in cancer treatment and will necessitate a multidisciplinary research team including oncologists, cancer researchers, TCM practitioners.

References

Abuaisha B, Costanzi J, Boulton AJ. Acupuncture for the treatment of chronic painful peripheral diabetic neuropathy: a long-term study. Diabetes Res Clin Pract. 1998;39:115–21.

Ahlemeyer B, Krieglstein J. Pharmacological studies supporting the therapeutic use of Ginkgo biloba extract for Alzheimer's disease. Pharmacopsychiatry. 2003;36:S8–14.

Ahles TA, Saykin AJ, Noll WW et al. The relationship of APOE genotype to neuropsychological performance in long-term cancer survivors treated with standard dose chemotherapy. Psychooncology. 2003;12:612–9.

Akihiro M, Tetsuo N, Yasuyoshi F et al. Efficacy of Keishi-bukuryo-gan for hot flushes caused by treatment with luteinizing hormone- releasing hormone agonist. Rinsho Hinyokika. 2006;60:139–42.

Al-Sadi M, Newman B, Julious SA. Acupuncture in the prevention of postoperative nausea and vomiting. Anaesthesia. 1997;52:658–61.

Alimi D, Rubino C, Pichard-Leandri E et al. Analgesic effect of auricular acupuncture for cancer pain: a randomized, blinded, controlled trial. J Clin Oncol. 2003;21:4120–6.

Amkraut A, Solomon GF. Stress and murine sarcoma virus (Moloney)-induced tumors. Cancer Res. 1972;32:1428–33.

Ang-Lee M, Moss J, Yuan CS. Herbal medicines and perioperative care. JAMA. 2001;286:208–16.

Bao HY, Zhang J, Yeo SJ et al. Memory enhancing and neuroprotective effects of selected ginsenosides. Arch Pharm Res. 2005;28:335–42.

Barlas P, Ting SL, Chesterton LS et al. Effects of intensity of electroacupuncture upon experimental pain in healthy human volunteers: a randomized, double-blind, placebo-controlled study. Pain. 2006;122:81–9.

Baxter LT, Jain RK. Transport of fluid and macromolecules in tumors. 1. Role of interstitial pressure and convection. Microvasc Res. 1989;37:77–104.

Billhult A, Lindholm C, Gunnarsson R et al. The effect of massage on immune function and stress in women with breast cancer – a randomized controlled trial. Auton Neurosci. 2009;150: 111–5.

Blom M, Dawidson I, Angmar-Mansson B. The effect of acupuncture on salivary flow rates in patients with xerostomia. Oral Surg Oral Med Oral Pathol. 1992;73:293–8.

Blom M, Dawidson I, Fernberg JO et al. Acupuncture treatment of patients with radiation-induced xerostomia. Eur J Cancer B Oral Oncol. 1996;32B:182–90.

Blom M, Lundeberg T. Long-term follow-up of patients treated with acupuncture for xerostomia and the influence of additional treatment. Oral Dis. 2000;6:15–24.

Blom M, Lundeberg T, Dawidson I et al. Effects on local blood flux of acupuncture stimulation used to treat xerostomia in patients suffering from Sjögren's syndrome. J Oral Rehab. 1993;20:541–8.

Boik J. Cancer and natural medicine: a textbook of basic science and clinical research. Rev ed. Princeton, MN: Oregon Medical Press; 1996a.

Boik J. Emerging trends in cancer research: development of a mechanism-based approach. Protocol J Botanic Med. 1996b;2:5–10.

Boon H, Brown JB, Gavin A et al. Breast cancer survivors' perceptions of complementary/alternative medicine (CAM): making the decision to use or not to use. Qual Health Res. 1999;9:639–53.

Bordeleau L, Pritchard K, Goodwin P et al. Therapeutic options for the management of hot flashes in breast cancer survivors: an evidence-based review. Clin Ther. 2007;29:230–41.

Borud EK, Alraek T, White A et al. The Acupuncture on Hot Flushes Among Menopausal Women (ACUFLASH) study, a randomized controlled trial. Menopause. 2009;16:484–93.

Braga FP, Sugaya NN, Hirota SK et al. The effect of acupuncture on salivary flow rates in patients with radiation-induced xerostomia. Minerva Stomatol. 2008;57:343–8.

Bressler R. Herb-drug interactions: interactions between Ginkgo biloba and prescription medications. Geriatrics. 2005;60:30–3.

Brizel DM, Sibley GS, Prosnitz LR et al. Tumor hypoxia adversely affects the prognosis of carcinoma of the head and neck. Int J Radiat Oncol Biol Phys. 1997;38:285–9.

Cai HB. A clinical audit of the treatment of 30 cases of cancer anorexia-cachexia syndrome with Buzhong Yiqi Tang. Xin Zhong Yi. 2003;3:25–6.

Campbell SS, Murphy PJ. Extraocular circadian phototransduction in humans. Science. 1998;279:396–9.

Cao GW, Yang WG, Du P. Observation of the effects of LAK/IL-2 therapy combining with *Lycium barbarum* polysaccharides in the treatment of 75 cancer patients. Zhonghua Zhong Liu Za Zhi. 1994;16:428–31.

Chang CC, Chang YC, Chang ST et al. Efficacy of near-infrared irradiation on intractable hiccup in custom-set acupoints: evidence-based analysis of treatment outcome and associated factors. Scand J Gastroenterol. 2008;43:538–44.
Chen JZ. Clinical effect of chemotherapy combined with Chinese herbs and Western drugs on leukocytes of gastric cancer patients. Zhong Xi Yi Jie He Za Zhi. 1990;10:717–9.
Cheng JH. Clinical study on prevention and treatment to chemotherapy caused nephrotoxicity with Jian-pi Yi-qi Li-shui Decoction. Zhongguo Zhong Xi Yi Jie He Za Zhi. 1994;14:331–3.
Cheung NK, Modak S, Vickers A et al. Orally administered xxb-glucans enhance anti-tumor effects of monoclonal antibodies. Cancer Immunol Immunother. 2002;51:557–64.
Cho WC, Chen HY. Clinical efficacy of traditional Chinese medicine as a concomitant therapy for nasopharyngeal carcinoma: a systematic review and meta-analysis. Cancer Invest. 2009a;27:334–44.
Cho WC, Chen HY. Transcatheter arterial chemoembolization combined with or without Chinese herbal therapy for hepatocellular carcinoma: meta-analysis. Expert Opin Investig Drugs. 2009b;18:617–35.
Cho JH, Chung WK, Kang W et al. Manual acupuncture improved quality of life in cancer patients with radiation-induced xerostomia. J Altern Complement Med. 2008;14:523–6.
Cho SH, Whang WW. Acupuncture for vasomotor menopausal symptoms: a systematic review. Menopause. 2009; 16:1065–73.
Coffey DS. Self-organization, complexity and chaos: the new biology for medicine. Nature Med. 1998;4:882–5.
Collins L, Zhu T, Guo J et al. Phellinus linteus sensitises apoptosis induced by doxorubicin in prostate cancer. Br J Cancer. 2006;95:282–8.
NIH Consensus Development. Panel on acupuncture. JAMA. 1998;280:1518–24.
Cumins SM, Brunt AM. Does acupuncture influence the vasomotor symptoms experienced by breast cancer patients taking tamoxifen? Acupunct Med. 2001;18:28–9.
Cuzick J, Holland R, Barth V et al. Electropotential measurements as a new diagnostic modality for breast cancer. Lancet. 1998;352:359–63.
Dai Y, Kato M, Takeda K et al. T-cell-immunity-based inhibitory effects of orally administered herbal medicine juzen-taiho-to on the growth of primarily developed melanocytic tumors in RET-transgenic mice. J Invest Dermatol. 2001;117:694–701.
DeFeudis FV. Bilobalide and neuroprotection. Pharmacol Res. 2002;46:565–8.
DeFeudis FV, Papadopoulos V, Drieu K. Ginkgo biloba extracts and cancer: a research area in its infancy. Fundam Clin Pharmacol. 2003;17:405–17.
Demark-Wahnefried W. Cancer survival: time to get moving? Data accumulate suggesting a link between physical activity and cancer survival. J Clin Oncol. 2006;24:3517–8.
Deng G, Hou BL, Holodny AI et al. Functional magnetic resonance imaging (fMRI) changes and saliva production associated with acupuncture at LI-2 acupuncture point: a randomized controlled study. BMC Complement Altern Med. 2008a;8:37.
Deng G, Rusch V, Vickers A et al. Randomized controlled trial of a special acupuncture technique for pain after thoracotomy. J Thorac Cardiovasc Surg. 2008b;136:1464–9.
Ding XF, Li DX, Zhao L. Rat study on the mucosa and nitric oxide levels of irradiated bowel after treatment with TCM. Zhongguo Xiandai Yixue Zhazhi. 2003;13:42–4.
Ding XF, Li DX, Zhao L. Clinical study of TCM on the treatment and prevention of radiation related bowel injury. Zhonghua Fangse Yixueyifangshu Zhazhi. 2004;24:49–51.
Dodge HH, Zitzelberger T, Oken BS et al. A randomized placebo-controlled trial of Ginkgo biloba for the prevention of cognitive decline. Neurology. 2008;70:1809–17.
Dong WH, Zhan LY, Chen F. The aetiology and management of acute urinary retention after rectal surgery. Xiandai Zhong Xi Yi Jiehe Zhazhi. 2003;12:2082–3.
Dundee JW, Chestnutt WN, Ghaly RG et al. Traditional Chinese acupuncture: a potentially useful antiemetic? BMJ. 1986;293:583–4.
Dundee JW, Ghaly RG, Fitzpatrick KT et al. Acupuncture prophylaxis of cancer chemotherapy-induced sickness. J R Soc Med. 1989;82:268–71.

Eldridge B, Hamilton K. Management of nutrition impact symptoms in cancer and educational handouts. Chicago: American Dietetic Association; 2004.
Ernst E, Cassileth BR. The prevalence of complementary/alternative medicine in cancer: a systematic review. Cancer. 1998;83:777–82.
Ezzo JM, Richardson MA, Vickers A et al. Acupuncture-point stimulation for chemotherapy-induced nausea or vomiting. Cochrane Database Syst Rev. 2006;2:CD002285.
Fan HG, Houédé-Tchen N, Yi QL et al. Fatigue, menopausal symptoms, and cognitive function in women after adjuvant chemotherapy for breast cancer: 1- and 2-year follow-up of a prospective controlled study. J Clin Oncol. 2005;23:8025–32.
Feng PF, Liu LM, Shen YY. Effect of Shenmai injection on sIL-2R, NK and LAK cells in patients with advanced carcinoma. Zhongguo Zhong Xi Yi Jie He Za Zhi. 1995;15:87–9.
Filshie J. Acupuncture for malignant pain. Acupunct Med. 1984;5:12–4.
Filshie J, Bolton T, Browne D et al. Acupuncture and self acupuncture for long-term treatment of vasomotor symptoms in cancer patients – audit and treatment algorithm. Acupunct Med. 2005;23:171–80.
Filshie J, Redman D. Acupuncture and malignant pain problems. Eur J Surg Oncol. 1985;11:389–94.
Flaws B. The classic of difficulties. Boulder: Blue Poppy Press; 1999.
Forman A. Peripheral neuropathy in cancer patients: incidence, features. Oncology (Huntington). 1990;4:57–62.
Frisk J, Carlhäll S, Källström AC et al. Long-term follow-up of acupuncture and hormone therapy on hot flushes in women with breast cancer: a prospective, randomized, controlled multicenter trial. Climacteric. 2008;11:166–74.
Fyles AW, Milosevic M, Wong R et al. Oxygenation predicts radiation response and survival in patients with cervix cancer. Radiother Oncol. 1998;48:149–56.
Gadsby JG, Flowerdew MW. Transcutaneous electrical nerve stimulation reduces pain and improves range of movement in chronic low-back pain. Cochrane Database Syst Rev. 2000;2:CD000210.
Gao YH, Dai XH, Chen GL et al. A randomized, placebo-controlled, multicenter study of *Ganoderma lucidum* (W. Curt.: Fr.) Lloyd (Aphyllophoromycetideae) polysaccharides (Ganopoly) in patients with advanced lung cancer. Int J Med Mushr. 2003;5:369–81.
Gill SK, Rieder MJ. Toxicity of a traditional Chinese medicine, Ganoderma lucidum, in children with cancer. Can J Clin Pharmacol. 2008;15:e275–85.
Girinsky T. Effects of ionizing radiation on the blood vessel wall. J Mal Vasc. 2000;25:321–4.
Glaus A. Fatigue and cachexia in cancer patients. Support Care Cancer. 1998;6:77–8.
Greif R, Laciny S, Mokhtarani M et al. Transcutaneous electrical stimulation of an auricular acupuncture point decreases anesthetic requirement. Anesthesiology. 2002;96:306–12.
Ha SW, Yi CJ, Cho CK et al. Enhancement of radiation effect by Ginkgo biloba in C3H mouse fibrosarcoma. Radiother Oncol. 1996;41:163–7.
Haines CJ, Lam PM, Chung TK et al. A randomized, double-blind, placebo-controlled study of the effect of a Chinese herbal medicine preparation (Dang Gui Buxue Tang) on menopausal symptoms in Hong Kong Chinese women. Climacteric. 2008;11:244–51.
Hammar M, Frisk J, Grimas O. Acupuncture treatment of vasomotor symptoms in men with prostatic carcinoma: a pilot study. J Urol. 1999;161:853–6.
Han JS. Electroacupuncture: an alternative to antidepressants for treating affective diseases. Int J Neurosci. 1986;29:79–92.
Harding C, Harris A, Chadwick D. Auricular acupuncture: a novel treatment for vasomotor symptoms associated with luteinizing-hormone releasing hormone agonist treatment for prostate cancer. BJU Int. 2009;103:186–90.
He JP, Friedrich M, Ertan AK et al. Pain-relief and movement improvement by acupuncture after ablation and axillary lymphadenectomy in patients with mammary cancer. Clin Exp Obstet Gynecol. 1999;26:81–4.

Hejna M, Raderer M, Zielinski CC. Inhibition of metastases by anticoagulants. J Natl Cancer Inst. 1999;91:22–36.

Hirata JD, Swiersz LM, Zell B et al. Does dong quai have estrogenic effects in postmenopausal women? A double-blind, placebo-controlled trial. Fertil Steril. 1997;68:981–6.

Hofseth LJ, Wargovich MJ. Inflammation, cancer, and targets of ginseng. J Nutr. 2007;137:183S–5S.

Hoppe RT, Fuks ZY, Strober S et al. The long term effects of radiation on T and B lymphocytes in the peripheral blood after regional irradiation. Cancer. 1977;40:2071–8.

Horie Y, Kato K, Kameoka S et al. Bu ji (hozai) for treatment of postoperative gastric cancer patients. Am J Chin Med. 1994;22:309–19.

Hou J, Liu S, Ma Z et al. Effects of Gynostemma pentaphyllum makino on the immunological function of cancer patients. J Tradit Chin Med. 1991;11:47–52.

Ikemi Y, Ikemi A. An oriental point of view in psychosomatic medicine. Advance. 1986;3:150–7.

Ikemoto S, Sugimura K, Yoshida N et al. Antitumor effects of scutellariae radix and its components baicalein, baicalin, and wogonin on bladder cancer cell lines. Urology. 2000;55:951–5.

Jane SW, Wilkie DJ, Gallucci BB et al. Effects of a full-body massage on pain intensity, anxiety, and physiological relaxation in Taiwanese patients with metastatic bone pain: a pilot study. J Pain Symptom Manage. 2009;37:754–63.

Jin R, Wan LL, Mitsuishi T et al. Effect of shi-ka-ron and Chinese herbs on cytokine production of macrophage in immunocompromised mice. Am J Chin Med. 1994;22:255–66.

Jing J, Zhang MZ. Clinical trial on Da An Wan reducing post colonic surgery chemotherapy nausea and vomiting. Zhongguo Zhongyiyao Newsletter. 2005;9:823–4.

Johnston MF, Yang C, Hui KK et al. Acupuncture for chemotherapy-associated cognitive dysfunction: a hypothesis-generating literature review to inform clinical advice. Integr Cancer Ther. 2007;6:36–40.

Johnstone PA, Peng YP, May BC et al. Acupuncture for pilocarpine-resistant xerostomia following radiotherapy for head and neck malignancies. Int J Radiat Oncol Biol Phys. 2001;50:353–7.

Jones RD. Depression and anxiety in oncology: the oncologist's perspective. J Clin Psychiatry. 2001;62:52–7.

Kang K, Kang B, Lee B et al. Preventive effect of epicatechin and ginsenoside Rb(2) on the inhibition of gap junctional intercellular communication by TP and H(2)O(2). Cancer Lett. 2000;152:97–106.

Kang JX, Liu J, Wang J et al. The extract of huanglian, a medicinal herb, induces cell growth arrest and apoptosis by upregulation of interferon-xxb and TNF-xxa in human breast cancer cells. Carcinogenesis. 2005;26:1934–9.

Kaplan R, Wiernik PH. Neurotoxicity of antineoplastic drugs. Semin Oncol. 1982;9:103–30.

Kastner J, Moje A. Chinese nutrition therapy: dietetics in traditional Chinese medicine. 1st ed. New York: Thieme Medical Publishers; 2004.

Kawakita T, Nakai S, Kumazawa Y et al. Induction of interferon after administration of traditional Chinese medicine, Xiao-Chai-Hu-Tang (shosaiko-to). Int J Immunopharmacol. 1990;12:515–21.

Kennedy DO, Scholey AB, Wesnes KA. Differential, dose dependent changes in cognitive performance following acute administration of a *Ginkgo biloba/Panax ginseng* combination to healthy young volunteers. Nutr Neurosci. 2001;4:399–412.

Kleijnen J, Knipschild P. *Ginkgo biloba*. Lancet. 1992;340:1136–9.

Kuang P, Tao Y, Tian Y. Radix Salviae miltiorrhizae treatment Results in decreased lipid peroxidation in reperfusion injury. J Tradit Chin Med. 1996;16:138–42.

Kurz A, Van Baelen B. Ginkgo biloba compared with cholinesterase inhibitors in the treatment of dementia: a review based on meta-analyses by the Cochrane collaboration. Dement Geriatr Cogn Disord. 2004;18:217–26.

Kutner JS, Smith MC, Corbin L et al. Massage therapy versus simple touch to improve pain and mood in patients with advanced cancer: a randomized trial. Ann Intern Med. 2008;149:369–79.

Lau BH, Ruckle HC, Botolazzo T et al. Chinese medicinal herbs inhibit growth of murine renal cell carcinoma. Cancer Biother. 1994;9:153–61.

Lebeau B, Chastang C, Brechot JM et al. Subcutaneous heparin treatment increases survival in small cell lung cancer. Petites Cellules Group Cancer. 1994;74:38–45.
Lee A, Done ML. The use of nonpharmacologic techniques to prevent postoperative nausea and vomiting: a meta-analysis. Anesth Analg. 1999;88:1362–9.
Lee A, Fan LT. Stimulation of the wrist acupuncture point P6 for preventing postoperative nausea and vomiting. Cochrane Database Syst Rev. 2009;2:CD003281.
Lee H, Schmidt K, Ernst E. Acupuncture for the relief of cancer-related pain: a systematic review. Eur J Pain. 2005a;9:437–44.
Lee MS, Chen KW, Sancier KM et al. Qigong for cancer treatment: a systematic review of controlled clinical trials. Acta Oncol. 2007a;46:717–22.
Lee MS, Kim KH, Shin BC et al. Acupuncture for treating hot flushes in men with prostate cancer: a systematic review. Support Care Cancer. 2009;17:763–70.
Lee MS, Pittler MH, Ernst E. Is tai chi an effective adjunct in cancer care? A systematic review of controlled clinical trials. Support Care Cancer. 2007b;15:597–601.
Lee TK, Johnke RM, Allison RR et al. Radioprotective potential of ginseng. Mutagenesis. 2005b;20:237–43.
Lerner JH. TCM/Kampo therapy also efficacious for menopause. Altern Ther Health Med. 2001;7:21.
Li NQ. Clinical and experimental study on Shen-qi Injection with chemotherapy in the treatment of malignant tumor of digestive tract. Zhongguo Zhong Xi Yi Jie He Za Zhi. 1992;12:588–92.
Li WX, Chen YR, Xu GZ. Treatment of nasopharyngeal carcinoma by combination therapy of radiotherapy and traditional Chinese medicine for invigorating blood circulation and eliminating blood stasis. Guangdong Med J. 2002;23:95–6.
Liang HL, Xue CC, Li CG. Regression of squamous cell carcinoma of the lung by Chinese herbal medicine: a case with an 8-year follow-up. Lung Cancer. 2004;43:355–60.
Lin ZB. Cellular and molecular mechanisms of immuno-modulation by *Ganoderma lucidum*. J Pharmacol Sci. 2005;99:144–53.
Lin YC. Acupuncture for persistent hiccups in a heart and lung transplant recipient. J Heart Lung Transplant. 2006;25:126–7.
Lin JG, Chen WL. Acupuncture analgesia: a review of its mechanisms of actions. Am J Chin Med. 2008;36:635–45.
Lin SY, Liu LM, Wu LC. Effects of Shenmai Injection on immune function in stomach cancer patients after chemotherapy. Zhongguo Zhong Xi Yi Jie He Za Zhi. 1995;15:451–3.
Lin H, She YH, Cassileth BR et al. Maitake xxb-glucan MD-Fraction enhances bone marrow colony formation and reduces doxorubicin toxicity in vitro. Int Immunopharmacol. 2004;4:91–9.
Ling HY, Wang NZ, Zhu HZ. Preliminary sudy of traditional Chinese medicine-Western medicine treatment of patients with primary liver carcinoma. Zhong Xi Yi Jie He Za Zhi. 1989;9:348–9, 325.
Lissoni P, Paolorossi F, Tancini G et al. Is there a role for melatonin in the treatment of neoplastic cachexia? Eur J Cancer. 1996;32A:1340–3.
Liu L, Ding Q, Dai XF. Study on the controlling effect of Shenqi Fuzheng Injection on plasma cytokine network in patients with thoracic tumor undergoing radiotherapy. Zhongguo Zhong Xi Yi Jie He Za Zhi. 2007;27:1082–5.
Liu X, Kirschenbaum A, Yao S et al. Inhibition of cyclooxygenase-2 suppresses angiogenesis and the growth of prostate cancer in vivo. J Urol. 2000;164:820–5.
Liu CL, Liu JX, Liu LP et al. Clinical observation on effect of nourishing-Yin and activating-blood circulation Recipe in reducing toxicity and enhancing therapeutic efficacy of radiotherapy in patients with nasopharyngeal carcinoma. Chin J Integr Tradit West Med. 2002;22:918–20.
Luo F, Wang JY. Modulation of central nociceptive coding by acupoint stimulation. Neurochem Res. 2008;33:1950–5.
Ma H, Zhang X, Bai M et al. Clinical effects of lianbai liquid in prevention and treatment of dermal injury caused by radiotherapy. J Tradit Chin Med. 2007;27:193–6.

Macek C. East meets west to balance immunologic yin and yang. JAMA. 1984;251:433–5.
Mao XL, Huang M. Clinical trial of the use of TCM to reduce side-effects of post-operative chemotherapy in colon cancer patients. Shandong Zhongyixue Daxuexuebao. 2005;29:128–9.
Martin L, Hagen N. Neuropathic pain in cancer patients: mechanisms, syndromes, and clinical controversies. J Pain Symptom Manage. 1997;14:99–117.
Matsui Y, Uhara J, Satoi S et al. Improved prognosis of postoperative hepatocellular carcinoma patients when treated with functional foods: a prospective cohort study. J Hepatol. 2002;37:78–86.
McCulloch M, See C, Shu XJ et al. Astragalus-based Chinese herbs and platinum-based chemotherapy for advanced non-small-cell lung cancer: meta-analysis of randomized trials. J Clin Oncol. 2006;24:419–30.
Meares A. Regression of osteogenic sarcoma metastases associated with intensive meditation. Med J Aust. 1978;2:433.
Meng MB, Cui YL, Guan YS et al. Traditional Chinese medicine plus transcatheter arterial chemoembolization for unresectable hepatocellular carcinoma. J Altern Complement Med. 2008;14:1027–42.
Menku A, Koc RK, Tayfur V et al. Effects of mexiletine, Ginkgo biloba extract (EGb 761), and their combination on experimental head injury. Neurosurg Rev. 2003;26:288–91.
Milosevic MF, Fyles AW, Wong R et al. Interstitial fluid pressure in cervical carcinoma. Within tumor heterogeneity, and relation to oxygen tension. Cancer. 1998;82:2418–26.
Mitomi T, Tsuchiya S, Iijima N et al. Randomized, controlled study on adjuvant immunochemotherapy with PSK in curatively resected colorectal cancer. The Cooperative Study Group of Surgical Adjuvant Immunochemotherapy for Cancer of Colon and Rectum (Kanagawa). Dis Colon Rectum. 1992;35:123–30.
Mok TS, Yeo W, Johnson PJ et al. A double-blind placebo-controlled randomized study of Chinese herbal medicine as complementary therapy for reduction of chemotherapy-induced toxicity. Ann Oncol. 2007;18:768–74.
Molassiotis A, Sylt P, Diggins H. The management of cancer-related fatigue after chemotherapy with acupuncture and acupressure: a randomised controlled trial. Complement Ther Med. 2007;15:228–37.
Morioka N, Akça O, Doufas AG et al. Electro-acupuncture at the Zusanli, Yanglingquan, and Kunlun points does not reduce anesthetic requirement. Anesth Analg. 2002;95:98–102.
Motoo Y, Sawabu N. Antitumor effects of saikosaponins, baicalin and baicalein on human hepatoma cell lines. Cancer Lett. 1994;86:91–5.
Murata P, Jase Y, Ishige A et al. The herbal medicine Dai-kenchu-to and one of its active components [6]-shogaol increase intestinal blood flow in rats. Life Sci. 2002;70:2061–70.
Myers CD, Walton T, Small BJ. The value of massage therapy in cancer care. Hematol Oncol Clin North Am. 2008;4:649–60.
National Center for Complementary and Alternative Medicine. Tai chi for health purposes. http://nccam.nih.gov/health/taichi . Accessed 2006.
Ning CH, Wang GM, Zhao TY et al. Therapeutical effects of jian pi yi shen prescription on the toxicity reactions of postoperative chemotherapy in patients with advanced gastric carcinoma. J Tradit Chin Med. 1988;8:113–6.
Oh B, Butow P, Mullan B et al. Medical qigong for cancer patients: pilot study of impact on quality of life, side effects of treatment and inflammation. Am J Chin Med. 2008;36:459–72.
Ohnishi Y, Fujii H, Hayakawa Y et al. Oral administration of a Kampo (Japanese herbal) medicine Juzen-taiho-to inhibits liver metastasis of colon 26-L5 carcinoma cells. Jpn J Cancer Res. 1998;89:206–13.
Ohnishi Y, Yasumizu R, Fan HX et al. Effects of juzen-taiho-toh (TJ-48), a traditional oriental medicine, on hematopoietic recovery from radiation injury in mice. Exp Hematol. 1990;18:18–22.
Oldenhave A, Jaszmann LJB, Haspels AA et al. Impact of climacteric on well-being. A survey based on 5213 women 39 to 60 years old. Am J Obst Gynec. 1993;168:772.

Patel M, Gutzwiller F, Paccaud F et al. A meta-analysis of acupuncture for chronic pain. Int J Epidemiol. 1989;18:900–6.
Phillips K, Skelton W, Hand G. Effect of acupuncture administered in a group setting on pain and subjective peripheral neuropathy in persons with human immunodeficiency virus disease. J Altern Complement Med. 2004;10:449–55.
Pomeranz B, Niznik G. Codetron: a new electrotherapy device overcomes the habituation problems of conventional TENS devices. Am J Electromed. 1987;2:22–6.
Porzio G, Trapasso T, Martelli S et al. Acupuncture in the treatment of menopause-related symptoms in women taking tamoxifen. Tumori. 2002;88:128–30.
Pyter LM, Pineros V, Galang JA et al. Peripheral tumors induce depressive-like behaviors and cytokine production and alter hypothalamic-pituitary-adrenal axis regulation. Proc Natl Acad Sci USA. 2009;106:9069–74.
Quasthoff S, Hartung H. Chemotherapy-induced peripheral neuropathy. J Neurol. 2002;249:9–17.
Rao XQ, Yu RC, Zhang JH. Sheng Xue Tang on immunological functions of cancer patients with spleen-deficiency syndrome. Zhong Xi Yi Jie He Za Zhi. 1991;11:218–9.
Roschke J, Wolf C, Muller MJ et al. The benefit from whole body acupuncture in major depression. J Affect Disord. 2000;57:73–81.
Rosenberg Z. Treating the undesirable effects of radiation and chemotherapy with Chinese medicine. J Chinese Med. 1997;55:29–30.
Rydholm M, Strang P. Acupuncture for patients in hospital-based home care suffering from xerostomia. J Palliat Care. 1999;15:20–3.
Sagar SM, Klassen GA, Barclay KD et al. Tumour blood flow: measurement and manipulation for therapeutic gain. Cancer Treat Rev. 1993;19:299–349.
Sagar SM, Singh G, Hodson DI et al. Nitric oxide and anti-cancer therapy. Cancer Treat Rev. 1995;21:159–81.
Sakamoto S. Recent advances in the pharmacology of Kampo (Japanese herbal) medicines. Excerpta Medica;1998:170–6.
Sancier KM. Medical applications of qigong. Altern Ther Health Med. 1996;2:40–6.
Santos RF, Galduroz JC, Barbieri A et al. Cognitive performance, SPECT, and blood viscosity in elderly non-demented people using Ginkgo biloba. Pharmacopsychiatry. 2003;36:127–33.
Satoh K, Hayakawa T, Kase Y et al. Mechanisms for contractile effect of Dai-kenchu-to in isolated guinea pig ileum. Dig Dis Sci. 2001;46:250–6.
Schipper H, Goh CR, Wang Tl. Shifting the cancer paradigm: Must we kill to cure? J Clin Oncol. 1995;13:801–7.
Schlager A, Offer T, Baldissera I. Laser stimulation of acupuncture point P6 reduces postoperative vomiting in children undergoing strabismus surgery. Brit J Anaesthesia. 1998;81:529–32.
Shi JL, Chen YQ, Wen L et al. Electroacupuncture in the treatment of urinary retention in postoperative period of rectal cancer patients. Zhongguo Zhong Xi Yi Jie He Za Zhi. 2008;28:158–9.
Shin HJ, Kim YS, Kwak YS et al. Enhancement of antitumor effects of paclitaxel (Taxol) in combination with red ginseng acidic polysaccharide (RGAP). Planta Med. 2004;70:1033–8.
Shoemaker M, Hamilton B, Dairkee SH et al. In vitro anticancer activity of twelve Chinese medicinal herbs. Phytother Res. 2005;19:649–51.
Shu X, McCulloch M, Xiao H et al. Chinese herbal medicine and chemotherapy in the treatment of hepatocellular carcinoma: a meta-analysis of randomized controlled trials. Integr Cancer Ther. 2005;4:219–29.
Sindrup H, Jensen T. Efficacy of pharmacological treatments of neuropathic pain: an update and effect related to mechanism of drug action. Pain. 1999;83:389–400.
Smith CA, Hay PPJ. Acupuncture for depression. Cochrane Database Syst Rev. 2005;2:CD004046.
So F, Guthrie N, Chambers A et al. Inhibition of proliferation of estrogen receptor-positive MCF-7 human breast cancer cells by flavonoids in the presence and absence of excess estrogen. Cancer Lett. 1997;112:127–33.

Song PR, Qiu BS, Wu YT. Clinical observation on TCM treatment according to syndrome differentiation in relieving acute radio-reaction in nasopharyngeal carcinoma patients. Zhongguo Zhong Xi Yi Jie He Za Zhi. 2007;27:452–5.

Stone P, Richards M, Hardy J. Fatigue in patients with cancer. Eur J Cancer. 1998;34:1670–6.

Sturgeon M, Wetta-Hall R, Hart T et al. Effects of therapeutic massage on the quality of life among patients with breast cancer during treatment. J Altern Complement Med. 2009;15:373–80.

Sun H, Duan S, Yu G. Free radical mechanism in enhancement of radiosensitization by SRSBR. J Tradit Chin Med. 1994;14:51–5.

Sun Y, Gan TJ, Dubose JW et al. Acupuncture and related techniques for postoperative pain: a systematic review of randomized controlled trials. Br J Anaesth. 2008;101:151–60.

Swarup AB, Barrett W, Jazieh AR. The use of complementary and alternative medicine by cancer patients undergoing radiation therapy. Am J Clin Oncol. 2006;29:468–73.

Syldona M, Rein G. The use of DC electrodermal potential measurements and healer's felt sense to assess the energetic nature of qi. J Alt Comp Med. 1999;5:329–47.

Taguchi A, Sharma N, Ali SZ et al. The effect of auricular acupuncture on anaesthesia with desflurane. Anaesthesia. 2002;57:1159–63.

Taixiang W, Munro AJ, Guanjian L. Chinese medical herbs for chemotherapy side effects in colorectal cancer patients. Cochrane Database Syst Rev. 2005;1:CD004540.

Takeda T, Kamiura S, Kimura T. Effectiveness of the herbal medicine daikenchuto for radiation-induced enteritis. J Altern Complement Med. 2008;14:753–5.

Talal N, Quinn JH, Daniels TE. The clinical effects of electrostimulation on salivary function of Sjögrens syndrome patients: a placebo controlled study. Rheumatol Int. 1992;12:43–5.

Tannock IF, Ahles TA, Ganz PA et al. Cognitive impairment associated with chemotherapy for cancer: report of a workshop. J Clin Oncol. 2004;22:2233–9.

Temoshok L. Biopsychosocial studies on cutaneous malignant melanoma: psychosocial factors associated with prognostic indicators, progression, psychophysiology, and tumor-host response. Soc Sci Med. 1985;8:833–40.

Temoshok L, Dreher H. The type C connection. New York: Random House; 1992.

Thomas JW, Lewis HS, Yuen A. Effect of therapeutic irradiation on lymphocyte transformation in lung cancer. Cancer. 1971;27:1046–50.

Thompson JW, Filshie J. Transcutaneous electrical nerve stimulation (TENS) and acupuncture. In: Doyle D, Hanks GW, MacDonald N, editors. Oxford Textbook of palliative medicine. 2nd edn. Oxford: Oxford University Press; 1998.

Tiller WA, Pecci EF. Science and human transformations: subtle energies, intentionality and consciousness. Walnut Creek, CA: Pavior; 1997.

Tode T, Kikuchi Y, Kita T et al. Inhibitory effects by oral administration of ginsenoside Rh2 on the growth of human ovarian cancer cells in nude mice. J Cancer Res Clin Oncol. 1993;120:24–6.

Tukmachi E. Treatment of hot flushes in breast cancer patients with acupuncture. Acupunct Med. 2000;18:22–7.

Uh S, Lee SM, Kim HT et al. The effect of radiation therapy on immune function in patients with squamous cell lung carcinoma. Chest. 1994;105:132–7.

Usichenko TI, Dinse M, Lysenyuk VP et al. Auricular acupuncture reduces intraoperative fentanyl requirement during hip arthroplasty – a randomized double-blinded study. Acupunct Electrother Res. 2006;31:213–21.

Vickers AJ, Straus DJ, Fearon B et al. Acupuncture for postchemotherapy fatigue: a phase ii study. J Clin Oncol. 2004;22:1731–5.

Wang GT. Treatment of operated late gastric carcinoma with prescription of strengthening the patient's resistance and dispelling the invading evil in combination with chemotherapy: follow-up study of 158 patients and experimental study in animals. Zhong Xi Yi Jie He Za Zhi. 1990;10:712–6.

Wang ZH, Guan WJ. Clinical Results of using TCM in treating chemotherapy related nausea. Shiyongquanke Yixue. 2004;2:254.

Wang JZ, Tsumura H, Shimura K et al. Antitumor activity of polysaccharide from a Chinese medicinal herb, *Acanthopanax giraldii* Harms. Cancer Lett. 1992;65:79–84.

Wefel JS, Kayl AE, Meyers CA. Neuropsychological dysfunction associated with cancer and cancer therapies: a conceptual review of an emerging target. Br J Cancer. 2004a;90:1691–6.

Wefel JS, Lenzi R, Theriault R et al. Chemobrain in breast carcinoma? A prologue. Cancer. 2004b;101:466–75.

Widerstrom-Noga E, Dyrehag LE, Borglum-Jensen L et al. Pain threshold responses to two different modes of sensory stimulation in patients with orofacial muscular pain: psychological considerations. J Orofac Pain. 1998;12:27–34.

Wiklund IK, Mattsson LA, Lindgren R et al. Effects of a standardized ginseng extract on quality of life and physiological parameters in symptomatic postmenopausal women: a double-blind, placebo-controlled trial. Swedish Alternative Medicine Group. Int J Clin Pharmacol Res. 1999;19:89–99.

Wong RKW, Jones GW, Sagar SM et al. A phase I/II study in the use of acupuncture-like transcutaneous nerve stimulation in the treatment of radiation-induced xerostomia in head and neck cancer patients treated with radical radiotherapy. Int J Radiat Oncol Biol Phys. 2003;57:472–80.

Wong RH, Lee TW, Sihoe AD et al. Analgesic effect of electroacupuncture in postthoracotomy pain: a prospective randomized trial. Ann Thorac Surg. 2006;81:2031–6.

Wong R, Sagar S. Acupuncture treatment for chemotherapy-induced peripheral neuropathy – a case series. Acupunct Med. 2006;24:87–91.

Wong R, Sagar SM. The treatment of persistent yawning with acupuncture. Acupunct Med. 2000;18:124–6.

Wong R, Sagar CM, Sagar SM. Integration of Chinese medicine into supportive cancer care: a modern role for an ancient tradition. Cancer Treat Rev. 2001;27:235–46.

Wu MH, Yuan B, Liu QF et al. Study of Qingre Liyan Decoction in treating and preventing acute radioactive oral mucositis. Chin J Integr Med. 2007;13:280–4.

Xu GZ, Cai WM, Qin DX et al. Chinese herb "destagnation" series i: combination of radiation with destagnation in the treatment of nasopharyngeal carcinoma (npc): a prospective randomized trial on 188 cases. Int J Radiat Oncol Biol Phys. 1989;16:297–300.

Xu BP, Long SX, Hu WH. Study on prevention and treatment of radiotherapy caused post-visual pathway injury in nasopharyngeal carcinoma patients by traditional Chinese medicine. Zhongguo Zhong Xi Yi Jie He Za Zhi. 2003;23:661–3.

Yan LS. Treatment of persistent hiccupping with electro-acupuncture at "hiccup-relieving" point. J Tradit Chin Med. 1988;8:29–30.

Yance DR, Sagar SM. Targeting angiogenesis with integrative cancer therapies. Integr Cancer Ther. 2006;5:9–29.

Yano H, Mizoguchi A, Fukuda K et al. The herbal medicine Sho-saiko-to inhibits proliferation of cancer cell lines by inducing apoptosis and arrest at the G0-G1 phase. Cancer Res. 1994;54:448–54.

Yeh SH, Chuang H, Lin LW et al. Regular tai chi chuan exercise enhances functional mobility and CD4 CD25 regulatory T cells. Br J Sports Med. 2006;40:239–43.

Yi WM, Li JJ, Lu XM et al. Effects of electroacupuncture on urinary bladder function after radical hysterectomy. Zhongguo Zhen Jiu. 2008;28:653–5.

Yin D, Tuthill D, Mufson RA et al. Chronic restraint stress promotes lymphocyte apoptosis by modulating *CD95* expression. JEM. 2000;191:1423–8.

Young DR, Appel LJ, Jee SH et al. The effects of aerobic exercise and tai chi on blood pressure in older people: Results of a randomized trial. J Am Geriatr Soc. 1999;47:277–84.

Yu RC, Guan CF, Zhang JH. Immune function of cancer patients with spleen-deficiency syndrome. Zhong Xi Yi Jie He Za Zhi. 1990;10:535–7.

Yu J, Liu C, Zhang X et al. Acupuncture improved cognitive impairment caused by multi-infarct dementia in rats. Physiol Behav. 2005;86:434–41.

Yu G, Ren D, Sun G et al. Clinical and experimental studies of JPYS in reducing side-effects of chemotherapy in late-stage gastric cancer. J Tradit Chin Med. 1993;13:31–7.

Zaborowska E, Brynhildsen J, Damberg S et al. Effects of acupuncture, applied relaxation, estrogens and placebo on hot flushes in postmenopausal women: an analysis of two prospective, parallel, randomized studies. Climacteric. 2007;10:38–45.

Zhang ZH. Effect of acupuncture on 44 cases of radiation rectitis following radiation therapy for carcinoma of the cervix uteri. J Tradit Chin Med. 1987;7:139–40.

Zhang WY. TCM (Fuzheng Peiben method) aids chemotherapy in 47 patients. Zhongyiyao Lingchuang Zhazhi. 2004;16:117–8.

Zhang LH, Fei GD. Clinical study on Fuzheng Peiben used preoperatively in 24 patients. Anhui Zhongyi Clin J. 2001;13:95–6.

Zhang M, Liu X, Li J et al. Chinese medicinal herbs to treat the side-effects of chemotherapy in breast cancer patients. Cochrane Database Syst Rev. 2007a;2:CD004921.

Zhang T, Ma SL, Yue JH. Clinical observation on treatment of radiation pneumonia by Qingjin Runfei Decoction combined with hormone and antibiotic. Zhongguo Zhong Xi Yi Jie He Za Zhi. 2007b;27:254–6.

Zheng W, Gao ZH, Wu LN. Clinical observation on treatment of radiative pneumonia in patients with lung cancer by integrative Chinese and Western medicine. Zhongguo Zhong Xi Yi Jie He Za Zhi. 2007;27:1121–3.

Zhou RF, Liu PX. Study progress in reversing multidrug resistance to breast cancer with Chinese herbs. Zhongguo Zhong Yao Za Zhi. 2005;30:1797–800.

Zhu YP. Chinese materia medica: chemistry, pharmacology and applications. Australia: Harwood Academic Publishers; 1998.

Chapter 2
Supportive Cancer Care with Acupuncture

Jaung-Geng Lin and Yi-Hung Chen

Abstract Acupuncture has many beneficial effects during cancer therapy and has proven efficacy in the management of side effects induced by chemotherapy and radiotherapy. The main merits are as follows:

(a) Pain: pain is the most debilitating symptom for cancer patients. Whereas opioid treatment is liable to cause drug dependency, acupuncture is able to suppress cancer pain without side effects and addiction problems. For cancer pain management, acupuncture on the Hegu (LI4) and Lieque (LU7) acupoints are effective for head and neck pain. Yanglingquan (GB34) and Weizhong (BL40) are appropriate acupoints for waist pain, while Zusanli (ST36) and Sanyangluo (TE8) are for abdominal and chest pain, respectively.
(b) Vomiting, nausea: most studies confirm excellent efficacy of acupuncture on symptoms of vomiting and nausea, including those induced by chemotherapy and radiotherapy. Neiguan (PC6), Zhigou (TE6) and Zusanli (ST36) are appropriate acupoints for treating vomiting and nausea induced by chemotherapy and radiotherapy.
(c) Xerostomia: head and neck cancer patients may receive radiotherapy and may develop xerostomia. Acupuncture on the Hegu (LI4) may relieve this symptom.
(d) Nervousness and insomnia: Acupuncture on the Shenmen (HT7) acupoints may cause sedative and hypnotic effects.

In addition to the above-mentioned acupoints, it is important to follow the classical Meridian theory when selecting acupoints.

In animal models, acupuncture has been shown to improve immune function that is weakened by tumour. However, whether similar beneficial effects are induced in humans remains to be clarified.

J.-G. Lin (✉)
Graduate Institute of Chinese Medical Science, China Medical University, Taichung, Taiwan
e-mail: jglin@mail.cmu.edu.tw

W.C.S. Cho (ed.), *Supportive Cancer Care with Chinese Medicine*,
DOI 10.1007/978-90-481-3555-4_2,

2.1 Introduction

Traditional Chinese acupuncture has a history of over 2,500 years (Wu 1996). Acupuncture has recently increased in popularity and is becoming more widespread throughout some Western countries (NIH Consensus Conference 1998). It is now known as "complementary medicine", because it is effective in the treatment of many conditions. In 1997, the US National Institutes of Health issued a report claiming that acupuncture is a useful method for treating many conditions and that it has fewer side effects compared with other medical procedures, such as surgery or pharmaceuticals (NIH Consensus Conference 1998).

The report concluded: *Acupuncture as a therapeutic intervention is widely practiced in the United States. While there have been many studies of its potential usefulness, many of these studies provide equivocal results because of design, sample size, and other factors. The issue is further complicated by inherent difficulties in the use of appropriate controls, such as placebos and sham acupuncture groups. However, promising results have emerged, for example, showing efficacy of acupuncture in adult post-operative and chemotherapy nausea and vomiting and post-operative dental pain. There are other situations such as addiction, stroke rehabilitation, headache, menstrual cramps, tennis elbow, fibromyalgia, myofascial pain, osteoarthritis, low back pain, carpal tunnel syndrome and asthma where acupuncture may be useful as an adjunct treatment or an acceptable alternative or be included in a comprehensive management programme. Further research is likely to uncover additional areas where acupuncture interventions will be useful.*

Furthermore, the WHO has published a guidance describing the efficacy of acupuncture in the cure or relief of 64 different symptoms (WHO 2003). For example, acupuncture has been successfully applied in cases of chronic pain, fatigue, nausea, arthritis, and digestive problems.

There are two different strategies used when performing acupuncture therapy; manual acupuncture (MA) and electroacupuncture (EA). EA is a modified form of traditional MA. The advantage of EA is in its combined therapeutic effects of transcutaneous electric nerve stimulation (TENS) and MA. Most studies use EA because EA can be standardized by frequency, voltage, wave form, length, etc. However, although standardization is essential for modern research, some experts do not agree that EA can be a substitution for MA (Lin and Chen 2008).

Obtaining qi (De qi or De chi) is a sensation of heaviness, soreness or numbness "recognized" by the cortex during acupuncture needling. Therefore, it is generally accepted that cortical involvement follows acupuncture stimulation (Kimura et al. 2006; Ernst et al. 2007; Kou et al. 2007).

2.2 Mechanism of Acupuncture

Many studies in animals and humans have demonstrated that acupuncture can cause multiple biological responses (Wang et al. 2001). From the neurophysiologic point of view, the mechanical action of needling or its electrical equivalent, i.e. EA, triggers a chain of events that can be understood through controlled experiments. For example, needling may cause receptors to send neural impulses to the spinal cord or act on ascending pathways to the brain, and cause the release of neurotransmitters that subsequently modulate functions in the brain as well as in the periphery (Sun and Li 2001; Liu et al. 2004; Middlekauff et al. 2004).

The best known mechanism is via endogenous opiates and their receptors. Early works have demonstrated the role that endogenous opiates play in the CNS in acupuncture analgesia. Different kinds of endogenous opiates, such as β-endorphin, enkephalin, endomorphin and dynophin, have been reported to be frequency-dependent factors of EA.

In the 1970s and early 1980s, acupuncture was regarded as a novel pain-killer. Naloxone, an opiate receptor antagonist, was shown to attenuate analgesic actions of acupuncture in humans (Mayer et al. 1977) and mice (Pomeranz and Chiu 1976); the release of a morphine-like substrate in the central nervous system was hypothesized to be a possible mechanism.

In the early 1980s, β-endorphin and enkephalin were purified and it was suggested that they play a role in acupuncture in humans and animals (Clement-Jones et al. 1980; Pert et al. 1981; Kiser et al. 1983). Elevated levels of endorphin in the cerebrospinal fluid (CSF) were observed in cats after auricular EA. In humans, elevated levels of β-endorphin in the CSF and also of plasma enkephalin were observed after acupuncture. Soon afterwards, the relationship between acupuncture analgesia and different kinds of endogenous opiates was explored in detail. For example, Pomeranz's group was the first to describe the possibility that there are different mechanisms of analgesia when EA is applied with different frequencies (Cheng et al. 1979).

In addition to opioids, researchers have focused on the role of central monoamimergic systems. Particular emphasis is given to serotonin, speculated to be an analgesic neurotransmitter (Cheng et al. 1979). Evidence suggests that serotonin levels increase in the spinal cord and that its precursor (5-hydroxytryptophan) responds to enhanced analgesia at 2 Hz EA (Chang et al. 2004).

As more studies are conducted worldwide, theories have been developed regarding serotonin and related descending pain inhibitory pathways. It is increasingly clear that EA evokes serotonin release from regions of the upper brain stem and hypothalamus, in addition to endogenous opiates (Lin and Chen 2008).

Acupuncture therapy is used not only to relieve pain but also to treat various medical conditions in traditional Chinese medicine (TCM). Some experiments have revealed a relationship between acupuncture and the autonomic nervous system (ANS) (Tracey 2002). The inflammatory reflex via the ANS could be a possible explanation for acupuncture's diverse therapeutic strategies. Many disorders are thought to be inflammation-related. It is hypothesized that acupuncture can modulate these inflammatory conditions through an inflammatory reflex (Sekido et al. 2003; Zhang et al. 2004). The hypothalamus is the modulator for both hormonal and neuronal systems. Therefore, the hypothalamus might play a key role in the mechanism of acupuncture (Chiu et al. 2003).

EA can modulate the imbalance between innate and acquired immune systems. EA has been shown to have the ability to adjust the pattern of leukocytes (granulocyte and lymphocyte) in human subjects (Mori et al. 2002). Several lines of evidence indicate that this effect is associated with the hypothalamus-pituitary-adrenal axis.

Although EA has been investigated extensively, these studies are of limited clinical relevance to traditional applications. Most Chinese medicine practitioners, especially in the East, use MA instead of EA. In those studies employing the EA method, it is not clear whether the analgesia effect is through needling itself or through electric stimulation. An investigator found that electrical stimulation of the peripheral nerve elicits an analgesic effect. Therefore, the fundamental question of acupuncture and the existence of specific points cannot be answered by results from studies which intend to explore the effect of EA.

2.3 Evaluation of Acupuncture's Curative Effect in the Treatment of Cancer Patients and the Side Effects of Chemotherapy and Radiotherapy

In recent years, cancer has been the leading cause of death in developed countries. Conventional cancer treatment still uses surgery, radiotherapy or chemotherapy as the main methods of treatment, assisted by hormone therapy and cancer immune therapy. However, since their side effects are associated with great amounts of pain and engender a sense of insecurity in patients, and as some cancer may have an incurable prognosis, the curative effects of these methods in cancer are remain less than ideal.

After British epidemiologists proposed evidence-based medicine (EBM; basing medical practice on the best available scientific evidence) in 1979, acupuncturists started to employ EBM standards in clinical randomized controlled trials (RCT) to evaluate the effects of acupuncture. In the PubMed and MEDLINE databases, much evidence attests to the benefits of acupuncture in clinical cancer therapy. Acupuncture can relieve cancer-related pain and side-effects after chemotherapy and radiotherapy, as detailed below.

2.3.1 Cancer Pain

Pain is the most debilitating symptom in cancer patients and is difficult for clinicians to treat, because analgesic drugs do not always procure complete relief (Portenoy and Lesage 1999; Alimi et al. 2003). After curative cancer treatment, pain often remains as a dominant symptom affecting the patient's physical and psychological states. Chronic pain in cancer patients is dominated by the neuropathic component, even when associated with nociceptive pain (Caraceni and Portenoy 1999). Neuropathic pain is the most difficult type of pain to treat in cancer patients, and in general, does not respond well to drug treatment (Filshie 1988).

Acupuncture activates central brain pathways, thus inhibiting the maladaptive reflex that contributes to neuropathic pain (Oleson 2002).

Although acupuncture analgesia has been studied in the laboratory and clinic for several decades (Lin et al. 2002; Lin and Chen 2008, 2009; Wu et al. 2009), few acupuncture clinical trials exist for cancer-specific pain. In a single-blind randomized controlled trial, 90 patients with cancer pain despite stable analgesic treatment were divided into three groups; one group received two courses of auricular acupuncture at points where an electrodermal signal had been detected, one group received auricular acupuncture at points with no electrodermal signal (placebo points) and the remaining group received auricular seeds fixed at placebo points (Alimi et al. 2003). Treatment efficacy was based on the absolute decrease in pain intensity using the visual analog score (VAS) measured 2 months after randomization. At 2 months, pain intensity had decreased by 36% from baseline in the group receiving acupuncture; there was little change for patients receiving placebo (2%). The difference between groups was statistically significant. The study represents a clear benefit from auricular acupuncture for cancer patients with ongoing pain despite analgesic therapy.

2.3.2 Nausea and Vomiting

Progress in the prevention and treatment of chemotherapy-induced nausea and vomiting has been achieved with the advent of 5-hydroxytriptamine 3 ($5HT_3$) receptor antagonists ondansetron and dexamethasone (Ioannidis et al. 2000). However, many patients still experience these symptoms. Chemotherapy-induced nausea and vomiting can impair a patient's quality of life (Osoba et al. 1997), cause emotional distress (Love et al. 1989), and aggravate cancer-related symptoms of cachexia, lethargy and weakness (Griffin et al. 1996; Roscoe et al. 2000).

In one study, 104 breast cancer patients who had received high-dose chemotherapy (HDC; cyclophosphamide, cisplatin, and carmustine) were randomly divided into three groups: low-frequency electroacupuncture at classic antiemetic acupuncture points (Neiguan and Zusanli) once daily for 5 days ($n = 37$); minimal needling at control points with mock electrostimulation on the same schedule ($n = 33$); or no adjunct needling ($n = 34$) (Vickers et al. 2004). The number of emesis episodes occurring during the 5 days was lower for patients receiving electroacupuncture compared with those receiving minimal needling or pharmacotherapy alone. The electroacupuncture group had fewer episodes of emesis than the minimal needling group, whereas the minimal needling group had fewer episodes of emesis than the antiemetic pharmacotherapy-alone group. The differences among groups were not significant during the 9-day follow-up period. The data suggest that in patients with breast cancer receiving high-dose chemotherapy, adjunct electroacupuncture was more effective in controlling emesis than minimal needling or antiemetic pharmacotherapy alone, although the observed effect was of limited duration.

However, another study has shown negative results of acupuncture on chemotherapy-induced nausea and vomiting. In this study, the researchers aimed to investigate an additional antiemetic effect to ondansetron with needle acupuncture at PC6 compared with non-skin-penetrating placebo acupuncture in patients undergoing high-dose chemotherapy and autologous peripheral blood stem cell transplantation (Streitberger et al. 2003). Eighty patients who were admitted to hospital for high-dose chemotherapy and autologous peripheral blood stem cell transplantation were included in a randomized placebo-controlled single-blind trial. The results of the study suggest that in combination with IV ondansetron, acupuncture at PC6 compared with non-skin-penetrating placebo acupuncture has no additional effect for the prevention of acute nausea and vomiting in high-dose chemotherapy.

2.3.3 Xerostomia

Xerostomia or dry mouth is a very common complication in patients treated with radiotherapy for head and neck cancer. The condition is caused by radiation damage to the salivary glands. It has been shown that the reduction in salivary flow depends on the radiation dose delivered and the volume of salivary glands irradiated. Even a low dose of radiation can cause a change in the quantity and quality of saliva, and up to 100% of patients who undergo radiotherapy for head and neck cancer develop some degree of xerostomia. The symptoms of radiation-induced xerostomia are often permanent and lead to difficulty in mastication, swallowing, and speaking. Other consequences include stomatitis, taste dysfunction, and increased susceptibility to dental caries (Dreizen et al. 1976; Franzen et al. 1992).

Oral pilocarpine hydrochloride treatment has been the most extensively studied and is commercially available for treating xerostomia. Despite a modest effectiveness with overall improvement in symptoms, adverse cholinergic effects, such as sweating, nausea, rhinitis and chills, limit the use of pilocarpine. In contrast, two clinical studies have demonstrated the efficacy of acupuncture in xerostomia.

In one study, a single treatment with eight needles of acupuncture was used. Three points were treated in each ear, and one in the radial aspect of each index finger. Patients were also administered a sugar-free lozenge in the mouth to further stimulate salivation. Response was measured by the xerostomia inventory (XI). Fifty patients underwent 318 treatments (Johnstone et al. 2002). Response (defined as improvement of 10% or better over baseline XI values) occurred in 35 patients (70%). Twenty-four patients (48%) experienced a benefit of 10 points or greater on the XI. In 13 patients (26%), the duration of treatment effect has exceeded 3 months. The results indicate that acupuncture palliates xerostomia for many patients. A regimen of 3 to 4 weekly treatments followed by monthly sessions is now recommended for cases of xerostomia.

The other study recruited 46 patients with symptomatic xerostomia and evidence of residual salivary function after radical radiotherapy for head and neck cancer. Two 6-week courses of an acupuncture-like transcutaneous nerve stimulation method (Codetron) without invasive needles were developed to mimic acupuncture treatment (Wong et al. 2003). Treatment of acupuncture points, preselected according to TCM principles, was administered with a 2-week break between each course.

Basal and citric acid-primed whole saliva production was measured at baseline and for up to 1 year after treatment completion. Xerostomia symptoms were assessed by a 5-item xerostomia symptom questionnaire with a VAS and quality of life was evaluated using the Head and Neck Radiotherapy Questionnaire. Improvement in xerostomia symptoms was noted, with a mean increase in the VAS score of 86 and 77 at 3 and 6 months after treatment completion, respectively. The treatment effects were sustained for at least 6 months after Codetron completion.

2.3.4 Nervousness and Insomnia

Insomnia is one of the most significant symptoms experienced by patients who have cancer, as well as nervousness. A small, non-cancer study found 5 weeks of acupuncture significantly reduced insomnia and anxiety, with accompanying significant increases in nocturnal melatonin secretion and in polysomnographic measure (Spence et al. 2004). A meta-analysis showed that the recovery and improvement rates produced by auricular acupuncture were significantly higher than those relating to diazepam (Chen et al. 2007). The rate of success was higher when auricular acupuncture was used to enhance sleeping hours by up to 6 hours in treatment subjects. The authors of this study concluded that ear acupuncture appears to be effective for treating insomnia.

However, in a Cochrane systematic review of acupuncture for insomnia, the authors found that acupuncture or its variants were not more significantly effective than a control (Cheuk et al. 2007). The authors concluded that the current evidence is not sufficiently extensive or rigorous enough to support the use of any form of acupuncture for treating insomnia. Larger high-quality clinical trials employing appropriate randomization, concealment, and blinding with longer follow-up are warranted to further investigate the efficacy and safety of acupuncture for treating insomnia.

2.3.5 Others

In animal models, acupuncture has been shown to improve immunity weakened by tumour growth. One suggests that moxibustion at the Guanyuan (CV4) acupoint can strengthen erythrocytic immunity and promote its regulative function (Wu et al. 2001).

According to the study by Yamaguchi et al. (2007), conducted with healthy volunteers, acupuncture did not affect leukocyte counts but significantly increased numbers of $CD2^+$ $CD4^+$, $CD8^+$, $CD11b^+$, $CD16^+$, $CD19^+$, $CD56^+$ cells as well as IL-4, IL-1β and IFN-γ levels in the cells.

One study suggest that moxibustion at the Shenque (CV8) acupoint can inhibit tumour growth, which is related to the increased serum IL-2 and IL-12 levels and the strengthening of NK cell activities (Qiu et al. 2004). Another study revealed that acupuncture was able to repress tumour growth in tumour-bearing mice (Hau et al. 1999).

In short, carefully chosen experiment designs, the number of research subjects, whether a trial is randomized and controlled or not, choice of acupuncture points, duration of needling, and temperature during moxibustion may all considerably affect the credibility of experimental data. We hope that in future, acupuncture research is aligned with international practice and clinical research becomes more objective, reliable, and convincing.

2.4 Clinical Practice

Acupuncture has many beneficial effects on cancer therapy and on the management of side effects induced by chemotherapy and radiotherapy. Regarding clinical practice, my personal experiences are detailed as follows.

2.4.1 Pain

Pain is the most debilitating symptom of tumour patients. Treatment with opioid medicine may result in drug dependency, whereas acupuncture is able to suppress cancer pain without side effects and addiction problems. For cancer pain management, acupuncture on the Hegu (LI4; Fig. 2.1) and Lieque (LU7; Fig. 2.2) acupoints are effective for head and neck pain. Yanglingquan (GB34; Fig. 2.3) and Weizhong (BL40; Fig. 2.4) are appropriate acupoints for waist pain, while Zusanli (ST36; Fig. 2.5) and Sanyangluo (TE8; Fig. 2.9) are for abdominal and chest pain, respectively.

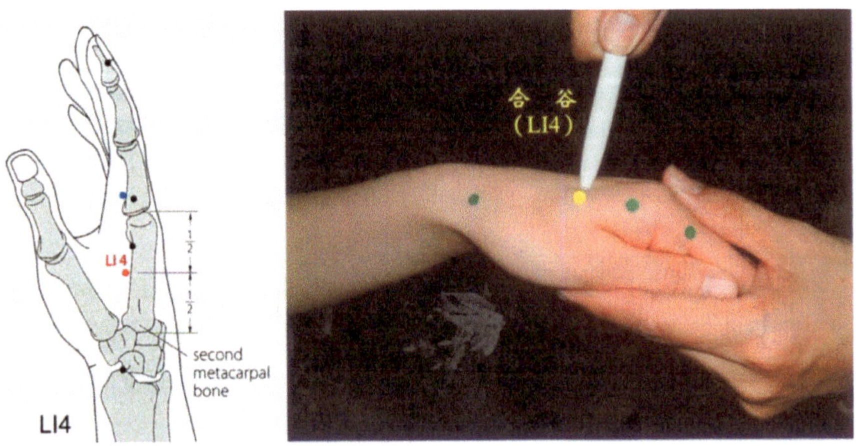

Fig. 2.1 LI4 (Hegu): On the dorsum of the hand, radial to the midpoint of the second metacarpal bone (WHO 2008)

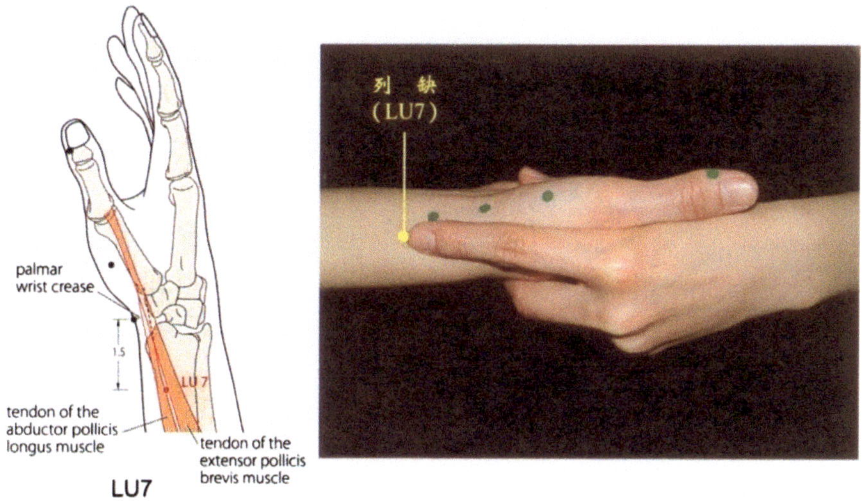

Fig. 2.2 LU7 (Lieque): On the radial aspect of the forearm, between the tendons of the abductor pollicis longus and the extensor pollicis brevis muscles, in the groove for the abductor pollicis longus tendon, 1.5 B-cun superior to the palmar wrist crease (WHO 2008)

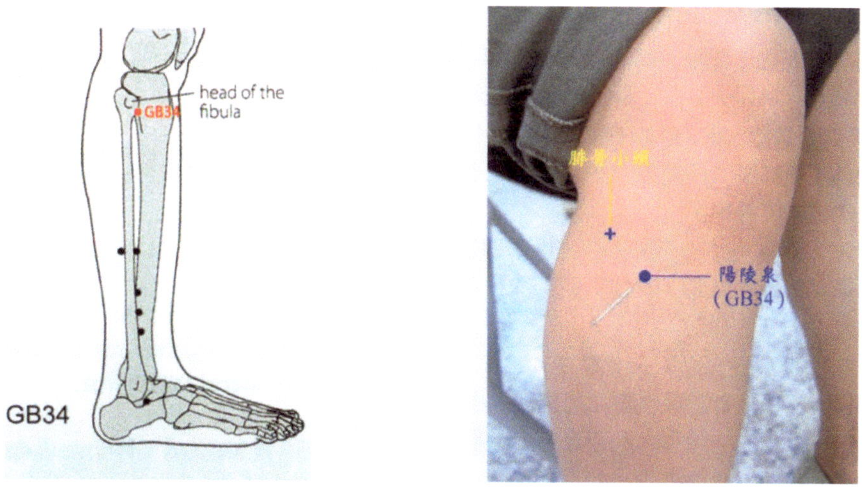

Fig. 2.3 GB34 (Yanglingquan): On the fibular aspect of the leg, in the depression anterior and distal to the head of the fibula (WHO 2008)

2.4.2 Vomiting, Nausea

Most studies confirm the excellent efficacy of acupuncture on vomiting and nausea, including that induced by chemotherapy and radiotherapy. Neiguan (PC6; Fig. 2.6), Zhigou (TE6; Fig. 2.7) and Zusanli (ST36; Fig. 2.5) are appropriate acupoints for treatment vomiting and nausea induced by chemotherapy and radiotherapy.

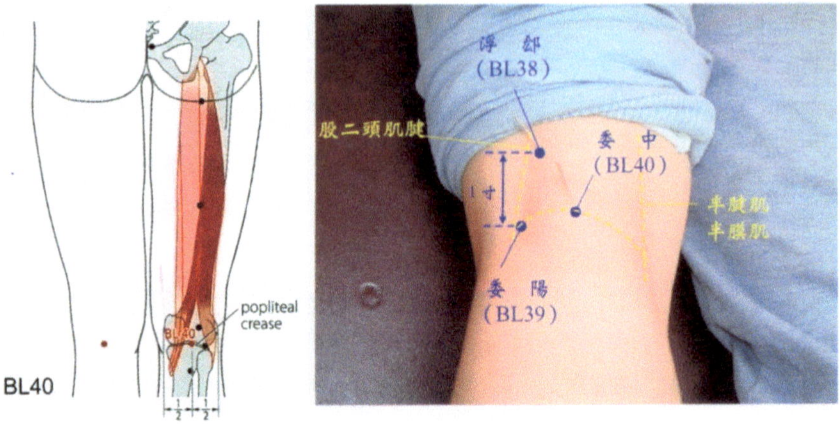

Fig. 2.4 BL40 (Weizhong): On the posterior aspect of the knee, at the midpoint of the popliteal crease (WHO 2008)

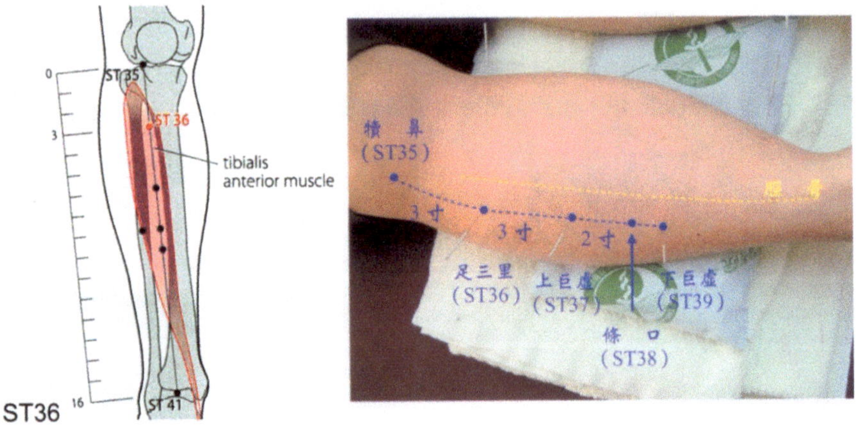

Fig. 2.5 ST36 (Zusanli): On the anterior aspect of the leg, on the line connecting ST35 with ST41, 3 B-cun inferior to ST35. Note: ST36 is located on the tibialis anterior muscle (WHO 2008)

2.4.3 Xerostomia

Head and neck cancer patients may receive radiotherapy and may develop xerostomia. Acupuncture on Hegu (LI4; Fig. 2.1) may relieve this symptom.

2.4.4 Nervousness and Insomnia

Acupuncture on Shenmen (HT7; Fig. 2.8) or Ximen (PC4; Fig. 2.10) may cause sedative and hypnotic effects.

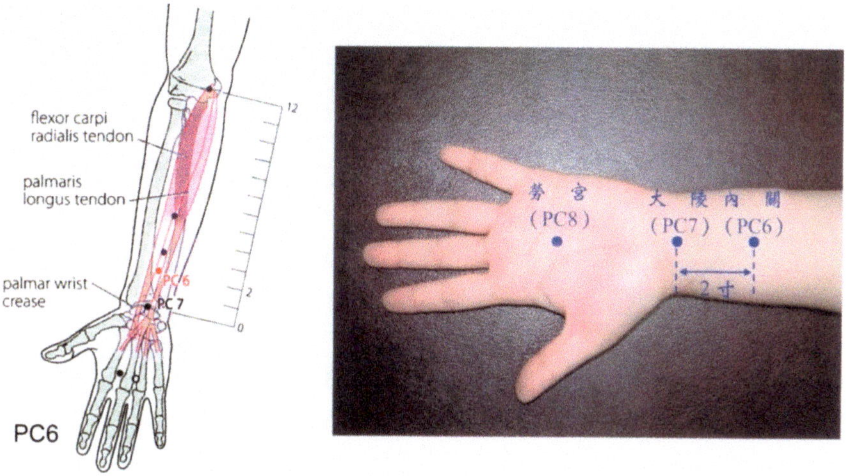

Fig. 2.6 PC6 (Neiguan): On the anterior aspect of the forearm, between the tendons of the palmaris longus and the flexor carpi radialis, 2 B-cun proximal to the palmar wrist crease. Note 1: With the fist clenched, the wrist supinated and the elbow slightly flexed, the two tendons become more prominent. PC6 is located 2 B-cun proximal to PC7. The posterial point corresponding to PC6 is TE5. Note 2: If the palmaris longus tendon is not present, PC6 is medial to the flexor carpi radialis tendon (WHO 2008)

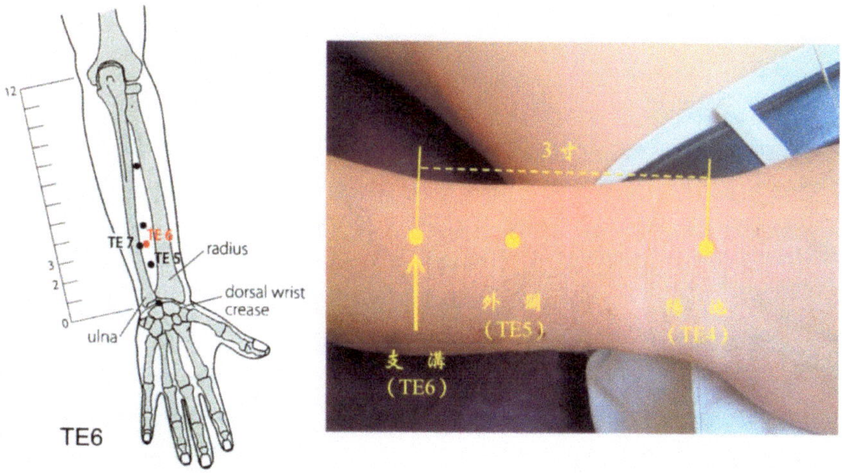

Fig. 2.7 TE6 (Zhigou): On the posterior aspect of the forearm, midpoint of the interosseous space between the radius and the ulna, 3 B-cun proximal to the dorsal wrist crease. Note 1: B-cun proximal to TE5, between the radius and the ulna, at the same level as TE7 (WHO 2008)

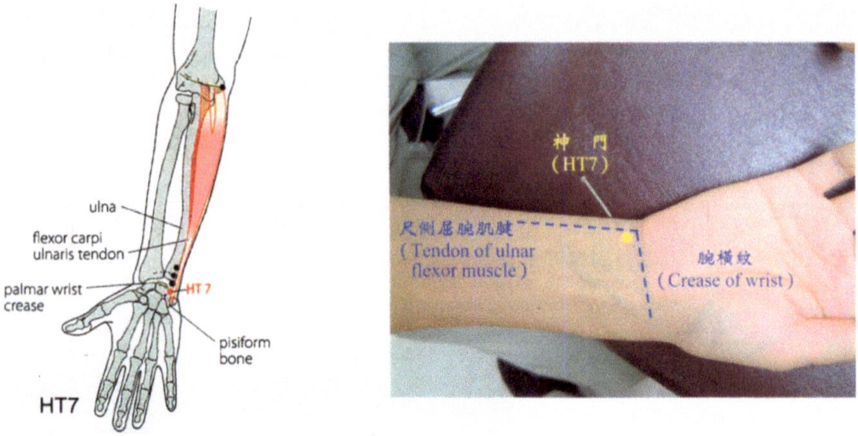

Fig. 2.8 HT7 (Shenmen): On the anteromedial aspect of the wrist, radial to the flexor carpi ulnaris tendon, on the palmar wrist crease. Note: In the depression radial to the proximal border of the pisiform bone, on the palmar wrist crease (WHO 2008)

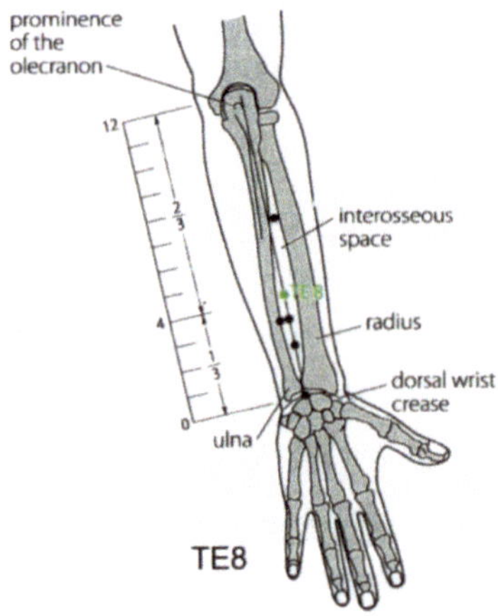

Fig. 2.9 TE8 (Sanyangluo): On the posterior aspect of the forearm, midpoint of the interosseous space between the radius and the ulna, 4 B-cun proximal to the dorsal wrist crease. Note: At the junction of the upper two thirds and lower one third of the line connecting TE4 with the tip of the elbow (WHO 2008)

Besides the above-mentioned advice on acupoints, it is important to follow the classical Meridian theory when choosing acupoints.

2.4.5 *Others*

2.4.5.1 Side Effects of Acupuncture

Serious complications associated with acupuncture are rare; most side effects are minor and include faintness and syncope, needle site bleeding, needle site pain,

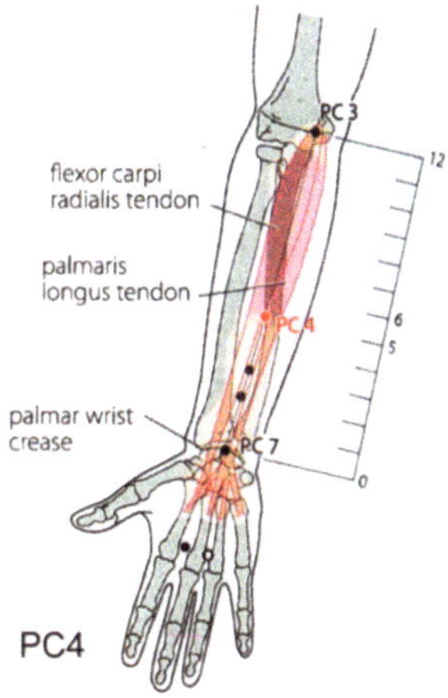

Fig. 2.10 PC4 (Ximen): On the anterior aspect of the forearm, between the tendons of the palmaris longus and the flexor carpi radialis, 5 B-cun proximal to the palmar wrist crease. Note 1: With the fist clenched, the wrist supinated, and the elbow slightly flexed, the two tendons become more prominent. PC4 is located 1 B-cun distal to the midpoint of the line connecting PC3 with PC7. Note 2: If the palmaris longus tendon is not present, PC4 is medial to the flexor carpi radialis tendon (WHO 2008)

initial aggravation of symptoms with subsequent improvement, infection, needle breakage, nerve damage, pneumothorax and abortion in pregnant women.

2.4.5.2 Precautions When Conducting Acupuncture

According to the report of Chung et al. (2003), patients with advanced liver disease may experience compromised clotting factor production and patients on anticoagulants may bleed for longer periods. Special attention should be paid to these patient populations because they are prone to bleeding during acupuncture treatment. Patients who taking high-dose steroids have suppressed immune systems and patients with diabetes are subject to poor wound healing. Special attention should be given to these patients because they are prone to infection. In addition, hypoglycemic, nervous, and fatigued patients might faint during acupuncture treatment.

Based on our experience, there are some precautions to be noted especially when conducting acupuncture in cancer patients.

1. Enlarged lymph node;
2. Anatomic change due to the tumour;
3. Leucopenia due to chemotherapy;
4. Thrombocytopenia due to chemotherapy.

References

World Health Organization. Acupuncture: review and analysis of reports on controlled clinical trials. Geneva, World Health Organization; 2003.

Alimi D, Rubino C, Pichard-Leandri E et al. Analgesic effect of auricular acupuncture for cancer pain: a randomized, blinded, controlled trial. J Clin Oncol. 2003; 21:4120–6.

Caraceni A, Portenoy RK. An international survey of cancer pain characteristics and syndromes. IASP Task Force on Cancer Pain. International Association for the Study of Pain. Pain. 1999;82:263–74.

Chang FC, Tsai HY, Yu MC et al. The central serotonergic system mediates the analgesic effect of electroacupuncture on ZUSANLI (ST36) acupoints. J Biomed Sci. 2004;11:179–85.

Chen HY, Shi Y, Ng CS et al. Auricular acupuncture treatment for insomnia: a systematic review. J Altern Complement Med. 2007;13:669–76.

Cheng R, Pomeranz B, Yu G. Dexamethasone partially reduces and 2% saline-treatment abolished electroacupuncture analgesia: these findings implicate pituitary endorphins. Life Sci. 1979;24:1481–6.

Cheuk DK, Yeung WF, Chung KF et al. Acupuncture for insomnia. Cochrane Database Syst Rev. 2007; 3:CD005472.

Chiu JH, Chung MS, Cheng HC et al. Different central manifestations in response to electroacupuncture at analgesic and nonanalgesic acupoints in rats: a manganese-enhanced functional magnetic resonance imaging study. Can J Vet Res. 2003;67:94–101.

Chung A, Bui L, Mills E. Adverse effects of acupuncture. Which are clinically significant? Can Fam Physician. 2003;49:985–9.

Clement-Jones V, McLoughlin L, Tomlin S et al. Increased beta-endorphin but not met-enkephalin levels in human cerebrospinal fluid after acupuncture for recurrent pain. Lancet. 1980;2:946–9.

Dreizen S, Brown LR, Handler S et al. Radiation-induced xerostomia in cancer patients. Effect on salivary and serum electrolytes. Cancer. 1976;38:273–8.

Ernst E, Pittler MH, Wider B et al. Acupuncture: its evidence-base is changing. Am J Chin Med. 2007;35:21–5.

Filshie J. The non-drug treatment of neuralgic and neuropathic pain of malignancy. Cancer Surv. 1988;7:161–93.

Franzen L, Funegard U, Ericson T et al. Parotid gland function during and following radiotherapy of malignancies in the head and neck. A consecutive study of salivary flow and patient discomfort. Eur J Cancer. 1992;28:457–62.

Griffin AM, Butow PN, Coates AS et al. On the receiving end. V: Patient perceptions of the side effects of cancer chemotherapy in 1993. Ann Oncol. 1996;7:189–95.

Hau DM, Lin IH, Lin JG et al. Therapeutic effects of moxibustion on experimental tumor. Am J Chin Med. 1999;27:157–66.

Ioannidis JP, Hesketh PJ, Lau J. Contribution of dexamethasone to control of chemotherapy-induced nausea and vomiting: a meta-analysis of randomized evidence. J Clin Oncol. 2000;18:3409–22.

Johnstone PA, Niemtzow RC, Riffenburgh RH. Acupuncture for xerostomia: clinical update. Cancer. 2002;94:1151–6.

Kimura K, Masuda K, Wakayama I. Changes in skin blood flow and skin sympathetic nerve activity in response to manual acupuncture stimulation in humans. Am J Chin Med. 2006;34: 189–96.

Kiser RS, Khatami MJ, Gatchel RJ et al. Acupuncture relief of chronic pain syndrome correlates with increased plasma met-enkephalin concentrations. Lancet. 1983;2:1394–6.

Kou W, Gareus I, Bell JD et al. Quantification of DeQi sensation by visual analog scales in healthy humans after immunostimulating acupuncture treatment. Am J Chin Med. 2007;35:753–65.

Lin JG, Chen WL. Acupuncture analgesia: a review of its mechanisms of actions. Am J Chin Med. 2008;36:635–45.

Lin JG, Chen WL. Review: acupuncture analgesia in clinical trials. Am J Chin Med. 2009;37:1–18.

Lin JG, Lo MW, Wen YR et al. The effect of high and low frequency electroacupuncture in pain after lower abdominal surgery. Pain 2002;99:509–14.
Liu JH, Yan J, Yi SX et al. Effects of electroacupuncture on gastric myoelectric activity and substance P in the dorsal vagal complex of rats. Neurosci Lett. 2004;356:99–102.
Love RR, Leventhal H, Easterling DV et al. Side effects and emotional distress during cancer chemotherapy. Cancer. 1989;63:604–12.
Mayer DJ, Price DD, Rafii A. Antagonism of acupuncture analgesia in man by the narcotic antagonist naloxone. Brain Res. 1977;121:368–72.
Middlekauff HR, Shah JB, Yu JL et al. Acupuncture effects on autonomic responses to cold pressor and handgrip exercise in healthy humans. Clin Auton Res. 2004;14:113–8.
Mori H, Nishijo K, Kawamura H et al. Unique immunomodulation by electro-acupuncture in humans possibly via stimulation of the autonomic nervous system. Neurosci Lett. 2002;320:21–4.
NIH Consensus Conference. Acupuncture. JAMA. 1998;280:1518–24.
Oleson T. Auriculotherapy stimulation for neuro-rehabilitation. NeuroRehabilitation. 2002;17: 49–62.
Osoba D, Zee B, Warr D et al. Effect of postchemotherapy nausea and vomiting on health-related quality of life. The Quality of Life and Symptom Control Committees of the National Cancer Institute of Canada Clinical Trials Group. Support Care Cancer. 1997;5:307–13.
Pert A, Dionne R, Ng L et al. Alterations in rat central nervous system endorphins following transauricular electroacupuncture. Brain Res. 1981;224:83–93.
Pomeranz B, Chiu D. Naloxone blockade of acupuncture analgesia: endorphin implicated. Life Sci. 1976;19:1757–62.
Portenoy RK, Lesage P. Management of cancer pain. Lancet. 1999;353:1695–700.
Qiu X, Chen K, Tong L et al. Effects of moxibustion at shenque (CV 8) on serum IL-12 level and NK cell activities in mice with transplanted tumor. J Tradit Chin Med. 2004;24:56–8.
Roscoe JA, Morrow GR, Hickok JT et al. Nausea and vomiting remain a significant clinical problem: trends over time in controlling chemotherapy-induced nausea and vomiting in 1413 patients treated in community clinical practices. J Pain Symptom Manage. 2000;20:113–21.
Sekido R, Ishimaru K, Sakita M. Differences of electroacupuncture-induced analgesic effect in normal and inflammatory conditions in rats. Am J Chin Med. 2003;31:955–65.
Spence DW, Kayumov L, Chen A et al. Acupuncture increases nocturnal melatonin secretion and reduces insomnia and anxiety: a preliminary report. J Neuropsychiatry Clin Neurosci. 2004;16:19–28.
Streitberger K, Friedrich-Rust M, Bardenheuer H et al. Effect of acupuncture compared with placebo-acupuncture at P6 as additional antiemetic prophylaxis in high-dose chemotherapy and autologous peripheral blood stem cell transplantation: a randomized controlled single-blind trial. Clin Cancer Res. 2003;9:2538–44.
Sun HL, Li XM. Clinical study on treatment of cerebral apoplexy with penetration needling of scalp acupoints [tou xue tou ci zhi liao nao zu zhong lin chuang yan jiu]. Zhongguo Zhen Jiu. 2001;21:275–8.
Tracey KJ. The inflammatory reflex. Nature. 2002;420:853–9.
Vickers AJ, Straus DJ, Fearon B et al. Acupuncture for postchemotherapy fatigue: a phase II study. J Clin Oncol. 2004;22:1731–5.
WHO standard acupuncture point locations in the Western Pacific region. World Health Organization; 2008.
Wang G, Jiang N, He Z. Effects of scalp acupuncture on plasma ET-1, MDA and NO contents in the patient of cerebral infarction. Chinese Acupuncture Moxibustion. 2001;21:241–2.
Wong RK, Jones GW, Sagar SM et al. A Phase I-II study in the use of acupuncture-like transcutaneous nerve stimulation in the treatment of radiation-induced xerostomia in head-and-neck cancer patients treated with radical radiotherapy. Int J Radiat Oncol Biol Phys. 2003;57:472–80.
Wu HC, Liu YC, Ou KL et al. Effects of acupuncture on post-cesarean section pain. Chin Med J. 2009;122:1743–48.

Wu JN. A short history of acupuncture. J Altern Complement Med. 1996;2:19–21.
Wu P, Cao Y, Wu J. Effects of moxa-cone moxibustion at Guanyuan on erythrocytic immunity and its regulative function in tumor-bearing mice. J Tradit Chin Med. 2001;21:68–71.
Yamaguchi N, Takahashi T, Sakuma M et al. Acupuncture regulates leukocyte subpopulations in human peripheral blood. Evid Based Complement Alternat Med. 2007;4:447–53.
Zhang SP, Zhang JS, Yung KK et al. Non-opioid-dependent anti-inflammatory effects of low frequency electroacupuncture. Brain Res Bull. 2004;62:327–34.

Chapter 3
Chinese Medicinal Herbs Use in Managing Cancer

Peter Dorsher and Zengfu Peng

Abstract For millennia, traditional Chinese medicine (TCM) practitioners have treated cancer with Chinese medicinal herbs (CMHs), which continue to be used in combination with conventional chemotherapy and radiotherapy in contemporary oncologic care in Asia. Recent advances in biochemistry and immunology have allowed discovery of the biologically active components of CMH and the mechanisms of their anti-cancer activities. This chapter provides an overview of CMH use in treating cancer, including discussion of the anti-cancer mechanisms for individual herbs that are commonly used to treat cancer in contemporary TCM practice. Most CMH cancer research studies have involved in vitro and in vivo animal studies, with a relative paucity of well designed, placebo-controlled human clinical trials. Despite this, there is evidence that CMH may mitigate immunosuppression from conventional chemotherapy and radiotherapy, reduce side effects from those treatments, and improve cancer patients' overall clinical status. Chinese medicinal herbs may produce tumour apoptosis, reduce metastases, and increase survival, either alone or in combination with conventional chemotherapy. Some CMHs interfere with conventional chemotherapy when administered simultaneously, yet enhance conventional chemotherapy efficacy when administered sequentially. Further controlled clinical trials of CMH with/without conventional chemotherapy and radiotherapy in cancer patients are needed to determine which herbs (and herb combinations) to use and the optimal timing of their administration to optimize cancer patients' survival, reduce tumour burden, enhance immunologic function and improve quality of life while minimizing the side effects (e.g. nausea/vomiting, anorexia and fatigue) of conventional radiotherapy or chemotherapy.

P. Dorsher (✉)
Mayo Clinic, Rochester, MN, USA
e-mail: dorsher.peter@mayo.edu

W.C.S. Cho (ed.), *Supportive Cancer Care with Chinese Medicine*,
DOI 10.1007/978-90-481-3555-4_3,

3.1 Introduction

Archeological evidence exists that ancient Chinese healers documented human tumours pictorially over 3,000 years ago, and approximately a thousand years later classical traditional Chinese medicine (TCM) texts described the causes of tumours as well as the principles of their treatment.

The Western diagnosis of cancer is called Ai in modern TCM terminology. Ai was first described in the Song Dynasty by Wei Ji Bao Shu circa 1171 AD (Mingji 1992). The original meaning of Ai referred to a hard, uneven surface, like a rock. Examples include breast cancer (Ru Ai) and kidney cancer (Shen Ai). Cancer was also termed Liu (meaning tumour) in inscriptions on oracle bones that are over 3,500 years old (Mingji 1992).

Western allopathic physicians have only (relatively) recently recognized that cancer represents many different disease entities influenced by both host and external/environmental factors. In contrast, those factors have always been fundamental to the diagnosis and treatment of all human illnesses including cancer since the principles of TCM were first formally described in the Huangdi's Internal Classic (Huangdi Neijing) ~200 BC (Zhu 2001). The use of Chinese medical herbs (CMHs) to treat illnesses including cancer has long been a part of TCM practice. A compendium of medicinal herbs, their formulations, and clinical uses was developed by the first century AD. Li Shizhen (1152–1578 AD) wrote the classic text delineating the use of 1,892 medicinal herbs and extracts during the Ming Dynasty (Porter and Stuart 2003). By 2005, the latest edition of The Pharmacopoeia of the People's Republic of China listed 1,146 single herbs or extracts (Pharmacopoeia Commission 2005).

Five principles organize the formulation of many herbal prescriptions for the treatment of cancer: supplement the qi and blood to strengthen host resistance; activate circulation to dispel blood stasis and ecchymosis; relieve pain; eliminate Heat and toxins; and soften lumps and dissolve masses. In simpler terms, a herbal treatment principle is both to 'strengthen the correct' meaning the body's general immunity (Fuzheng) while simultaneously regenerating and repairing the body (Guben) (Dawes 2004). Chinese medicinal herbal formulations to treat cancer may also be thought of as strengthening healthy qi to eliminate pathogens.

3.2 Principles of Herbal Treatments

Fundamental to the use of CMH to treat cancer is accurate diagnosis of the patient's condition using the four diagnostic methods. The herbal prescription is formulated to normalize any bodily excesses or deficiencies noted on the four diagnostic methods that have led to the stagnation and accumulation of qi and blood as tumour (phlegm) in the patient. Further, treatment of the root causes of the cancer must be addressed in the herbal prescription to prevent tumour recurrence.

According to TCM theory (Abbate 2006), the causes of tumour are the deficiency of Zheng qi (a concept that can be considered analogous to the Western concept of immune system competency/strength) and the excess of Xie qi (pathogenic factors). Tumour is a type of Ji Ju (meaning accumulation of things; or something gathered). In the early stages of cancer, the Xie qi is considered the main causative factor in cancer patients, while in the middle and advanced stages of the disease, the deficiency of Zheng qi is the main issue to address in cancer patients. Traditional Chinese medicine practitioners believe that the lack of Zheng qi is the inevitable result from the intrusion of Xie qi and toxin that in turn results in their accumulation, leading to the formation of tumours by the turbid phlegm and toxin in the body. Further, allopathic cancer treatment using radiotherapy and chemotherapy kills not only tumour cells but also normal cells (including T-cell and B-cell lymphocytes) leading to immune system suppression (further reduction of Zheng qi) that favors tumour growth and spread.

In CMH therapy for cancer in early stages, then, the prescription must address clearing the excess of Xie qi, but it should also address protection of the Zheng qi to maximize the cancer patient's immunity (Lahans 2008). Traditional Chinese medicine theory describes that the early stages of tumour development are mainly caused by qi stagnation and blood stasis that heat, cold and phlegm may indirectly contribute to. Thus, the CMH prescription for tumours in their early stages should primarily focus on promoting circulation of qi and blood, though it optimally should include herbs that clear heat and phlegm, reduce phlegm, and resolve masses in accordance with the individual patient's status based on the four diagnostics examination.

Experimental studies of CMH prescriptions for promoting blood circulation (Huo Xue Hua Yu) have demonstrated several anti-cancer effects. First, huoxuehuayu prescriptions produce direct inhibition and apoptosis of tumour cells. Second, these CMH prescriptions produce reduced blood coagulability and viscosity, including inhibition of platelet activation and increased fibrinolysis. This enhancement of microcirculation may serve to prevent tumour cell metastases, increase the efficiency of chemotherapy and radiotherapy, and reduce radiotherapy induced tissue fibrosis. Third, the huoxuehuayu prescriptions improve humoral antibody and complement levels, which allow the immune system to more optimally inhibit tumour growth and spread. Finally, huoxuehuayu prescriptions also have analgesic, anti-inflammatory, and anti-infective properties. Most TCM scholars in China believe that these herbal prescriptions can reduce hematogenous spread of tumour and enhance immune function. In theory, allopathic chemotherapy, via production of cell lysis, may produce increased blood viscosity which in turn would create more favorable conditions for hematogenous spread of tumour cells.

Herbs used to specifically treat a tumour (via breaking up stagnant blood and qi) are often chosen based on the location of the tumour. Herbal anti-toxin therapies are added using herbs that inhibit tumour growth by a variety of mechanisms. *Sargassum pallidum* (sargasum) and *Phytolacca acinosa* (poloborry root) are among the herbs described to dissolve tumours in Chinese herbal therapy. The most highly praised blood tonic in the East, *Angelica sinensis* (Chinese angelica root), has been used clinically in China to treat cancer of the esophagus and liver with good results. The Chinese have claimed success using this herb both alone and in combination with other medicinal agents to treat cervical cancer and less frequently breast cancer in women (Walters 1993). Chinese angelica root can be administered by either infusion or douche preparations.

In treating tumours in later stages of the disease process, the cancer patient's Zheng qi is the primary factor to be addressed in the CMH prescription so as to maximize their immune status. This is essential to assist the body to attack the tumour which is essential to achieve optimal clinical results.

A commonly used CMH formulation used in treating cancer to boost nonspecific immunity and increase T-cell function is Fuzheng, whose principal herbs include *Astragalus membranaceus* (astragalus root), *Ligustrum lucidum* (glossy privet fruit), *Panax ginseng* (ginseng), *Codonopsis pilosula* (dangshen), *Atractylodes macrocephala* (bighead atractylodes rhizome) and *Ganoderma lucidum* (lucid ganoderma) (Walters 1993) (Table 3.1). Studies of Fuzheng therapy in the United States and China have demonstrated its value in treating a wide range of immune-compromised conditions, including cancer and leukemia. In a study of 76 patients with Stage II primary liver cancer, 29 of the 46 people receiving Fuzheng therapy in combination with radiation or chemotherapy survived for a year, and 10 survived for 3 years. Only 6 of the 30 patients who received radiation or chemotherapy alone survived 1 year, and all died by the third year (Li and Lien 1986). In laboratory studies, Fuzheng herbs have prevented the growth of transplanted tumours.

Herbs to treat toxicity related to the use of conventional chemotherapy are also frequently included as part of the herbal prescription for cancer. Finally, the CMH prescription often includes herbs that serve to enhance absorption of the cancer fighting herbs.

3.3 Individual Herbs Commonly Used to Treat Cancer

Table 3.2 delineates some of the more commonly used CMH and their traditional indications, while Table 3.3 delineates which herbs may often be used for treating specific cancers. A more detailed discussion of the allopathic medical studies of many of these herbs and their purported scientific mechanisms and evidence will follow.

Table 3.1 Immune system effects of selected Chinese medicinal herbs

Common name	Species	Immune system effects
Spreading hedyotis herb	*Hedyotis diffusa*	↑ Phagocytosis (Shan et al. 2001), ↑ adrenal cortex function, inhibits cancer growth and metastases, and ↑ cancer cell apoptosis (Gupta et al. 2004)
Bighead atractylodes rhizome	*Atractylodes macrocephala*	↑ Phagocytosis (Lee and Jeon 2005), lymphocyte transformation (Lee et al. 2007), rosette formation and serum IgG post chemotherapy (Bakuridze et al. 1993)
Astragalus root	*Astragalus membranaceus*	↑ CD4/CD8 ratio and phagocytosis after chemotherapy (Duan and Wang 2002), ↑ production of IL-2, IL-3, IL-6, TNFα and IFN-γ (Upton 2005), ↑ T-cell mitosis (Cho and Leung 2007)
Prepared rehmannia root	*Rehmannia glutinosa*	↑ Lymphocyte DNA synthesis, protein synthesis, IL-2 production, T- lymphocyte proliferation, NK and CTL activity in mouse spleen (Zhang et al. 2008), ↓ immunosuppression in mice caused by cyclophosphamide and steroids
Glossy privet fruit	*Ligustrum lucidum*	↓ Leukopenia secondary to chemotherapy or radiation (Gaeddert 2005)
Barbat skullcap	*Scutellaria barbata*	↑ Caspase-dependent apoptosis and cytotoxicity in vitro (Cha et al. 2004), ↑ macrophage function in mouse model (Wong et al. 2009)
Dangshen	*Codonopsis pilosula*	Slight ↑ IgM (Zneg et al. 1992), ↑ macrophage and granulocyte function (Byeon et al. 2009)
Tuckahoe	*Poria cocos*	↑ Monocyte GM-CSF production, rosette formation, lymphocyte transformation and IgG levels (Yu and Tseng 1996). Enhanced bone marrow recovery in mice after radiation.
Wolfberry fruit	*Lycium barbarum*	↑ Non-specific immunity, macrophage phagocytosis, and T-lymphocyte production, ↑ hematopoiesis, ↑ cytotoxicity of CTL and NK cells in mice (Cao et al. 1994)

Table 3.1 (continued)

Common name	Species	Immune system effects
American ginseng	*Panax quinquefolium*	↑ TNF, IL-2 and IFN-g production in mice after cyclophosphamide with simultaneous reversal of suppression of cytokine production (Shin et al. 2000)
Babylon weeping willow twig	*Salix babylonica*	↑ Regeneration of bone marrow post chemotherapy (Cohen et al. 2002)
Lucid ganoderma	*Ganoderma lucidum*	↑ Macrophage phagocytosis, alter the levels of TNF and interleukins, and ↑ non-specific immune response (Gao et al. 2005)
Dandelion herb	*Taraxacum mongolicum*	Induce cytotoxicity through TNF-α and IL-1α secretion (Koo et al. 2004)

Table 3.2 Herbs commonly used to treat cancer

Strengthen immunity	Blood and/or qi invigoration	General anti-tumour effects
Astragalus membranaceus (astragalus root)	*Curcuma zedoaria* (zedoary)	Various mushrooms e.g. *Ganoderma lucidum* (lucid ganoderma)
Panax quinquefolium (American ginseng)	*Citrus aurantium* (immature bitter orange)	*Solanum nigrum* (black nightshade)
Glycyrrhiza uralensis (licorice root)	*Sparganium stoloniferum* (burreed tuber)	*Scutellaria barbata* (barbat skullcap)
Rehmannia glutinosa (prepared rehmannia root)	*Carthamus tinctorius* (safflower)	*Rabdosia rubescens* (blushred rabdosia)
Angelica sinensis (Chinese angelica root)	*Prunus Persica* (peach seed)	*Hedyotis diffusa* (spreading hedyotis herb)
Amyda sinensis (fresh-water turtle shell)	*Trogopterus xanthipes* (flying squirrel feces)	*Polistes mandarinus* (wasp's nest)
Ligustrum lucidum (glossy privet fruit)	–	–

Table 3.3 Herbs used for specific cancer sites

Traditional Chinese medicinal herbs	Cancer type						
	Liver	Lung	Ovarian	Colon	Breast	Stomach	Esophageal
Hedyotis diffusa (spreading hedyotis herb)	✓	✓	✓	✓	✓	✓	✓
Scutellaria barbata (barbat skullcap)	✓	✓	✓	✓	✓	✓	✓
Imperata cylindrical (lalanggrass rhizome)	–	–	–	–	–	✓	✓
Taraxacum mongolicum (dandelion herb)	–	✓	–	–	✓	–	–
Solanum nigrum (black nightshade)	–	–	✓	✓	–	–	–
Phragmites communis (reed rhizome)	✓	–	–	–	–	–	–
Citrus aurantium (immature bitter orange)	–	–	–	–	✓	–	–
Curcuma longa (common turmeric)	–	–	–	–	✓	–	–
Gossypium herbaceum (levant cotton root)	–	–	–	–	–	–	✓
Sanguisorba officinalis (garden burnet root)	–	–	–	✓	–	–	–
Viola yedoensis (Tokyo violer herb)	–	–	–	✓	–	–	–
Amyda sinensis (fresh-water turtle shell)	–	–	✓	–	–	–	–
Ophiopogon japonicus (dwarf lilyturf tuber root)	–	✓	–	–	–	–	–
Paeonia lactiflora (white peony root)	✓	–	–	–	–	–	–

Other herbs that are frequently used in CMH preparations to treat cancer (Schreck 2008) include *Coix lacryma-jobi* (coix seed), *Imperata cylindrica* (lalang-grass rhizome), *Taraxacum mongolicum* (dandelion herb), *Phragmites communis* (reed rhizome), *Ostrea gigas* (oyster shell) and *Spatholobus suberectus* (suberect stem).

3.4 Individual Herbs

Panax quinquefolium (American ginseng), derived from the plant root, inhibits tumour growth in vitro and enhances cellular and humoral immunity (MSK 2009). The biologically active ingredients appear to be saponin glycosides. Beyond the anti-cancer effects of American ginseng, it also may cause stimulation of the central nervous system and alter cardiovascular tone. A North Central Cancer Treatment Group study reported by Mayo Clinic randomized, placebo-controlled study of 282 patients over an 8 week period demonstrated that higher doses (1–2 gm/day) of American ginseng improved energy level as well as mental, physical, spiritual, and emotional health (Barton et al. 2009). American ginseng may improve blood sugar regulation in diabetics, but it may reduce the effectiveness of warfarin and increase the hypoglycemic effect of insulin and sulfonylureas (MSK 2009).

Astragalus root has traditionally been used in combination with other herbs to strengthen and enhance the immune system. Definitive scientific evidence for using astragalus for any health condition is limited, with results from a few studies showing its potential benefits for using astragalus root along with another herb, glossy privet fruit, as an adjunctive therapy for cancer. The true benefit of this therapy is uncertain as generally those studies were not well designed (NCCAM 2009). Astragalus root extracts, though, appear to inhibit tumour growth, and delayed the onset of chemically induced hepatic cancers in rat models. It may also reduce immunosuppression caused chemotherapy agents. Astragalus root works by stimulating the immune system. In vitro, its polysaccharides potentiate the anti-tumour activity of interleukin-2 in vitro, improve lymphocyte responses of lymphocytes in healthy and cancer patients, increase the natural killer (NK) cell activity of healthy subjects, potentiate the activity of monocytes, and increase phagocytosis perhaps via regulating tumour necrosis factor (TNF) production. Its saponins also potentiate NK cell activity beyond restoring steroid-inhibited NK cell activity in vitro. No adverse effects have been reported (MSK 2009).

Atractylodes lancea (atractylodes rhizome) derives from its rhizome (rootstalk). Its major chemical constituents include atractylone, atractylol, butenolide B, acetoxyatractylon, hydroxyatractylon, and vitamin A. Lactone I from atractylodes rhizome can be beneficial for treating cancer cachexia. A randomized, non-blinded pilot study of the therapeutic efficacy of giving atractylenolide I in one study group compared to fish oil extract in the comparison group for management of gastric cancer cachexia over 7 weeks. Effects on mid-arm muscle circumference, body weight, and tumour necrosis factor (TNF)-α increases and concomitant IL-1 decreases were statistically significant in both groups, but atractylenolide I treatment was statistically significantly more effective than fish oil in improving appetite and Karnofsky performance status with only mild symptoms of nausea or dry mouth with either intervention that did not interrupt treatment (Liu et al. 2005). A study of the effects of atractylodes rhizome on mouse splenocytes demonstrated that it markedly stimulated lymphocyte proliferation, antibody production, and cytokine secretion in mouse splenocytes. There was preferential stimulation of Th1 rather than Th2 lymphocytes, and production of glycoprotein(s) with molecular weights of around 30 kDa that may play critical roles in modulating immune-response induction (Lee et al. 2007).

Scutellaria barbata (barbat skullcap) has been used to treat hepatic and other cancers in CHM. Data from in vitro studies suggest that barbat skullcap has anti-mutagenic and anti-cancer properties thought related to its flavonoid components (MSK 2009). The safety and efficacy of this herb have not been evaluated in humans. Barbat skullcap produces caspase-dependent apoptosis and cytotoxicity in vitro, and in a murine cancer cell line reduces tumour growth by increasing macrophage function. Barbat skullcap also affects the metabolism of mutagenic compounds such as benzopyrene so as to reduce their ability to bind DNA. A derivative of barbat skullcap, BZL101, caused cell apoptosis of breast cancer cells in vitro and in animal studies; and a Phase I trial in 21 women with progressive stage IV metastatic breast cancer refractory to conventional chemotherapy were given 12 grams per day of barbat skullcap (~triple the amount in a cup of brewed tea) for about a year. Twenty-five percents of the women had stabilization of their disease for 90 days, and 19% for 180 days. BZL101 appears to prevent cancer cells from undergoing glycolysis that accounts for as much as 85% of cancer cells' energy supply (Rugo et al. 2007).

Collocalia esculenta (edible birds nest) is made from the nests of swiftlets; it contains mainly glycoproteins, carbohydrates, amino acids and mineral salts. Sialic acid, the major carbohydrate in edible birds nest, may enhance immune function by stimulating immune cell division (Ng et al. 1986). In vitro, an aqueous extract of edible birds nest has epidermal growth factor (EGF)-like activity which stimulates the fibroblast DNA synthesis in a dose-dependent manner (Kong et al. 1987). EGF appears to have an important role in cellular processes including proliferation, differentiation and development. EGF receptors are highly expressed in a number of solid tumours, including breast, head and neck, non-small-cell lung, renal, ovarian and colon cancers (Herbst and Langer 2002). Despite lack of evidence, there is concern that edible birds nest use in these cancer types could theoretically induce tumour progression and cause tumour cells to be resistant to chemotherapy or radiotherapy. An in vitro study of the effects of aqueous extract of edible birds nest on the viability on human breast and liver cancer cell lines compared to no treatment demonstrated no observable effect on cancer cell viability (Chan 2009).

Codonopsis (*Codonopsis lanceolata* or *Codonopsis pilosula*), or Dangshen, is used as a tonic for the lung and spleen and to strengthen and nourish the blood and balance metabolic function. A biologically active component of dangshen, codonoposide 1c, is a potent inducer of apoptosis of cancer cells. It leads to caspase activation, providing a potential mechanism for its cytotoxic activity. Most of this work has been done in test tubes and on small laboratory animals, and large-scale controlled human studies have yet to be done. The hematologic and immunologic protective effects of dangshen for 76 cancer patients compared to those not receiving this herb showed no effect on hemoglobin or leukocyte counts, a reduction of the immunosuppressive effect of radiotherapy on delayed hypersensitive reaction, and lymphocyte response to PHA and IL-2. There were no significant differences between subjects treated with the herb and control groups in most humoral immune indices such as IgG, IgA and C3 though there was a slight increase in IgM in treated patients compared to a significant decrease of IgM in controls (Zneg et al. 1992).

Cordyceps sinensis (cordyceps) is derived from a vegetable caterpillar and a fungus that grows on it. Cordyceps contains multiple constituents including amino acids, polyamines, saccharides, fatty acids, sterols (ergosterol), and the nucleoside 3-deoxyadenosine (cordycepin). In vitro studies of cordyceps demonstrate that it increases T-helper cell numbers, increases NK cell activity, and increases lymphocyte survival. Cordyceps down-regulates MHC class II antigen expression and increases production of TNF-α and interleukin 1 (MSK 2009).

Coix seed is commonly used in CMH cancer treatment formulas. Recent studies have shown coix seed extracts significantly inhibit growth of breast cancer xenografts in mice through mechanisms including downregulation of cyclooxygenase-2 (COX-2) and matrixmetalloproteinases genes that are considered to be important in neoplasia. Coix seed also influences cellular pathways that are important in cancer including a dose-dependent inhibition of NF-κB signaling that inhibits activity of protein kinase C, a major mediator of signal transduction and activator of NF-κB (Woo et al. 2007). Coix seed extract also produces significant dose dependent inhibition of fatty acid synthase FAS activity via inhibition of β-ketoacyl reductases and enoyl reductase sites, and affected G6PD activity (Yu et al. 2008).

Lucid ganoderma is used as an immune system stimulant in cancer treatment and its active constituents are thought to include both β-glucan polysaccharides and triterpenes. Extracts of lucid ganoderma can stimulate macrophages, alter the levels of TNF and interleukins, and enhance immune responses in advance-stage cancer patients. It may inhibit tumour invasion by reducing matrix metalloproteinase expression and tumour metastases by limiting attachment to endothelial cells. A number of its polysaccharides, such as β-glucans, have demonstrated antitumour and immune stimulating activities. Lucid ganoderma extracts can inhibit 5α-reductase, an important enzyme that converts testosterone to dihydrotestosterone and is upregulated in benign prostatic hyperplasia. Adverse events reported include dry nose and throat, nausea, vomiting and other GI symptoms. Also, in vitro studies suggest that high doses may induce cellular toxicity. Theoretically, lucid ganoderma can interfere with the actions of immunosuppressant medications, anticoagulants, and certain chemotherapeutic agents. Furthermore, lucid ganoderma polysaccharides inhibit CYP2E1, CYP1A2 and CYP3A, potentially interfering with the metabolism of drugs that use these pathways (MSK 2009).

Glossy privet fruit has been used in CHM preparations to treat chemotherapy side effects and boost immunity. Though in vitro studies have shown that its fruits have immune stimulating, anti-mutagenesis, and anti-tumour activities, the data from in vivo human studies is lacking. No adverse effects from the use of this herb are reported (MSK 2009).

Lalanggrass rhizome extracts are described to have viricidal and anti-cancer activities (Duke and Ayensu 1985).

Smilax glabra (glabrous greenbrier rhizome) inhibits the activity of JTC26 in vitro, and in vivo inhibits sarcoma-180 and liver cancer in mice. Glabrous greenbrier rhizome is frequently used in China for the treatment of brain tumours (including meningioma), osteosarcoma, nasopharyngeal carcinoma, lung cancer, cervical cancer and lymphoma (Tang et al. 2006).

Sargasum is large brown algae that are a type of seaweed. Limited, mostly in vitro evidence hints that sargasum possesses cancer preventative effects on toxin induced breast cancer in rats, through it also has described anti-tumour effects of its fucoidan fraction as well as immunomodulatory effects on human lymphocytes (BHS 2009). Some sargasum supplements have been found to contain toxic levels of arsenic. Seawater contains highly diluted arsenic, but sargasum may concentrate arsenic in its tissues. There are reports of two people who developed symptoms of arsenic poisoning after consuming sargasum. Researchers have also found that the rats' estrous cycles increased from an average of 4.3 to 5.4 days for the low dose sargasum group, and to 5.9 days for the high dose sargasum group. Overall, dietary sargasum resulted in a 37% increase in the length of the rat estrous cycle. Studies in humans have linked longer menstrual cycle lengths to lower risk of breast, ovarian and endometrial cancers (Skibola et al. 2005).

Glycyrrhiza uralensis (licorice root) is thought to strengthen immunity and combat bacterial infections, including hepatitis. Licorice root, though, in large amounts can lead to elevated blood pressure, salt and water retention, and low potassium levels that can lead to cardiac problems, though for deglycyrrhizinated licorice (DGL) products do not appear to have those side effects (NCCAM 2009). DGL preparations have been shown to lead to a decrease in serum testosterone and an increase in 17-hydroxyprogesterone have been shown. Licorice root has recently been shown to have chemopreventive effects in human breast cancer cells and colon carcinogenesis. Thus, its estrogenic effects may underlie the use of licorice root in CHM preparations for prostate cancer (MSK 2009).

Millettia (*M. pachycarpa* and *M. reticulata*), or Suberect stem, has been demonstrated to contain flavonoid compounds that have anti-estrogenic activities, which may account for its cancer use in CMH therapy (Okamoto et al. 2006). There are many species of suberect stem, which may reflect why there are many differing reports in the literature regarding its constituents and pharmacology. Besides their primary flavonoid constituents, suberect stem species also contain other biologically active substances including saponins (such as triterpenes) and alkaloids. Suberect stem contains isoflavones, chalcones, coumestans, tannins, triterpenes, sterols and phenolic organic acids.

Hedyotis diffusa (spreading hedyotis herb) is the most common CMH used for treating cancer. It can be used for many tumour types, especially tumours of the liver or digestive tract, though it is used for breast, ovarian, lung, laryngeal cancers, as well as lymphosarcoma. It benefits cancer patients who have pleural effusions and ascites with soft bowels. It is also very effective to minimize the side effects produced by radiotherapy and chemotherapy (Tang et al. 2006). Spreading hedyotis herb exerts an inhibitory effect on various kinds of human leukemia cells in vitro and in vivo inhibits liver cancer in mice, Walker carcinoma 256, cervical carcinoma 14, sarcoma 180, and liver cancer of parenchymal type. It inhibits the mitosis of sarcoma 180 cells, and promotes the activity of mononuclear macrophages and adrenal cortex function (AAMD 2009).

Phragmites (*Rhizoma phragmites*), or Reed rhizome, is aquatic grass species whose rhizomes are used in herbal preparations and contain multiple vitamin A, several B vitamins, ascorbic acid, and several triterpenes, which may account for its anti-cancer activities (NCCAM 2009).

Poloborry root is derived from the root of the pokeweed plant. Patients have used this herb to treat cancer. Poloborry root causes significant toxicity following oral or topical administration. Reported adverse effects include nausea, diarrhea, protracted vomiting, hypotension, convulsions, dyspnea and death. Due to the toxic nature of this herb, it is not recommended for sale by the US Herbal Trade Association. Poloborry root mitogens and glycosidic saponins are known toxins that possess mitogenic and irritant properties (MSK 2009).

Glycine max (soy bean), a product has been used to treat breast and prostate cancer. Soy bean contains isoflavones, which have chemical similarity to estrogen. Soy bean theoretically could stimulate development of breast cancer or other hormone-sensitive conditions (such as ovarian or uterine cancer), so until a better understanding of how soy bean effects estrogen levels, women who are increased risk of developing these cancers should consult with their health care providers before utilizing soy bean preparations (NCCAM 2009). Soy bean may reduce risk of prostate, lung and endometrial cancers, but may increase the risk of bladder cancer and endometrial hyperplasia. Phytochemicals in soy bean have anti-carcinogenic and anti-oxidant activity. Genistein demonstrates cell anti-proliferative effects in estrogen receptor positive and negative breast cancers, androgen sensitive and insensitive prostate cancers, neuroblastoma, sarcoma and retinoblastoma. Genistein may also act as an anti-estrogen by competing for receptor binding, thus reducing estrogen-induced stimulation of breast cell proliferation. Other soy bean isoflavones such as daidzein demonstrate weaker growth inhibition of breast cancer cell lines. Soy bean isoflavones may also reduce endogenous ovarian steroid levels. In prostate cancer, soy protein extracts appear to reduce the progression of established tumours independent of the estrogenic effects of genistein and reduce androgen receptor expression in prostate tumours. Other proposed mechanisms of prostate cancer prevention include genistein-induced reduction of prostate cancer cell adhesion and induction of apoptosis. Flatulence and occasionally allergic reactions have occurred with soy bean preparations (MSK 2009).

Dandelion herb may induce cytotoxicity through TNF-α and IL-1α secretion in cancer cells (Koo et al. 2004). The anti-tumour activities of dandelion herb are thought to be similar to that of tumour polysaccharides such as lentinan. Dandelion herb has been shown to decrease human hepatoma cell line viability by increasing TNF-α and interleukin-1α production. Other research, however, has shown that the presence of luteolin and luteolin 7-glucoside in dandelion herb extract exhibits cytotoxic activities against the colon adenocarcinoma cell line (Caco-2). Still other studies have isolated an active compound identical to lupeol, a lupane-type triterpene, that inhibited cell growth and induced melanogenesis of a mouse melanoma cell line (B16 2F2). Another study has demonstrated that taraxinic acid induces differentiation in HL-60, a promyelocytic leukemia cell line (MSK 2009).

Curcuma longa (common turmeric) is used in CHM preparations for treating cancer. Common turmeric oil and water soluble curcuminoids, including curcumin, are thought to be the biologically active ingredients. In vitro and animal studies suggest it has cancer anti-proliferative and preventative effects, and curcumin induces apoptosis in human colon cancer and promyelocytic leukemia cells (MSK 2009). Curcumin potentiated gemcitabine action in both in vitro and in vivo studies of pancreatic cancer. In a phase II trial in pancreatic cancer patients, down-regulation of NF-κB and COX-2 were observed. Recent animal studies indicate that dietary common turmeric may inhibit the anti-tumour action of chemotherapeutic agents such as cyclophosphamide in treating breast cancer, so it is advisable for cancer patients undergoing chemotherapy to limit intake of common turmeric until research further clarifies this matter. In vitro and animal models of breast cancer showed that common turmeric may inhibit chemotherapy-induced apoptosis via inhibition of the JNK pathway and generation of reactive oxygen species (ROS). In vitro and in vivo studies report that NF-kB-mediated resistance of cancer cells to gemcitabine and gamma-radiation was reduced by curcumin administration. In laboratory tests, the anti-tumour actions of common turmeric appear to be due to interactions with arachidonate metabolism and its in vivo anti-angiogenic properties (NCCAM 2009).

Sun's Soup has been promoted as a potential treatment for cancer based on preliminary favorable tumour responses in mice. It is a combination of *Lentinus edodes* (Shiitake mushroom), *Phaseolus radiatus* (mung bean), spreading hedyotis herb and barbat skullcap. A dietary supplement Selected Vegetables contains similar vegetables and herbs including soy bean, Shiitake mushroom, mung bean, *Ziziphus jujuba* (red date), *Allium ascalonicum* (scallion), *Allium satirum* (garlic), *Allium tuberosum* (leek), *Lens culinaris* (lentils), *Crataegus cuneata* (hawthorn fruit), *Allium cepa* (onion), ginseng, *Angelica dahurica* (angelica root), licorice root, *Taraxacum officinale* (dandelion root), *Polygala tenuifolia* (thinleaf milkwort root), *Zingiber officinale* (ginger), *Olea europaea* (olive), *Sesamum indicum* (sesame seed) and *Petroselinum crispum* (parsley). Tumour growth in the mice was slowest when they received both Shiitake mushroom and mung bean in their diet. Many of the vegetables and herbs chosen to include in Selected Vegetables and Sun's Soup were chosen based on previous allopathic and TCM research that suggested they contain anticancer phytochemicals including protease inhibitors, plant sterols, and isoflavones that may block the growth of cancer cells and/or improve the body's immune system ability to respond to cancer cells. A few small, non-controlled clinical trials have been done with Selected Vegetables/Sun's Soup. Most patients receiving the vegetable mixtures lived longer, were better able to carry out their daily activities, and either gained weight or did not lose weight. In some patients who ate Selected Vegetables/Sun's Soup, tumour growth slowed or the tumour completely went away. The patients were also receiving other treatments including chemotherapy, so it is not clear whether their favorable responses were due to Selected Vegetables/Sun's Soup, the allopathic cancer treatments, or both. The National Cancer Institute has approved a prospective randomized clinical trial of this vegetable-herb mixture in patients with advanced lung cancer but the protocol has not been activated by the investigators for over a year now (NCI 2009).

3.5 Issues with Cancer Research Using Chinese Herbal Medicine

3.5.1 Purity

An example of the potential problems with purity of the herbal products studied is the PC-SPES, which was introduced in the United States in 1997 as a non-prescription herbal treatment to slow the growth of prostate cancer (NCI 2009). The preparation contained barbat skullcap, licorice root, lucid ganoderma, *Isatis tinctoria* (indigowoad root), ginseng or *Panax notoginseng* (notoginseng), *Chrysanthemum morifolium* (chrysanthemum flower), *Rabdosia rubescens* (blushred rabdosia) and *Serenoa repens* (Juzonglu). PC-SPES when put through independent chemical analysis was also found to contain DES (an estrogen analog), warfarin (a blood thinner) and the anti-inflammatory drug indomethacin; and different batches of the product were found to have varying ingredient compositions. The National Center for Complementary and Alternative Medicine halted four clinical studies of PC-SPES once these issues were found, and the company manufacturing PC-SPES subsequently withdrew the product from market and closed. Patients who took PC-SPES had responses similar to those of patients treated with DES, The phytoestrogenic properties of some of the herbs in PC-SPES serve to suppress testicular testosterone production, which in turn inhibits the growth of some prostate cancers. PC-SPES also demonstrated anti-cancer effects that were not due to estrogen-like effects, and beneficial effects on other cancer types.

Similar concerns have been raised about Chinese herbal products for other diseases, which have been found to contain toxic contaminants and prescription drugs such as diazepam (Valium). Tests of Chinese herbal remedies by the California Department of Health found that nearly one third contained prescription drugs or were contaminated with toxic metals such as mercury, arsenic and lead. Concerns about Chinese herbal products have been raised in other countries as well. The Japanese Ministry of Health, Labour and Welfare reported that some Chinese herbal products contained contaminants that caused severe and sometimes fatal liver and thyroid problems (ACS 2009).

As previously mentioned, some sargasum supplements also have been found to contain toxic levels of arsenic (BHS 2009).

3.5.2 Herb-Drug Interactions

Some of the CMH substances are metabolized by the same liver pathways that conventional chemotherapy and allopathic prescription medications are. This could potentially lead to increased or decreased serum levels of these pharmaceutical preparations and lead to toxicity issues or lack of efficacy, respectively. For example, lucid ganoderma polysaccharides inhibit CYP2E1, CYP1A2 and CYP3A pathways which could potentially interfere with the metabolism of drugs that use these pathways (MSK 2009). Most of these potential herb-pharmaceutical potential interactions have not been studied to date, and should be a focus of future herbal research.

The timing of administration of CMH and conventional chemotherapy agents may have clinical importance as well. A study that examined the in vitro anticancer activity of 12 CMHs alone and in combination with doxorubicin found that while most of the herbs showed additive activity when administered simultaneously with doxorubicin, a few had antagonistic effects (Campbell 2009). Simultaneous in vivo administration of *Vaccaria segetalis* (cow-fat seed), *Anemarrhena asphodeloides* (wind-weed rhizome) or barbat skullcap with doxorubicin antagonizes that chemotherapy agent's anti-cancer activity. This in vitro study with these three herbs found similar results, while these herbs produced additive tumour cell growth inhibition when they were administered sequentially with doxorubicin (Campbell 2009). One CMH, cow-fat seed was demonstrated to enhance the uptake of doxorubicin into the cancer cells. Several CMHs with growth inhibitory effects on a drug-sensitive human breast cancer cell line (MCF-7) were also effective against a drug-resistant cell line (NCI/ADR-RES), suggesting that the active compounds in these herbs may be potentially useful in treating drug resistant breast cancer (Campbell 2009). These findings may have important clinical implications for the use of Chinese medicinal herbs in conjunction with standard chemotherapeutic agents.

3.5.3 Herb Toxicity

Eighteen patients experienced severe renal failure as a result of taking a combination of two CMHs, *Stephania tetrandra* (fourstamen stephania root) and *Magnolia officinalis* (magnolia bark), that led to their needing kidney dialysis or kidney organ transplants (deJonge and Vanrenterghem 2008). Another CMH, *Aristolochia fangchi* (Guangfangji), also has been linked to kidney failure and may cause cancer as well. Patients at a Belgian weight loss clinic were inadvertently given this herb for approximately a year (possibly due to a manufacturing error), in a preparation that was supposed to include only fourstamen stephania root. Of the patients who accidentally received the herb, 18 developed cancers of the urinary system (Nortier et al. 2000). The Chinese name for Guangfangji is similar to that for fourstamen stephania root, and it is often substituted for fourstamen stephania root. Though the Guangfangji was a contaminant, it appears to have significant toxicity and mutagenic potential if administered incorrectly.

3.5.4 Evidence-Based Medicine Reviews

Unfortunately there have not been enough well designed, placebo-controlled, double-blind studies performed to date to allow meta-analyses of CMH preparations either as single herb or herb combination to allow definitive statements about their efficacy or appropriate use in treating cancer either as first-line treatments or as adjunctive treatments to conventional chemotherapy.

In fact, a 2007 evidence-based review of individualized herbal medicine found only three moderate to good quality (Jadad score) randomized, double-blind placebo-controlled trials among 1,360 studies examined (Guo et al. 2007). The authors of this review queried 15 professional bodies representing the interests of different practitioner bodies from around the world but those organizations were unable to contribute any further studies. The authors concluded that individualized CMH and Ayurvedic herbal medicine has an extremely sparse evidence base with no convincing evidence supporting its use in any indication. Only one of the three studies, which examined CMH for treating irritable bowel syndrome, indicated that individualized CMH treatment was superior to placebo though it was less efficacious than standard allopathic treatment.

A limited number of Cochrane reviews for CMH use in cancer have been performed to date. One Cochrane review of the use of astragalus root species to treat chemotherapy side effects in colorectal cancer patients found only four studies of low methodological quality. These studies overall did show astragalus root administration significantly reduced the frequency of nausea and vomiting due to chemotherapy, reduced the incidence of clinically significant leucopenia, enhanced T-cell lymphocyte counts for certain subsets (CD3, CD4 and CD8) and did not affect immunoglobulin levels (Wu et al. 2005). A 2007 systematic review of the use of CMH for esophageal cancer concluded there were no authentic randomized controlled trials to analyze and thus no scientific evidence that CMH is beneficial in treating esophageal cancer either as standalone treatment or with radiotherapy or chemotherapy (Wei et al. 2007). Another 2007 systematic review of the use of CMH in treating chemotherapy side-effects of breast cancer treatment found only seven randomized controlled trials of low quality that examined the used of CMH with chemotherapy versus chemotherapy alone. Use of CMH did not statistically significantly improve alopecia, phlebitis, renal or hepatic toxicity from chemotherapy in any of the studies. Only one study found improvement in nausea, vomiting and fatigue; and two herbal compounds appeared to improve quality of life. Three studies demonstrated improvement in white blood cell counts and only one study found statistically significant improvement in CD3, CD4 and CD8 T-cell lymphocyte counts. The evidence was not considered conclusive and well designed clinical trials were recommended as needed before making any statements about the safety or efficacy of CMH in managing breast cancer patients (Zhang et al. 2007). Protocols are in progress to examine the evidence for symptom palliation in lung cancer, induction of remission in advanced or late gastric cancer and treating gastric precancerous lesions.

Other evidence-based medicine reviews have found potential efficacy of CMH in treating cancer. A review of CMH use in nasopharyngeal carcinoma examined 18 controlled trials that suggest CMH increases survival, improves functional status and enhances immune status while reducing side effects of conventional treatment, though rigorously designed controlled trials are needed to confirm those findings (Cho and Chen 2009b). A meta-analysis of CMH in combination with arterial chemoembolization of hepatocellular carcinoma found that addition of CMH to this mode of chemotherapy enhances survival and performance status, reduces side effects of conventional therapy, and also results in higher leukocyte (including T-cell and natural killer cell) levels with lower α-fetoprotein levels. Limited data and heterogeneity of the studies examined made definitive recommendations difficult, with further trials needed (Cho and Chen 2009a). A review of CMH for lung cancer (Liang et al. 2003) concluded that CMH alone may have efficacy (improved survival and quality of life) in treating lung cancer, may have an additive or synergistic effect when combined with chemotherapy or radiotherapy, and may reduce side effects from conventional therapy. Most clinical studies reviewed had methodological flaws, so it was not possible to draw definitive conclusions regarding the efficacy of CMH in treating lung cancer, and more rigorously designed studies were recommended to evaluate the efficacy and safety of CMH to treat lung cancer (Table 3.3).

3.6 Summary

The use of individualized CMH for treating cancer has been in clinical use, particularly in Asia, for thousands of years. Modern biochemistry and immunology techniques have helped isolate biologically active constituents of individual CMH. The preponderance of research into the use of CMH to treat cancer to date has consisted of in vitro studies or in vivo animal studies. Despite the widespread use of CMH in treating cancer and/or its side effects, there unfortunately have been very few well designed (by contemporary Western research standards) double-blinded, placebo-controlled human clinical trials with single, standardized (e.g. Fuzheng), or individualized CMH.

Issues with purity of herbal preparations in general (e.g. PC-SPES) are critical for clinical research and practice, and strict labeling of CMH constituents and enforced standards for purity of CMH including active and inert ingredients is needed.

Despite this, there is some evidence that CMH may mitigate immunosuppression from conventional chemotherapy and radiotherapy, reduce side effects from those treatments, and improve cancer patients' overall clinical status. Chinese medicinal herbs may also produce tumour apoptosis, reduce metastases and increase survival (either alone or in combination with conventional chemotherapy). Some CMHs interfere with conventional chemotherapy when administered simultaneously, yet enhance conventional chemotherapy efficacy when administered sequentially.

Further well designed, double-blinded, placebo-controlled clinical trials of CMH with/without conventional chemotherapy and radiotherapy in cancer patients are needed to provide definitive scientific evidence as to which Chinese medicinal herbs (and herb combinations) have efficacy in treating cancer as well as to determine the optimal doses and timing of CMH administration that will optimize cancer patients' survival, tumour burden reduction, immunologic function and quality of life while minimizing the side effects (e.g. nausea/vomiting, anorexia and fatigue) of conventional radiotherapy or chemotherapy.

References

Abbate S. Advanced techniques in oriental medicine. Stuttgart: Georg Thieme Verlag; 2006.

About herbs, botanicals, and other products. Memorial Sloan Kettering Cancer Center. http://www.mskcc.org/mskcc/html/69128.cfm.

American Cancer Society. Chinese herbal medicine. http://www.cancer.org/docroot/ETO/content/ETO_5_3x_Chinese_Herbal_Medicine.asp

Asian Anti-Cancer Materia Database. http://asiancancerherb.info/bai%20hua%20she%20she%20cao.htm

Bakuridze AD, Kurtsikidze MS, Pisarev VM et al. Immunomodulators of plant origin. Pharm Chem J. 1993;27:589–95.

Baptist Health Systems (Jackson, Mississippi). Kelp information. http://www.mbhs.org/healthgate/GetHGContent.aspx?token=9c315661–83b7–472d-a7ab-bc8582171f86&chunkiid=21786

Barton DL, Soori GS, Bauer BA et al. Pilot study of *Panax quinquefolius* (American ginseng) to improve cancer-related fatigue: a randomized, double-blind, dose-finding evaluation: NCCTG trial N03CA. Support Care Cancer. 2009;doi: 10.1007/s00520-009-0642–2

Byeon SE, Lee YG, Cho JY. Regulatory effects of *Codonopsis lanceolata* on gene expression of GM-CSF in macrophage-like cells. J Ethnopharmacol. 2009;123:185–9.

Campbell M. Chinese herb/chemotherapy interactions in breast cancer. California Breast Cancer Research Program Research Portfolio. http://www.cbcrp.org/research/PageGrant.asp?grant_id=2568

Cao GW, Yang WG, Du P. Observation of the effects of LAK/IL-2 therapy combined with Lycium barbarum polysaccharides in the treatment of 75 cancer patients. Chunghua Chung Liu Tsa Chih. 1994;16:428–31.

Cha YY, Lee EO, Lee HJ et al. Methylene chloride fraction of *Scutellaria barbata* induces apoptosis in human U937 leukemia cells via the mitochondrial signaling pathway. Clin Chim Acta. 2004;348:41–8.

Chan SW. Review of scientific research on edible bird's nest. http://www.hkfsta.com.hk/articles/special/article7.htm. Accessed 2009

Cho WC, Chen HY. Transcatheter arterial chemoembolization combined with or without Chinese herbal therapy for hepatocellular carcinoma: meta-analysis. Expert Opin Invest Drugs. 2009a;18:617–35.

Cho WC, Chen HY. Clinical efficacy of traditional Chinese medicine as a concomitant therapy for nasopharyngeal carcinoma: a systematic review and meta-analysis. Cancer Invest. 2009b;27:334–44.

Cho WC, Leung KN. In vitro and in vivo immunomodulating and immunorestorative effects of *Astragalus membranaceus*. J Ethnopharmacol. 2007;113:132–41.

Cohen I, Tagliaferri M, Tripathy D. Traditional Chinese medicine in the treatment of breast cancer – part three. http://www.cancerlynx.com/chinesemedicine3.html.

Dawes N. Constitutional treatment 'fortify the righteous, secure the root'. http://www.pacificcollege.edu/alumni/newsletters/summer2004/30.html.

DeJonge H, Vanrenterghem Y. Aristolochic acid: the common culprit of Chinese herbs nephropathy and Balkan endemic nephropathy. Nephrol Dial Transplant. 2008;23:39–41.

Duan P, Wang ZM. Clinical study on effect of Astragalus in efficacy enhancing and toxicity reducing of chemotherapy in patients of malignant tumor. Zhongguo Zhong Xi Yi Jie He Za Zhi. 2002;22:515–7.

Duke JA, Ayensu ES. Medicinal plants of China. Algonac: Reference Publications Inc.; 1985.

Gaeddert A. Chinese herbs for immune disorders. http://www.pacificcollege.edu/alumni/newsletters/summer2005/herbs.html.

Gao Y, Tang W, Dai X et al. Effects of water soluble *Ganoderma lucidum* polysaccharides on the immune function of patients with advanced lung cancer. J Med Food. 2005;8:159–68.

Guo R, Canter P, Ernst E. No evidence supporting the use of individualised herbal medicine in any indication. Focus Altern Complement Ther. 2007;12:244–7.

Gupta S, Zhang D, Yi J et al. Anticancer activities of *Oldenlandia diffusa*. J Herb Pharmacother. 2004;4:21–33.
Herbs at a Glance: National Center for Complementary and Alternative Medicine. http://nccam.nih.gov/health/herbsataglance.htm.
Herbst RS, Langer CJ. Epidermal growth factor receptors as a target for cancer treatment: the emerging role of IMC-C225 in the treatment of lung and head and neck cancer. Semin Oncol. 2002;29:27–36.
Kong YC, Keung WM, Yip TT et al. Evidence that epidermal growth factor is present in swiftlet's (collocalia) nest. Comp Biochem Physiol B. 1987;87:221–6.
Koo HN, Hong SH, Song BK et al. Taraxacum officinale induces cytotoxicity through TNFα and IL-1α secretion in Hep G2 cells. Life Sci. 2004;74:1149–57.
Lahans T. The treatment of colorectal cancer using chemotherapy and Chinese herbal medicine. Chin Med Times. 2008;3:4.
Lee KY, Jeon YJ. Macrophage activation by polysaccharide isolated from Astragalus membranaceus. Int Immunopharmacol. 2005;5:1225–33.
Lee J, Lee K, Son Y et al. Stimulating effects on mouse splenocytes of glycoproteins from the herbal medicine *Atractylodes macrocephala* Koidz. Phytomedicine. 2007;14:390–5.
Li W, Lien EJ. Fu-zhen herbs in the treatment of cancer. Orient Heal Arts Int Bull. 1986;11:1–8.
Liang HL, Xue CC, Zhou DH et al. Chinese herbal medicine for lung cancer: a critical literature review (continued). Chin J Integr Med. 2003;9:232–6.
Liu Y, Ye F, Qiu GU et al. Effects of lactone I from Atractylodes macrocephala Koidz on cytokines and proteolysis-inducing factors in cachectic cancer patients. Di Yi Jun Yi Da Xue Bao. 2005;25:1308–11.
Mingji P. Cancer treatment with Fuzheng Peiben principle. Fuzhou: Fujian Science and Technology Press; 1992.
National Cancer Institute Cancer topics. PC-SPES PDQ. http://www.cancer.gov/cancertopics/pdq/cam/pc-spes/healthprofessional/allpages.
National Cancer Institute Cancer Topics. Selected Vegetables/Sun's Soup PDQ. http://www.cancer.gov/cancertopics/pdq/cam/vegetables-sun-soup/healthprofessional/allpages.
Ng MH, Chan KH, Kong YC. Potentiation of mitogenic response by extracts of the swiftlet's (collocalia) nest. Biochem Int. 1986;13:521–31.
Nortier JL, Muniz Martinez MC et al. Urothelial carcinoma associated with the use of a Chinese herb (*Aristolochia fangchi*). NEJM. 2000;342:1686–92.
Okamoto Y, Suzuki A, Ueda K et al. Anti-estrogenic activity of prenylated isoflavones from *Millettia pachycarpa*: Implications for pharmacophores and unique mechanisms. J Health Sci. 2006;52:186–91.
Pharmacopoeia Commission. Pharmacopoeia of the People's Republic of China. Beijing: Chemical Industry Press; 2005.
Porter SF, Stuart GA. Chinese medicinal herbs: a modern edition of a classic 16th edition manual. Mineola, NY: Dover Press; 2003.
Rugo H, Shtivelman E, Perez A et al. Phase I trial and antitumor effects of BZL101 for patients with advanced breast cancer. Breast Cancer Res Treat. 2007;105:17–28.
Schreck JH. A patient's guide to Chinese medicine: Dr Shen's handbook of acupuncture & herbs. Port Richmond, CA: Bay Tree Publishing; 2008.
Shan BE, Zhang JY, Du XN. Immunomodulatory activity and anti-tumor activity of *Oldenlandia diffusa* in vitro. Zhongguo Zhong Xi Yi Jie He Za Zhi. 2001;21:370–4.
Shin HR, Kim JY, Yun TK et al. The cancer-preventive potential of Panax ginseng: a review of human and experimental evidence. Cancer Causes Control. 2000;11:565–76.
Skibola CF, Curry JD, VandeVoort C et al. Brown kelp modulates endocrine hormones in female Sprague-Dawley rats and in human luteinized granulosa cells. J Nutrition. 2005;135:296–300.
Tang XP, Guo FL, Wang ZQ. Clinical oncology guidelines for commonly used Chinese medicine. Scientific and Technical Literature Publishing House; 2006.

Upton R. Astragalus. In: Coates P, Blackman M, Cragg G, et al., editors. Encyclopedia of dietary supplements. New York: Marcel Dekker; 2005. pp. 25–30.

Walter R. Options: the alternative cancer therapy book. New York: Avery Publishing Group; 1993.

Wei X, Chen Z, Yang X et al. Medicinal herbs for esophageal cancer. Cochrane Database Syst Rev. 2007;2:CD004520.

Wong BY, Nguyen DL, Lin T et al. Chinese medicinal herb *Scutellaria barbata* modulates apoptosis and cell survival in murine and human prostate cancer cells and tumor development in TRAMP mice. Eur J Cancer Prev. 2009;18:331–41.

Woo JH, Li D, Wilsbach K et al. Coix seed extract, a commonly used treatment for cancer in China, inhibits NFkappaB and protein kinase C signaling. Cancer Biol Ther. 2007;6:2005–11.

Wu T, Munro AJ, Guanjian L et al. Chinese medical herbs for chemotherapy side effects in colorectal cancer patients. Cochrane Database Syst Rev. 2005;1:CD004540.

Yu F, Gao J, Zeng Y et al. Inhibition of Coix seed extract on fatty acid synthase, a novel target for anticancer activity. J Ethnopharmacol. 2008;119:252–8.

Yu SJ, Tseng J. Fu-Ling, a Chinese herbal drug, modulates cytokine secretion by human peripheral blood monocytes. Int J Immunopharmacol. 1996;18:37–44.

Zhang RX, Li MX, Jia ZP. Rehmannia glutinosa: review of botany, chemistry and pharmacology. J Ethnopharmacol. 2008;117:199–214.

Zhang M, Liu X, Li J et al. Chinese medicinal herbs to treat the side-effects of chemotherapy in breast cancer patients. Cochrane Database Syst Rev. 2007;2:CD004921.

Zhu M. translator. The medical classic of the yellow emperor. Beijing: Foreign Languages Press; 2001.

Zneg XL, Li XA, Zhang BY. Immunological and hematopoietic effect of *Codonopsis pilosula* on cancer patients during radiotherapy. Zhongguo Zhong Xi Yi Jie He Za Zhi. 1992;12:607–8.

Chapter 4
Supportive Cancer Care with Qigong

Myeong Soo Lee, Kevin W. Chen and Edzard Ernst

Abstract The objective of this chapter is to systematically review the evidence for the effectiveness of qigong in supportive cancer care. Fifteen databases were searched from inception through May 2009. Controlled trials testing qigong in patients with cancer of any origin that assessed clinical outcome measures were considered. The selection of studies, data extraction, and validations were performed independently by two reviewers. Risk of bias was assessed using Cochrane criteria. Six randomized clinical trials (RCTs) and 5 non-randomized controlled clinical trials (CCTs) met our inclusion criteria. The six RCTs tested the effects of qigong as supportive cancer care compared with usual care or herbal medicine and showed no significant differences in most outcome measures. All of the 5 CCTs showed favourable effects of qigong. Two trials suggested effectiveness in prolonging life of cancer patients while one failed to do so. All of the CCTs had a high risk of bias. Collectively, the existing trial evidence does not show convincingly that qigong is effective for supportive cancer care. Future studies should be of high quality with a particular emphasis on designing an adequate control intervention.

4.1 Introduction

Cancer is a leading cause of global mortality and is responsible for 13% (7.9 million people in 2007) of all deaths (World Health Organization). However, the estimated 5-yr survival rate across all cancers has risen to about 66% (American Cancer Society 2009). These successes have been achieved largely as a result of aggressive interventions including surgery, chemotherapy and radiation therapy (Courneya 2003). The frequently experienced and severe adverse events associated with such treatments lead patients to seek supportive complementary and alternative medicine (CAM), which many patients use as adjuncts to conventional treatments (National

M.S. Lee (✉)
Division of Standard Research, Korea Institute of Oriental Medicine, Daejeon, 305-811, South Korea
e-mail: drmslee@gmail.com; mslee@kiom.re.kr

W.C.S. Cho (ed.), *Supportive Cancer Care with Chinese Medicine*,
DOI 10.1007/978-90-481-3555-4_4,

Center for Complementary and Alternative Medicine 2009). The results of the 2007 National Health Interview Survey showed that rates of CAM usage are especially high among US patients with serious illnesses, such as cancer (National Center for Complementary and Alternative Medicine 2009). Several surveys reported CAM usage by 53–88% of cancer patients (Dy et al. 2004; Frenkel et al. 2005; Richardson et al. 2000) and showed that CAM is usually combined with conventional treatments (Richardson et al. 2000).

Qigong (pronounced chee-gong) is a general term for all mind-body exercises that integrate the adjustments of body posture, breathing and mind into oneness. Internal and external qigong can be distinguished. Internal qigong is self-directed and involves the use of movements and meditation. It can be performed with or without the presence of a teacher. Two main characteristics of qigong practice are controlled breathing with slow body movements as an aerobic exercise and relaxation (Ernst et al. 2008). External qigong is performed by a trained practitioner using their hands or any part of their body to direct qi energy onto the patient. Unlike taichi, a martial art related to exercise routine, internal qigong is self directed and actively engages people in their personal health and well-being. It is best practiced on a daily basis to promote health maintenance and disease prevention. In external qigong a practitioner is involved in the treatment. Although neither qigong itself nor the mechanism of its effects is understood within the paradigm of medical science, there are increased reports of its effects on human health. Several reviews claim that qigong offers therapeutic benefits for cancer patients (Sancier 1996, 1999; Chen and Yeung 2002). However, these reviews are not systematic and therefore open to selection bias. The aim of this systematic review is to summarise and critically evaluate clinical trial evidence regarding the effectiveness of any type of qigong in supportive cancer care.

4.2 Methods

4.2.1 Data Sources

The following databases were searched from their inception through May 2009: MEDLINE, AMED, EMBASE, CINAHL, five Korean Medical Databases (Korean Studies Information, DBPIA, Korea Institute of Science and Technology Information, KoreaMed, and Research Information Center for Health Database), Chinese Medical Databases (China National Knowledge Infracture: CNKI), qigong Database (Qigong Institute, Menlo Park, version 7.4) and The Cochrane Library 2009, Issue 2. The search terms used were based on two concepts. Concept one included terms for qigong and concept two included terms for cancer. The two were combined using the Boolean operator "AND". Korean and Chinese terms for qigong and cancer were used in the Korean and Chinese databases. We also performed electronic searches of relevant journals [FACT (Focus on Alternative and Complementary Therapies) and Research in Complementary Medicine (Forschende

Komplementarmedizin) up to May 2009]. In addition, reference lists of all papers were searched. Further, our own personal files were manually searched. Hardcopies of all articles were obtained and read in full.

4.2.2 Study Selection

All prospective clinical trials were included if they investigated patients with cancer who received qigong alone or combined with other treatments. No language restrictions were imposed. Trials with designs that did not allow for an evaluation of the effectiveness of the intervention (e.g., by using a treatment of unproven efficacy in the control group or comparing two different forms of qigong) were excluded. Dissertations and abstracts were also included. Case series and case reports were excluded.

4.2.3 Data Extraction

All clinical endpoints were considered, but the main outcome measures were effectiveness of qigong for treating symptoms in cancer patients and cancer survivors. Secondary outcome measures included survival rate and quality of life. Trials were excluded from this review if the outcomes were related only to immunological or other surrogate endpoints. All articles were read by two independent reviewers and data from the articles were validated and extracted according to the pre-defined criteria listed in Table 4.1. Discrepancies between reviewers were resolved by a third independent reviewer.

4.2.4 Assessment of Risk of Bias

Risk of bias was assessed using the Cochrane classification based on four criteria: randomization, blinding, withdrawals and allocation concealment (Julian and Douglas 2008). Taking into account that patients are difficult to blind to treatment, we only evaluated assessor blinding. Disagreements were resolved by discussions between the two reviewers and, if necessary, through discussion with the author. There were no disagreements between the three reviews.

4.3 Results

4.3.1 Study Description

The searches identified 242 potentially relevant articles (Fig. 4.1). There were 231 excluded because they were duplicate articles ($n = 3$), not related to cancer ($n = 35$), not related to the efficacy of qigong ($n = 45$), not clinical trials ($n = 55$), animal or

Table 4.1 Summary of randomized clinical studies of qigong for supportive cancer care

Reference Country	Sample size Type of cancer	Intervention (Regimen)	Control (Regimen)	Main outcome measures	Results	Adverse events	Comments
Oh et al. (2008) Australia	30 Various cancers	(A) Qigong (90 min, 1 or 2 times weekly for 8 weeks, n=14), plus usual medical care	(B) Usual medical care (n=16)	(1) Quality of life (EORTC QLQ-30) (2) Side effects of cancer (3) Inflammation	(1) NS (2) P=0.037 (consTipation) in favour of qigong (3) NS	n.r.	Drop-out rate (40%) Lack of standard deviation value
Wang et al. (1993) China	62 Late stage cancer	(A) Qigong (n.r., n.r.), plus chemotherapy (n=32)	(B) Chemotherapy (n=0)	(1) Response rate (Health state)	(1) A(29/32, 91%); B(12/30, 40%), P=0.0004	n.r.	Proceeding
Fu and Zou (1995) China	20 Gastric cancer	(A) Qigong (n.r., 3 times daily for 4 weeks, n=10), plus chemotherapy	(B) Chemotherapy (MMC+UFT,4 weeks, n=10)	(1) Response rate (short term) (2) Symptoms improvement	(1) A(9/10,90%); B(8/10,80%), P=0. 54 (2) A: 80%; B:70%, NS	n.r.	Book

Table 4.1 (continued)

Reference Country	Sample size Type of cancer	Intervention (Regimen)	Control (Regimen)	Main outcome measures	Results	Adverse events	Comments
Fu and Wang (1995) China	40 Late stage stomach cancer	(A) Qigong (n.r, once daily for 3 months, n=22), plus herbal medicine	(B) Herbal medicine (n=18)	(1) Response rate (2) X-ray, CT or Ultra-sound to measure tumour size (3) symptoms checklist & quality of life index	(1) A(7/22, 32%); B(6/18, 33%), P=0.92 (2) NS (3) P<0.05	n.r.	Book
Fu et al. (1996) China	186 Cardiac adeno-carcinoma (Stage I–III)	(A) Qigong (n.r., daily, n.r., n=50), plus herbal treatment and surgery	(B) Surgery (n=48) (C) chemotherapy, plus surgery (n=42) (D) Herbal treatment, plus surgery (n=46)	(1) Survival rate (%, after 1, 3, 5 year) (2) Mean survival time (months)	(1) A(86, 64, 36); B(80, 37, 21); C(86, 45,25); D(85, 44, 26), A vs. B, P<0.01 (2) A:48; B:30; C:36; D:36.5	n.r.	Proceeding

Table 4.1 (continued)

Reference Country	Sample size Type of cancer	Intervention (Regimen)	Control (Regimen)	Main outcome measures	Results	Adverse events	Comments
Lam (2004) China	58 Hepatocellular carcinoma	(A) Qigong (2 hr, twice weekly for 6 weeks in class and 3.5–5 h once daily for 24 weeks, n=29), plus TACE	(B) TACE (n=29)	(1) Survival rate (2) Quality of life (SF-36)	(1,2) NS	A: 11 in 8 subjects B: 13 in 12 subjects All AE were not related with qigong	Thesis

AE: adverse events; CT: computed tomography; EORTC-QoL: European Organization for Research and Treatment of Cancer Quality of Life Questionnaire; MMC: Mitomycin; n.r.: not reported; NS: no significance; TACE: Transcatheter arterial chemoembolization; UFT: uracil.

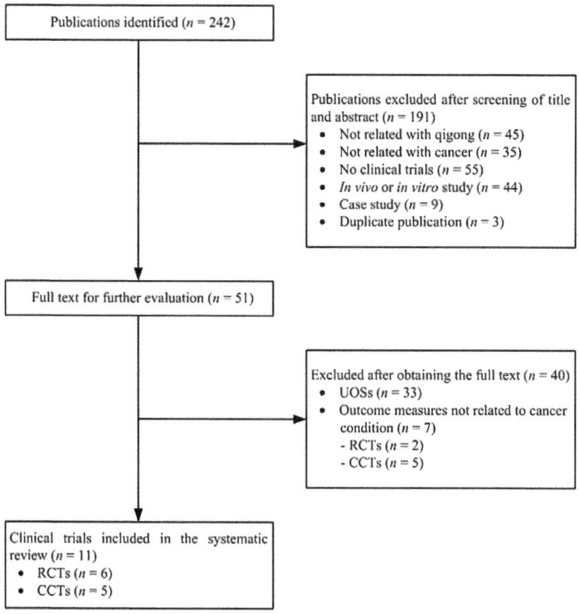

Fig. 4.1 Flowchart of trial selection process. RCT: randomized clinical trial; CCT: controlled clinical trial; UOS: uncontrolled observational study

in vitro studies ($n = 44$), and case reports ($n = 9$). Two independent reviewers read 51 articles in full, of which 40 were excluded. There were 33 uncontrolled observational studies (UOSs), and 2 RCTs and 5 non-randomized clinical trials (CCTs) were excluded because outcome measures were not directly related with cancer care.

Eleven studies, which included six RCTs (Wang et al. 1993; Fu and Wang 1995; Fu and Zou 1995; Fu et al. 1996; Lam 2004; Oh et al. 2008) and 5 CCTs (Sun and Zhao 1988; Zheng 1990; Wang and Ye 2002; Hong 2003; Lee et al. 2006), with a total of 921 participants met our inclusion criteria. Key data are listed in Tables 4.1 and 4.2. One of the included RCTs was conducted in Australia (Oh et al. 2008) and the other five were from China (Wang et al. 1993; Fu and Wang 1995; Fu and Zou 1995; Fu et al. 1996; Lam 2004). One CCT was conducted in Korea (Hong 2003), one in Taiwan (Lee et al. 2006) and three in China (Sun and Zhao 1988; Zheng 1990; Wang and Ye 2002). Ten of the included trials had a two-armed, parallel group design (Sun and Zhao 1988; Zheng 1990; Wang et al. 1993; Fu and Wang 1995; Fu and Zou 1995; Wang and Ye 2002; Hong 2003; Lam 2004; Lee et al. 2006; Oh et al. 2008) and one RCT used a 4-armed parallel group design (Fu et al. 1996). The types of cancer treated within the trials were gastric cancer (Fu and Wang 1995; Fu and Zou 1995; Hong 2003), cardiac adenocarcinoma (Fu et al. 1996), hepatocellular carcinoma (Lam 2004), breast cancer (Lee et al. 2006), and various cancers (Sun and Zhao 1988; Zheng 1990; Wang et al. 1993; Wang and Ye 2002; Oh et al. 2008). The subjective outcome measures were quality of life (QoL)

Table 4.2 Summary of non-randomized controlled studies of qigong for supportive cancer care

Reference Country	Sample size Type of cancer	Intervention (Regimen)	Control (Regimen)	Main outcome measures	Intergroup difference	Adverse events	Comments
Sun and Zhao (1988) China	123 Advance stage of various cancer (Stage III, IV)	(A) Qigong (2 hr daily for 3 months), plus same drug as control group	(B) Drug (n.r.)	(1) Strength (2) Appetite (3) Diarrhea or defection	(1–3) Significant difference (no *P* value reported)	n.r.	Proceeding
Zheng (1990) China	100 Various cancer (liver, lung and gastric)	(A) Qigong (n.r.)	(B) Other therapies (n.r.)	(1) Survival rate (%, 1,5 year) (2) Mean survival time (months)	(1) Lung cancer: A (83, 17); B (n.r., 7) stomach cancer: A(83, 23); B (n.r., 12) (2) A: 20.7; B: 3.5, $P<0.01$	n.r.	Proceeding
Wang and Ye (2002) China	211 Various cancer	(A) Qigong (n.r.), plus radiotherapy, chemotherapy, and herbal medicine	(B) Radiotherapy, chemotherapy, and herbal medicine	(1) Anxiety (SAS) (2) Depression (SDS) (3) Personality (EPQ)	(1) $P<0.01$ (2,3) NS	n.r.	–

Table 4.2 (continued)

Reference Country	Sample size Type of cancer	Intervention (Regimen)	Control (Regimen)	Main outcome measures	Intergroup difference	Adverse events	Comments
Hong (2003) Korea	24 Advanced gastric cancer	(A) Qigong (15–20 min, twice daily for 8 weeks), plus same chemotherapy received by control group	(B) Chemotherapy (5-FU+ Sunpla or Epirubicin)	(1) Fatigue (2) Physical functioning (MOS SF-36) (3) Index of nausea and vomiting (4) Occurrence of stomatitis	(1) P=0.018 at week 4, P=0.0013 at week 8 in favour of qigong (2) P=0.058 at week 4, P=0.0005 at week 8 in favour of qigong (3) P=0.025 at week 4, P=0.051 at week 8 in favour of qigong (4) P=0.64 at week 4, P=0.0029 at week 8 in favour of qigong	n.r.	Thesis Sample size calculation

n.r.: notl reported; NS: no significance.

(Lam 2004; Oh et al. 2008) with EORTC QoL-30 or SF-36, response rate (Wang et al. 1993; Fu and Wang 1995; Fu and Zou 1995), survival rate (Zheng 1990; Fu et al. 1996; Lam 2004), several psychological symptoms, (Wang and Ye 2002; Lam 2004; Lee et al. 2006) and fatigue (Hong 2003).

4.3.2 Risk of Bias

The included trials had a high risk of bias, except for two recent RCTs. Six RCTs (Wang et al. 1993; Fu and Wang 1995; Fu and Zou 1995; Fu et al. 1996; Lam 2004; Oh et al. 2008) were randomized and two (Lam 2004; Oh et al. 2008) described the methods of randomization, but none adopted both assessor and subject blinding. Details of drop-outs and withdrawals were described in two trials (Lam 2004; Oh et al. 2008). Only one RCT reported details about allocation concealment (Lam 2004). Adverse events were mentioned in one study (Lam 2004).

4.3.3 Detailed of Included Studies

4.3.3.1 Randomized Clinical Trials

Oh et al. (2008) evaluated the efficacy of qigong on quality of life and inflammation biomarkers in various cancer patients (Table 4.1). Thirty patients were randomly divided into two groups receiving qigong with usual medical care ($n = 14$) or usual medical care ($n = 16$) only. The main outcomes were QoL, as measured by the European Organization for Research and Treatment of Cancer Quality of Life Questionnaire, (EORTC QLQ-30) and improvement of side effects of usual medical care including chemotherapy. The progress of disease was assessed by the inflammation biomarker C – reactive protein (CRP). Quality of life was improved in the qigong group but there was no significant difference compared with control. ConsTipation was improved significantly compared with the control group ($P = 0.034$). However, there was no significant difference in CRP between the two groups.

Wang et al. (1993) conducted an RCT to evaluate the effects of qigong in late stage cancer patients. Sixty-one patients were randomly divided to receive chemotherapy only ($n = 29$) or chemotherapy plus qigong ($n = 32$). The main outcome measures were improvement in health and white blood cell (WBC) count. The experimental group experienced improved health and a stable WBC counts, whereas 12 of 30 patients in the control group reported worse health with more cancer-related symptoms, and all control patients showed a decline in WBC count.

Fu and Zou (1995) investigated the effects of qigong combined with chemotherapy on short-term response rates and symptom improvement in patients with gastric cancer. Twenty patients were randomized into two groups receiving qigong plus chemotherapy ($n = 10$) and chemotherapy only ($n = 10$). Qigong exercises were performed three times daily for 4 weeks. The main outcome measures were the response rate and symptom improvement. The differences between the qigong and the control groups were not statistically significant for either response rate or symptom improvement.

Fu and Wang (1995) conducted an RCT to evaluate the short-term effects of a special Chinese herbal medicine *versus* qigong therapy plus the herbal medicine in elderly patients with late-stage stomach cancer. Forty patients with late-stage stomach cancer with confirmed tumour size with imagery or pathological measures (such as X-ray, CT scan, biopsy, and/or ultra-sound) were recruited for this special study. Most of the patients (80%) were either too old or too far along in their diagnosis to undergo surgery. The patients were randomly assigned into two treatment groups: herbal medicine alone ($n = 18$) and qigong plus herbal medicine ($n = 22$). After three months of intensive treatment with daily herbal medicine or herbal plus qigong, the majority of patients reported various degrees of improvement with 22–23% of patients reporting complete release (measurable tumour reduction), but there was no significant difference between the two treatment groups in terms of proportion of tumour decrease. However, they found that the qigong plus herbal group reported significantly more symptom reduction ($P < 0.05$) and increases in immune functioning ($P < 0.01$) measured after the treatment.

Fu et al. (1996) carried out an RCT to assess the effectiveness of combined qigong and herbal treatment on survival rates in 186 post-surgery patients with cardiac adenocarcinoma (155 men and 31 women; mean age = 59.8 ± 8.8 years). Patients were randomized into four groups: surgery only (control; $n = 48$), chemotherapy only (etoposide, doxorubicin and cisplatin: EAP, $n = 42$), herbal therapy only (not specified, $n = 46$), and qigong combined with herbal treatment ($n = 50$). The main outcomes were survival rate and median survival period. The survival rates were 80.1, 36.5, and 20.8% for the control group at 1, 3 and 5 years respectively; 85.7, 45.2, and 25.1% for the chemotherapy group; 84.5, 43.5, and 26.1% for the herbal group; and 86.0, 64.0, and 36.0% for the qigong combined with herbal treatment group. There were significant differences between the qigong combined with herbal treatment and the control group ($P < 0.01$). The median survival period was 30 months for the control group, 36 and 36.5 months for chemotherapy and herbal groups, respectively, and 48 months for the qigong combined with herbal therapy group.

Lam (2004) investigated the effect of qigong combined with transcatheter arterial chemoembolization (TACE) on survival rate and QoL in patients with hepatocellular carcinoma. Patients were randomized into two groups receiving qigong combined with TACE and TACE only. Qigong exercises lasted 2 h per session, and were performed twice weekly for 6 weeks in class and 3.5–5 h daily for 24 weeks at home. The main outcome measures were survival rate and QoL, measured with the SF-36. The survival rate was 52.6% for the qigong group and 29.0% for controls. The median survival time was not provided for the qigong group (overall survival rate was higher than 50%) and 242 days for the control group. The differences between the intervention and the control group were not statistically significant for either survival rate or QoL.

4.3.3.2 Non-randomized Controlled Trial

Sun and Zhao (1988) conducted a CCT to assess the effectiveness of qigong on symptoms of cancer patients (Table 4.2). Patients were divided non-randomly into two parallel groups: qigong (two hours daily for three months) combined with drugs ($n = 97$, types of drug were not specified) and drug therapy only ($n = 30$). The outcome measures included physical strength, appetite, diarrhoea, defecation, and body weight. At the end of the trial, 82% of patients from the group receiving qigong therapy had improved physical strength, 63% improved appetite, and 33% were free of diarrhoea or irregular defecation. The corresponding rates for the control group were 10, 10, and 6%, respectively. All these parameters yielded significant inter-group differences.

Zheng (1990) tested the effects of qigong on survival rates of various late-stage cancer patients. One hundred patients were compared with patients in the same hospital who underwent other therapies without qigong. This study did not mention the type of qigong (regimen) nor the interventions administrated in the control group. The main outcomes were survival rate and median survival time. One and five year survival rates were 83 and 17% for lung cancer patients (survival rate was 7% at 5 years for the control group,) and 83 and 23% for stomach cancer patients (controls: 12% at 5 years). The median survival time favoured the group receiving qigong therapy (20.7 vs. 3.5 months, $P < 0.01$).

Wang and Ye (2002) investigated the therapeutic effects of qigong on psychological symptoms during rehabilitation of cancer patients. They recruited 104 cancer patients from a qigong rehabilitation unit as the experimental group and 107 cancer patients with similar a demographic distribution and types of cancer from a regular cancer clinic. They evaluated all patients using the Eysenck Personality Questionnaire and Zung's Self-evaluating Anxiety Scale and Depression Scale before and three months after treatment. Patients who chose to go to qigong rehabilitation were more likely to be extroverts and have lower anxiety and depression levels at baseline than controls. Compared to the controls more patients in the qigong group reported relief of anxiety and depression.

Hong (2003) evaluated the efficacy of qigong on adverse events of chemotherapy in advanced stomach cancer patients. Twenty-four patients were non-randomly divided into two groups receiving either qigong with chemotherapy (5-FU plus Sunpla or Epirubicin) or chemotherapy only. The main outcome was the level of fatigue as measured by the Piper fatigue scale. The difficulty with daily activities was assessed according to the Physical functioning subscale of Medical Outcome Study-36. The frequencies of nausea and vomiting for the preceding 12 h were evaluated with an index ranging from 0 (none) to 5 (for more than 7 times). Fatigue was lower in the qigong group compared to controls. There were also significant differences between the two groups in the level of difficulty with daily activities, nausea, vomiting and stomatitis.

Lee et al. (2006) conducted a CCT to evaluate the effects of qigong on symptoms and psychological distress in 67 breast cancer patients receiving chemotherapy. Patients were divided into two groups, one receiving qigong with chemotherapy and another receiving chemotherapy only. Primary outcome measures were symptom distress (measured with McCorkle and Young's symptom distress scale) and psychological distress (measured with symptom checklist-90-revision; SCL-90-R). The results showed significant differences between the groups with respect to symptom distress after 21 days but not at 5, 8 or 15 days. No significant differences between the intervention and control groups were noted with regard to psychological distress.

4.3.4 Safety

Adverse events were reported in one study (Lam 2004), while others did not report them. However, they were related with TACE but not qigong.

4.4 Discussion

This systematic review shows that there are some promising reports on positive effect of qigong for supportive cancer care, but its value and efficacy has not been adequately investigated. There are no large-scale rigorous RCT studies which could provide a definitive answer. Six RCTs (Wang et al. 1993; Fu and Wang 1995; Fu and Zou 1995; Fu et al. 1996; Lam 2004; Oh et al. 2008) tested the effects of qigong as supportive cancer care compared with usual care or herbal medicine and showed no significant differences in most outcome measures, whereas all five CCTs (Zheng 1990; Sun and Zhao 1988; Wang and Ye 2002; Hong 2003; Lee et al. 2006) showed favourable effects of qigong. Two RCTs suggested effectiveness in prolonging life of cancer patients, and one failed to do so (Fu et al. 1996; Lam 2004). Most of the trials have a high risk of bias. Of course, it is methodologically challenging to design rigorous trials for qigong. In CCTs, the nature of the control intervention deserves consideration. A placebo for qigong, effectively, does not exist. In the present set of studies, an absence of adequate statistical analysis of the variability of therapeutic protocols and poor quality of reporting are frequent methodological problems. The current evidence from RCTs on qigong as supportive cancer care is not convincing. However, the number of trials and the total sample size are too small to draw firm conclusions.

The risk of bias in the studies was assessed based on the descriptions of randomization, blinding, withdrawals and allocation concealment (Julian and Douglas 2008). All of the studies were burdened with a high risk of bias due to the fact that traditional double-blind randomized control trial may not be the best model to investigate a self-applied behavior therapy. Only one RCT (Lam 2004) employed allocation concealment and none of the RCTs made an attempt to blind assessors. Two RCTs (Lam 2004; Oh et al. 2008) reported details of drop-outs and withdrawals that may have led to exclusion or attrition biases. Only one RCT employed intention-to-treat analysis (Lam 2004). Thus the reliability of the evidence presented is clearly limited. Among the 11 studies we included, only 6 were randomized (Wang et al. 1993; Fu and Wang 1995; Fu and Zou 1995; Fu et al. 1996; Lam 2004; Oh et al. 2008). The rest were wide open to selection bias, which can generate false positive findings. Four studies (Sun and Zhao 1988; Wang et al. 1993; Zheng 1990; Fu and Zou 1995) were published in proceedings without adequate reporting of essential details. Two were unpublished theses (Hong 2003; Lam 2004) and two were published in a book (Fu and Wang 1995; Fu and Zou 1995), which had not gone through the formal peer review process. One RCT (Lam 2004) failed to show an effect of qigong on survival rate and QoL in hepatocellular carcinoma patients when compared with TACE. This trial lacked details in the reporting of methodological features such as carcinoma staging and co-interventions. Another RCT (Fu et al. 1996) suggested some survival advantages in cardiac adenocarcinoma cancer patients receiving qigong. However, its methodology was not clearly described. The third RCT showed significant symptom reduction and increases in immune function, but failed to show total response rates in patients with gastric cancer. The fourth RCT (Fu and Zou 1995) also failed to show favourable effects of qigong with respect to response rates and symptom improvement. The two RCTs (Fu and Wang 1995; Fu and Zou 1995) that were published in a book had not gone through the process of formal peer review. The fifth RCT (Wang et al. 1993) reported that qigong has favourable effects on health state and WBC. Unfortunately, it was only published as an abstract and was without essential details. The sixth RCT (Oh et al. 2008) tested qigong as adjuvant to usual medical care in various cancer patients and failed to showed favourable effects on QoL and inflammation biomarkers. The compliance rate of this trial was 60% and the author did not conduct intent-to-analysis. All of included RCTs have small sample sizes and therefore their results are prone to type II errors.

Two excluded RCTs (Luo and Tong 1988; Luo et al. 1991) failed to report exact outcome measures for cancer care. One RCT comparing qigong plus radiotherapy with conventional drug therapy plus radiotherapy showed favourable effects of qigong on haemoglobin, RBC and WBC cell counts. The other RCT reported beneficial effects of qigong plus chemotherapy on haemoglobin, RBC and WBC cell counts compared with qigong only or chemotherapy only. Collectively, even if we consider these excluded trials, the evidence is not sufficiently convincing to suggest that qigong is an effective treatment for supportive cancer care.

In the absence of a sufficient number of controlled clinical trials, other types of evidence might be helpful. Uncontrolled trials and case reports imply that qigong is beneficial for symptom management of various cancers. Unfortunately, such data are highly susceptible to bias and hence, they provide little useful information on the specific effects of qigong as it relates to supportive cancer care.

One could argue that currently there are not enough RCTs to do a conclusive systematic review. However, it is not only a matter of the number of RCTs but also one of methodological rigor, including features such as appropriate sample size, subject, practitioner, or assessor blinding, and adequate allocation concealment. Currently there is one ongoing RCT, funded by the UTMD. Anderson Cancer Center is testing the effectiveness of pre-surgical qigong therapy for women with breast cancer. Perhaps this RCT will help to clarify the issue.

Taichi is an intervention that shares many characteristics with qigong; it might therefore be helpful to consider the findings of systematic reviews of taichi in supportive cancer care. A recent review (Lee et al. 2007) identified three controlled studies, two of which were RCTs. The authors concluded that the evidence is insufficient to suggest that taichi is an effective supportive treatment for cancer.

The fact that there is no good trial evidence in support of qigong therapy is in line with several different interpretations. Qigong may be ineffective, the studies may have been incorrectly designed or the treatment may not have been administered optimally in the existing studies. For instance, the number of qigong sessions could have been too small to generate a significant effect, or the type of qigong or the applied protocol might not have been suitable for cancer care. A clinical study is only truly useful if the intervention used can be replicated, and hence, the type of qigong employed and a full description are important. There are significant differences between the numerous forms of qigong, which pose difficulties in establishing quality standards of treatment. A clear description of the qigong intervention used should be provided together with a description of the level of expertise of the instructors.

The next question that arises is that of the safety of qigong. None of the reviewed studies reported any adverse events related with qigong. Qigong appears to be generally safe, and serious adverse effects have not been reported. Some studies (Ng 1999; Lee 2000; Kemp 2004) reported adverse events, including headache, dizziness, nausea, mental disorders and psychosis, in individuals who practice qigong incorrectly, although these risks have not been formally studied. Adverse effects were not the focus of this review; regardless, the safety of qigong needs further research.

Assuming that qigong is a potentially beneficial option for cancer patients, the mechanism may be of interest. One possible mechanism is an improvement in immune function through modulating the level of cytokine and hormone, which may counteract the immune deficiency experienced by most of cancer patients (Jones 2001; Chen 2004; Lee et al. 2005). Others have postulated that qigong improves microcirculatory function, including changes in blood viscosity, elasticity of blood vessel, and platelet function(Chen 2004). A third proposed mechanism is an increase in pain threshold as a result of the relaxation effects (Chen 2004). Further possible mechanism suggested that qigong induces apoptosis in pancreatic cancer cells and increase or repress PI3K activity of highly enriched PI3K preparations, suggesting that external qigong could regulate enzymes (such as Akt and Erk1/2) positively or negatively in different settings (e.g., in cancer cells vs. normal cells) (Yan et al. 2006, 2008). If these theories were confirmed, they may explain how qigong leads to clinical improvements in patients.

4.4.1 Limitation of This Review

Limitations of our systematic review and any systematic review in general pertain to the potential incompleteness of the evidence reviewed. We aimed to identify all

RCTs and CCTs on the topic. The distorting effects on systematic reviews and meta-analyses arising from publication bias and location bias are well documented (Ernst and Pittler 1997; Egger and Smith 1998; Pittler et al. 2000). In this review, there were no restrictions in terms of publication language and a large number of different databases were queried. We are confident that our search strategy has located all relevant data, however, a degree of uncertainty remains. Moreover, selective publishing and reporting can be major causes of bias. It is conceivable that several negative RCTs remain unpublished, thus distorting the overall picture. Another possible source of bias is the fact that most of the included trials were carried out in China and Korea, regions which have been shown to produce almost no negative studies (Vickers et al. 1998). Further limitations of our review are the potentially poor quality of the primary data and poor reporting of results, which were highly heterogeneous in virtually every respect. To establish the role of qigong in the management of cancer patients, adequately designed trials are required.

4.4.2 Recommendations for Future Research

Future RCTs of qigong for supportive cancer care should adhere to accepted standards of trial methodology. The studies included in this review show a number of problems that have been noted by other reviews of trials examining the efficacy of qigong or taichi, e.g., expertise of qigong practitioners, the pluralism of qigong, frequency and duration of treatment, employing validated primary outcome measures and adequate statistical tests, and heterogeneous comparison groups (Chen and Yeung 2002; Wayne and Kaptchuk 2008). Furthermore, even though it is difficult to blind subjects to treatment, employing assessor blinding and allocation concealment are important for reducing bias.

4.4.3 Perspectives

This review of RCTs and CCTs focused on the effects of qigong as supportive cancer care. Collectively, the existing trial evidence is not convincing and does not show qigong to be an effective modality for supportive cancer care. Future studies should be of high quality with a particular emphasis on designing adequate and appropriate control groups.

Acknowledgement The authors specially thank Dr Tae-young Choi of the Korea Institute of Oriental Medicine (KIOM) for extensively searching the Chinese Databases. MS Lee was supported by KIOM (K09050).

References

American Cancer Society. Cancer facts and figures 2008. http://www.cancer.org/downloads/STT/2008CAFFfinalsecured.pdf. Accessed 15 June 2009 2009:18.

Chen KW. An analytic review of studies on measuring effects of external qi in China. Altern Ther Health Med. 2004;10:38–50.
Chen K, Yeung R. Exploratory studies of qigong therapy for cancer in China. Integr Cancer Ther. 2002;1:345–70.
Courneya KS. Exercise in cancer survivors: an Overview of research. Med Sci Sports Exerc. 2003;35:1846–52.
Dy GK, Bekele L, Hanson LJ et al. Complementary and alternative medicine use by patients enrolled onto phase I clinical trials. J Clin Oncol. 2004;22:4810–5.
Egger M, Smith GD. Bias in location and selection of studies. BMJ. 1998;316:61–66.
Ernst E, Pittler MH. Alternative therapy bias. Nature. 1997;385:480.
Ernst E, Pittler M, Wider B et al. Oxford handbook of complementary medicine. Oxford, UK: Oxford University Press; 2008.
Frenkel M, Ben-Arye E, Baldwin CD et al. Approach to communicating with patients about the use of nutritional supplements in cancer care. South Med J. 2005;98:289–94.
Fu JZ, Fu SL, Qin JT. Effect of qigong and anticancer body-bulding herbs on the prognosis of postoperative patients with cardiac adenocarcinoma. Third World Conference on Medical Qigong 1996.
Fu JZ, Wang SM. Qigong plus herbal medicine in treating late-stage stomach cancer in the elderly. In: Lin ZP editors. Understanding of true qi cultivation and sublimation. Beijing, China: Chinese Publisher of Constructive Materials; 1995. 155–57.
Fu JZ, Zou ZK. Qigong combined with chemotherapy in the treatment of gastric cancer. In: Lin ZP editors. Understanding of true qi cultivation and sublimation. Beijing, China: Chinese Publisher of Constructive Materials; 1995. 157–8.
Hong EY. The effect of Yudongkong exercise in fatigue, difficulty of daily activities and symptoms of side effect in advanced gastric cancer patients receiving chemotherapy (Doctorial dissertation). Seoul, Korea: Yonsei University; 2003. 83.
Jones BM. Changes in cytokine production in healthy subjects practicing Guolin qigong: a pilot study. BMC Complement Altern Med. 2001;1:8.
Julian PTH, Douglas GA. Assessing risk of bias in included studies. In: Julian PT, Green S editors. Cochrane handbook for systematic reviews of interventions. West Sussex, England: Wiley-Blackwell; 2008. 187–241.
Kemp CA. Qigong as a therapeutic intervention with older adults. J Holist Nurs. 2004;22: 351–73.
Lam SWY. A randomized, controlled trial of Guolin qigong in patients receiving transcatheter arterial chemoembolisation for unresectable hepatocellular carcinoma (Master). Hong Kong: University of Hong Kong; 2004. 130.
Lee S. Chinese hypnosis can cause qigong induced mental disorders. BMJ. 2000;320:803.
Lee TI, Chen HH, Yeh ML. Effects of chan-chuang qigong on improving symptom and psychological distress in chemotherapy patients. Am J Chin Med. 2006;34:37–46.
Lee MS, Kim MK, Ryu H. Qi-training (qigong) enhanced immune functions: what is the underlying mechanism?. Int J Neurosci. 2005;115:1099–104.
Lee MS, Pittler MH, Ernst E. Is taichi an effective adjunct in cancer care? A systematic review of controlled clinical trials. Support Care Cancer. 2007;15:597–601.
Luo JF, He CW, Lu HH et al. Analysis of the impact of qigong for patients with nasopharyngeal carcinoma. Chin J Cancer. 1991;10:343–4.
Luo S, Tong T. Effects of vital gate qigong on malignant tumor. 1st World Conf Acad Exch Med Qigong, Beijing, China; 1988.
National Center for Complementary and Alternative Medicine. Cancer and complementary and alternative medicine. http://nccam.nih.gov/health/cancer/camcancer.htm . Accessed 15 June 2009.
Ng BY. Qigong-induced mental disorders: a review. Aust N Z J Psychiatry. 1999;33:197–206.
Oh B, Butow P, Mullan B et al. Medical qigong for cancer patients: pilot study of impact on quality of life, side effects of treatment and inflammation. Am J Chin Med. 2008;36:459–72.

Pittler MH, Abbot NC, Harkness EF et al. Location bias in controlled clinical trials of complementary/alternative therapies. J Clin Epidemiol. 2000;53:485–89.
Richardson MA, Sanders T, Palmer JL et al. Complementary/alternative medicine use in a comprehensive cancer center and the implications for oncology. J Clin Oncol. 2000;18:2505–14.
Sancier KM. Medical applications of qigong. Altern Ther Health Med. 1996;2:40–46.
Sancier KM. Therapeutic benefits of qigong exercises in combination with drugs. J Altern Complement Med. 1999;5:383–89.
Sun QZ, Zhao L. Clinical observation of qigong as a therapeutic aid for advanced cancer patients. First World Conference for Academic Exchange of Medical Qigong, Beijing, China; 1988.
Vickers A, Goyal N, Harland Rm et al. Do certain countries produce only positive results? A systematic review of controlled trials. Control Clin Trials. 1998;19:159–66.
Wang CH, Wang BR, Shao MY et al. Clinical study if the routine treatment if cancer coordinated by qigong. 2nd World Conference for Academic Exchange of Medical Qigong, 1993.
Wang Y, Ye M. Analysis of psychological err factors in assessment of therapeutic effect of qigong rehabilitation in cancer patients. Acta Universitatis Traditionis Medicalis Sinensis Pharmacologiaeque Shanghai. 2002;16:20–22.
Wayne PM, Kaptchuk TJ. Challenges inherent to t'ai chi research: part II-defining the intervention and optimal study design. J Altern Complement Med. 2008;14:191–7.
World Health Organization. Cancer. http://www.who.int/cancer/en/. Accessed 15 June 2009.
Yan X, Shen H, Jiang H et al. External qi of Yan Xin qigong differentially regulates the Akt and extracellular signal-regulated kinase pathways and is cytotoxic to cancer cells but not to normal cells. Int J Biochem Cell Biol. 2006;38:2102–13.
Yan X, Shen H, Jiang H et al. External qi of Yan Xin qigong induces G2/M arrest and apoptosis of androgen-independent prostate cancer cells by inhibiting Akt and NF-kappa B pathways. Mol Cell Biochem. 2008;310:227–34.
Zheng RR. Observation of 100 cases with comprehensive qigong therapy for treating later-stage cancer. World Qigong. 1990;3:19.

Chapter 5
Traditional Chinese Medicine in the Reduction of Discomfort and Side-Effects of Surgery

Kok-Yang Tan, Xiaoxiu Wu and Francis Seow-Choen

Abstract Surgery for cancer has made significant progression in recent years and these developments have been in tandem with various adjuvant treatments including chemotherapy and radiotherapy. The concurrent use of traditional Chinese medicine (TCM), a 5,000-year-old art, with surgery has not been popular among those who practice Western style medicine. This is largely due to the different philosophies and relatively lack of scientific evidence of TCM. There is however current intense research on TCM as novel or additional treatment methods for cancer surgery. This chapter reviews the current use of TCM in cancer surgery and the intention is not to coerce the surgeon into using TCM but to increase the awareness of surgeons and provide a stimulus for research. The pathogenesis of cancer according to TCM is discussed. Traditional Chinese medicine has been used successfully during the perioperative period to relieve intestinal obstruction, reduce postoperative ileus and reduce urinary retention after rectal surgery. Traditional Chinese medicine has also been shown to modulate the inflammatory response of surgical stress. Although the reported results of TCM have been exciting thus far, problems of lack of consensus on treatment regimes and questions on the reliability, validity and applicability of published studies prevent its widespread use and these issues will be discussed in this chapter. There is thus a pressing need for surgeons to work with TCM physicians in the continuing research on this area in order to unleash its full potential for our patients.

5.1 Introduction

Surgery for cancer has made significant progression in recent years and these developments have been in tandem with various adjuvant treatments including chemotherapy and radiotherapy. Molecular therapy, immunotherapy and gene

K.-Y. Tan (✉)
Department of Surgery, Colorectal Service, Alexandra Hospital, Singapore
e-mail: kokyangtan@gmail.com

W.C.S. Cho (ed.), *Supportive Cancer Care with Chinese Medicine*,
DOI 10.1007/978-90-481-3555-4_5, © Springer Science+Business Media B.V. 2010

therapy are hot on the heels of more traditional adjuvant treatment. There has been much research on perioperative processes over the years with elucidation of physiological concepts that are the backbone of current perioperative guidelines and protocols. The recent emphasis on evidence-based practices has somewhat contributed to this progression where some traditional practices were debunked as myths and practices streamlined. With the progression of evidence-based practices in Western medicine, it is easy to see why the concurrent use of traditional Chinese medicine (TCM) with surgery has not been popular among those who practice Western style medicine. This is largely due to the different philosophies and relatively lack of understanding of TCM by Western medicine.

There is no doubt however that TCM, which is a 5,000-year-old art, has been used to treat cancer with a certain amount of success. What is interesting is that while many ancient traditional concepts remain the cornerstone of the practice of TCM, there has also been a shift in the paradigm to more scientific practices. Traditional Chinese medicine use in cancer is currently an area of intense research.(He 2006; Zhou and Su 2007; Hsu et al. 2008; Konkimalla and Efferth 2008; Cho and Chen 2009) Some of which on colorectal cancer treatment were recently highlighted (Tan et al. 2008). There is now some insight into the physiological basis behind TCM and TCM now has become an exciting entity that may well offer novel or additional treatment methods of cancer surgery.

Interestingly, a very recent survey found Western oncologists to be as likely to combine complementary or alternative medicine with conventional treatment as oncologists from China and Taiwan (Lee et al. 2008). Indeed, the growing interest in the use of alternative modalities is occurring as a worldwide phenomenon.

Another study in Singapore on 2,010 subjects aged 65 and above found that 25.3% of those studied were taking Chinese herbal medicine and of these 52% were on Western prescription medicines (Ng et al. 2004). This ancient art is actually much more widely accepted and used in the community than what doctors who practice Western medicine think.

As cancer surgeons in the interest of medical advancement, we cannot pass off TCM treatments as myths without first acquiring a proper understanding or study into it. An attempt should be made to understand the basics of TCM and the principles behind it. This chapter reviews the current use of TCM in cancer surgery and the intention is not to coerce the surgeon into using TCM but to increase the awareness of surgeons and provide a stimulus for research. Perhaps we can see better then, the advantages of combining Western and Eastern medicine in surgery.

5.2 Pathogenesis of Cancer According to Traditional Chinese Medicine

The concepts of TCM have been passed down from nearly 5,000 years ago. Many of the medical writings regard the ancient writings of Huangdi's Internal Classic (Huangdi Neijing) to be the most authoritative. The main focus of TCM is the use of an extensive variety of plant, animal products and minerals, many of which were compiled by Li Shizhen in the Compendium of Materia Medica (Bencao Gangmu) in the 16th century.

Most of the concepts of TCM revolve around the concepts of qi and the internal balance in the body of complementary forces (yin and yang). The concept of qi is interesting. The ancient Chinese writings define that qi is the most basic substance constituting the world. Accordingly, TCM also believes that qi is the most fundamental substance in the construction of the human body and in the maintenance of its life activities. Qi of the human body takes 2 forms. The first is coagulated qi which is manifested as various structural components of the body, such as viscera, body figure, sense organs, blood and body fluids; the second is diffused qi which is manifested as the energy and life force that flows in the body, but takes no certain form. It flows within a fixed network of twelve invisible pathways or meridians in the body. This is the most important concept of Chinese medicine. Qi has the function of promoting the growth and development of the body and the distribution and discharge of blood and body fluids. Qi also has the function of warming, defense and homeostasis in the human body (Huangdi's Internal Classic).

Yin (feminine – cool, moist, nutritive, quiet) and yang (masculine – warm, dry, energetic, active) are complementary yet opposite forces that are important in the achievement of wellness. When they are in balance, unobstructed flow of qi is promoted. An imbalance of qi, yin and yang are believed to result in sickness. All treatments aim to balance a person's qi. Several methods are used to promote, maintain and restore qi, including herbal remedies for nourishment, acupuncture, moxibustion (heat therapy), diet, massage, meditation and exercises such as qigong and taichi (Tan et al. 2008).

Although, like in Western medicine, there are different concepts to the pathogenesis of cancer according to TCM, one common theme is that cancer is a systemic disease and the tumour is but the local manifestation. Some manifestations have been associated with particular problems for example the accumulation of phlegm is associated with enlarged lymph nodes or cancer metastasis and blood stasis with tumours of the abdomen.

The cause of the systemic disease can be divided into external environmental forces and internal problems that interact. External forces include exposure to a cold and wet environment, poor eating habits and ingestion of toxins and alcohol which gives rise to poor flow of qi and accumulation of toxins. Internal problems include mental stress and depression, weakened internal organs and an imbalance of the forces in the body including qi (Sun 2001).

An example of the concepts behind cancer can be illustrated with the entity of colorectal cancer. The main pathophysiology behind the development of colorectal cancer is that of the accumulation of toxins. The excess toxic fluids and heat in the body cause an imbalance in the body which is relatively deplete of qi. The combination of these effects is further aggravated by a weak spleen and kidney allowing the flow of toxins into the intestines where it accumulates. A deficiency of qi is also thought to be the major driving force resulting in colorectal cancer. As such some herbs are making progress as main remedies, these herbs are mainly used to promote circulation, eliminate blood stasis, clear toxins and heat, invigorate the spleen and kidney and most importantly replenish qi (Sun 2001; Tan et al. 2008).

5.3 Rationale of Using Herbal Therapy in Cancer Surgery Treatment

The modality of open surgery has not been well accepted by TCM as the act of "opening one up" is actually thought to allow escape of vital qi. One wonders then if minimally invasive surgery would then be advantages in preserving the qi in the body! With advancement in surgical techniques and results, TCM practitioners are becoming more receptive to the idea that surgery is the best treatment option in some patients. The focus of the use of TCM during the perioperative period is then complementary in nature. This practice is now becoming more widespread with many hospitals practicing Western medicine having input from TCM physicians as well. In some hospitals in China, surgical patients are freely referred to the TCM department of the same hospital during the perioperative period.

The complementary role of TCM to surgery is focused on how to use TCM to reduce the extent of the trauma and stress of surgery. At the same time, there is also focus on how to replenish and repair the leakage of vital energy due to surgery (Liu and Xu 2000). Although some of these concepts may seem difficult to understand, there are now emerging clinical studies on these areas and there are also some studies that may offer some insight into the molecular basis of the use of TCM in the perioperative period. Indeed this ancient art is now fast becoming a science.

Described perioperative roles of TCM include treatment of anaemia, low serum albumin, poor circulation and electrolyte imbalances (Sun 2001). Traditional Chinese medicine has also been used to raise immunity and improve the endurance for surgical stress. There are also roles in the reduction of operative pain, bleeding, infection, intestinal ileus and poor urinary flow. These will be discussed in the following sections.

5.4 Role of Herbal Therapy At the Preoperative Phase of Treatment

The role of herbal therapy in the preoperative period involves improving the overall condition of the patient as much as possible before undergoing surgery. These involve the reduction of the symptoms and complications caused by the primary pathology, improving the internal milieu of the body and also the psychological status of the patient.

5.4.1 Treatment of Complications Arising from the Primary Pathology

The presentation of acute malignant intestinal obstruction is invariably associated with a higher perioperative surgical morbidity and mortality. There may also be poorer long term prognosis even after successful surgery. The use of TCM in patients with acute malignant intestinal obstruction is well documented (Liu and Xu 2000). In TCM, malignant bowel obstruction is considered much more serious than non-malignant obstruction. The reason is that malignant obstruction does not only involve mechanical obstruction of the bowel but there are other deleterious effects. The impaired flow of qi, blood stasis and accumulation of toxins that occurs in malignant bowel obstruction are thought to be important factors that contribute to poor outcomes of surgery. It is thought that these issues have severe impact on surgical outcome and need to be resolved to achieve uncomplicated surgery (Liu and Xu 2000).

The usual formulas used are derived from an ancient formula that consists of *Rheum palumatum* (rhubarb) and *Natrium sulfuricum* (mirabilite) which has a purgative effect and *Magnolia officinalis* (magnolia bark) which is qi regulating.

Peng reported a series of 45 patients who presented with acute bowel obstruction (Peng 2003). The treatment regime included a concoction comprising: *Citrus aurantium* (immature bitter orange), magnolia bark, fried *Raphanus sativus* (radish root), *Codonopsis pilosula* (dangshen), rhubarb, *Paeonia veitchii* (red peony root), mirabilite and *Patrinia villosa* (patrinia herb). Of the 45 patients, 35 experienced relief of the obstruction before surgery and subsequently underwent surgery with no complications. The obstruction was not resolved in the remaining 10 who underwent emergency surgery.

Zhou (2004) treated 30 patients with acute colonic obstruction using rhubarb, mirabilite, immature bitter orange, magnolia bark, *Angelica sinensis* (Chinese angelica root), red peony root and *Aucklandia lappa* (aucklandia root). Obstruction was alleviated in 14 patients, they underwent complication free curative surgery with good survival on follow-up. Of the remaining 16 who underwent emergency surgery, 6 underwent curative surgery while the remaining 10 underwent non-curative surgery. All did not have major surgical complications. These herbs used have been thought to be able to reduce inflammation, improve circulation to the bowel wall and thus have a protective effect on bowel anastomosis.

The accompanying problems of blood loss, frequency of bowel actions and abdominal discomfort can be treated with Yunnan Baiyao and Peach Seed and Safflower Decoction of Four Ingredients (Taohong Siwu Decoction) which have been reported to be useful in this setting (Liu and Xu 2000).

5.4.2 Improving the Overall Condition to Facilitate Surgery

The Chinese physicians believe that cancer is a consumptive disease giving rise to malnutrition, anaemia, lethargy and inactivity, hypoproteinaemia and electrolyte

Table 5.1 Herbs used in the preoperative phase to improve the overall condition for surgery

Herb (Latin name)	Herb (Common name)
Panax ginseng	Ginseng
Astragalus membranaceus	Astragalus root
Angelica sinensis	Chinese angelica root
Salvia miltiorrhiza	Red sage root
Poria cocos	Tuckahoe
Atractylodes macrocephala	Bighead atractylodes rhizome
Ganoderma lucidum	Lucid ganoderma
Cornus officinalis	Asian cornelian cherry fruit
Cistanche deserticola	Desertliving cistanche
Agrimonia pilosa	Hairy vein agrimony herb
Rehmannia glutinosa	Rehmannia dried root

imbalances. In the modern setting, comorbidities of hypertension, heart disease, diabetes and other chronic illnesses may coexist, especially in older patients. All these may have a negative effect on the outcome of surgery in the patients (Liu and Xu 2000). These concepts are in fact not dissimilar to that of Western medicine. *Panax ginseng* (ginseng), dangshen, Chinese angelica root or combinations including the Decoction of Six Noble Drugs (Liujunzi Decoction) and the Decoction of Eight Precious Drugs (Babao Decoction) have been used to enhance the patients' overall condition prior to surgery (Sun 2001). Common herbs used in the preoperative period are listed in Table 5.1.

5.4.3 Improving the Overall Mental State Prior to Surgery

The implication of harbouring cancer is very serious and weighs heavily in a patient's mind. Management of this psychological stress may improve the outcomes of cancer patients (Liu and Xu 2000). Traditional Chinese medicine has methods to regulate the flow of qi and to calm the nerves. Herbs that have been used for this function include *Cyperus rotundus* (natgrass galingale rhizome), *Curcuma longa* (common turmeric), *Bupleurum chinense* (thorowax root), immature bitter orange and *Panax notoginseng* (notoginseng) (Sun 2001). The use of these herbs may alleviate the patients' tense anxious mood giving rise to a better mental condition going into surgery.

5.5 Role of Herbal Therapy in the Postoperative Phase of Treatment

Cancer surgery is usually accompanied by pain, blood loss and other discomforts. There are also risks of complications including susceptibility to infection, altered homeostasis including intestinal ileus and poor wound healing. Traditional Chinese medicine may offer some solutions to these problems. These are discussed in the following sections.

5.5.1 Reducing Postoperative Intestinal Ileus

While postsurgical ileus is treated with nutrition and supportive treatment in Western centres, TCM offers an extra dimension with a combination of acupuncture and herbal enemas. Acupuncture has been used in combination with rhubarb and mirabilite formulas. The most clearly reported study on using herbal medicine on postsurgical ileus came however from the Japanese (Suehiro et al. 2005). Sixty-six patients who underwent colorectal surgery were studied. Patients who were given 7.5 g of Dai-kenchu-to and 6.0 g of Keishi-bukuryo-gan on the first operative day were compared to control who did not take herbal medicines. Dai-kenchu-to is used in Kampo medicine used by the Japanese and consists of *Zanthoxylum bungeanum* (Sichuan pepper), ginseng and *Saccharum granorum* (malt extract). Keishi-bukuryo-gan consists of *Cinnamomum cassia* (cinnamom twig), *Paeonia lactiflora* (white peony root) and *Prunus persica* (peach seed). Those on the herbal treatment were found to have a faster time to flatus compared to control (63.1 ± 22.8 h vs. 95.4 ± 33.0 h). The time to tolerance of regular diet was also significantly shorter (2.53 ± 1.93 days vs. 6.25 ± 1.50 days). There were similar complications of nausea, vomiting, anastomotic leak and wound infection in both groups.

5.5.2 Reducing Postoperative Adhesion Formation

The role of TCM in reducing postsurgical ileus was then extrapolated to the prevention of post-surgical adhesions. The basis is to increase the motility and thus mobility of the gut at an early stage, preventing the formation of adhesions to paralyzed and immobile bowel. These formulas are mainly rhubarb based. A study compared patients treated with such a formula to control and found that bowel sounds and function returned many hours earlier in treated patients (Su 2000). The incidence of adhesions determined by typical symptoms of adhesions appearing within the next 3 years was also lowered. The adverse effects of using purgatives just hours after surgery were however not reported. Nonetheless, many surgical departments in China do practice this with believe that these formulations also promote circulation of qi and reduce blood stagnation.

5.5.3 Inflammatory Response and Immunity Associated with Surgery

The effect of TCM on the inflammatory response to surgery was studied by Cai et al. (2005) in a prospective, single-blinded, randomized controlled clinical trial on patients who underwent surgery for gastric cancer. Seventeen patients were randomized to the study group while 14 patients were in the control group. Patients in the study group were given rhubarb before operation, and at 1 day and 2 days after operation. Enteral diet (isocaloric and isonitrogenous in both groups) was started 36 hours after operation, and continued for 6 days. They found that patients in both groups had acute inflammatory response, and the indexes of nutritional status decreased after operation. Interleukin (IL)-6, C-reactive protein (CRP) and Tumour necrosis factor-alpha (TNF-α) tested at 3 and 7 days after operation were lower in the study group as compared with those in the control group, and the recovery time of gastrointestinal motility was shorter in the study group as compared with that in the control group (Table 5.2). They concluded that rhubarb can positively modulate the acute inflammatory response, promote the recovery of postoperative gastrointestinal motility, and benefit enteral nutrition support in patients who have undergone major operations.

Liang et al. (2005) studied the effects of early intestinal application of Decoction of Four Noble Drugs (Sijunzi Decoction, SJZD) on the immune function in post-operational patients of gastrointestinal tumour. The main 4 constituents of this decoction are ginseng, *Atractylodes macrocephala* (bighead atractylodes rhizome), *Poria cocos* (tuckahoe) and *Glycyrrhiza uralensis* (licorice root). Ninety-two patients with malignant gastrointestinal tumour were randomized. Patients in both groups were given the isocaloric and isonitrogenous enteral nutritional support starting from the first day after operation for 1 week, but to the tested group, SJZD was given additionally. Serum levels of IL-1, IL-2, IL-6 and TNF-α, the peripheral blood cell counts of total lymphocyte, T-lymphocyte, B-lymphocyte and T-lymphocyte subsets (CD3, CD4, CD8, CD4/CD8) as well as the levels of IgA, IgG, IGM and CRP were measured on the day before operation, the first morning after operation and at the end of study. They found the concentrations of IgA, IgG, 1gM, number of total lymphocyte, CD3, CD4 and CD4/CD8, and serum IL-2 were significantly higher ($P < 0.05$), and levels of IL-6, TNF-α and CRP were significantly lower in the tested group than those in the control group ($P < 0.05$). Liang et al concluded

Table 5.2 Inflammatory markers and gastrointestinal motility in the study by Cai et al. (2005)

	Study group $n = 17$	Control group $n = 14$
3 Days post surgery		
CRP (mg/L)	12.63 ± 7.81	29.62 ± 19.03
TNF-α (ng/L)	53.41 ± 18.97	66.23 ± 15.94
IL-6 (ng/L)	20.08 ± 5.85	26.84 ± 10.67
7 Days post surgery		
CRP (mg/L)	5.14 ± 2.37	17.58 ± 11.62
TNF-α (ng/L)	45.84 ± 17.83	62.45 ± 25.89
IL-6 (ng/L)	15.82 ± 6.44	22.57 ± 8.03
Gastrointestinal motility		
Time to borborygmus (h)	43.2 ± 13.4	56.5 ± 16.8
Time to gas passage (h)	52.6 ± 12.7	80.6 ± 18.2
Time to defaecation (h)	67.4 ± 17.8	87.4 ± 21.5

that the application of SJZD on the base of enteral nutritional therapy can lessen the degree of post-operational stress and inflammatory response, and enhance the immune function of patients.

5.5.4 Reducing Urinary Dysfunction

Urinary dysfunction following rectal surgery is a recognized complication. Careful sharp dissection of the mesorectal plane and preservation of the pelvic nerves are important technical aspects that have improved results. The problem however still remains in some patients. The modality of TCM had been reported to be an effective treatment of urinary dysfunction after rectal surgery. Acupuncture can be used to improve the flow of blood and qi, regulate water flow and invigorate the bladder. Acupuncture after recto-anal surgery had been used with an efficacy reported as high as 94% (Dong and Zhan 2003). However at the moment there is still a lack of standard protocol, inadequate data from different centers and minimal basic research.

5.5.5 Reducing Chronic Pain After Surgery

While modern Western medicine has innovated excellent methods of pain control for acute postoperative pain. However some patients continue to suffer from chronic pain secondary to tissue fibrosis, scarring of muscular tissue and damage to nerve endings. Traditional Chinese medicine also believes that one of the contributing factors to chronic pain after cancer surgery is the persistence of the internal problems associated with cancer even after removal of the cancer. Poor circulation of qi and stagnation of blood then result in the persistent manifestation of pain. Continuing efforts to correct these problems are required to ensure the patient does not have continuing pain. Table 5.3 lists some herbs used for these effects.

Table 5.3 Herbs used to reduce chronic pain after cancer surgery

Mode of action	Herb (Latin name)	Herb (Common name)
Invigorating spleen and tonifying	Glycyrrhiza uralensis	Licorice root
	Astragalus membranaceus	Astragalus root
	Codonopsis pilosula	Dangshen
	Atractylodes macrocephala	Bighead atractylodes rhizome
	Poria cocos	Tuckahoe
Promoting blood circulation and removing blood stasis	*Paeonia lactiflora*	White peony root
	Angelica sinensis	Chinese angelica root
	Corydalis turtschaninovii	Corydalis tuber
	Sparganium stoloniferum	Burreed tuber
	Curcuma zedoaria	Zedoary

5.6 Potential Toxicities

The presence of potential toxicities of TCM is real and is an area of concern for most practitioners of Western medicine. A study from Europe revealed that at least 5% of patients receiving complementary therapy develop side-effects and the actual figure may be higher (Molassiotis et al. 2005). Very often these therapies are used in combination with Western medicines and thus interpretation of the adverse effects may be very difficult. For example, many plant derived herbal medications interact in a major way with the hepatic P_{450} cytochrome system. It is thus difficult to determine whether some adverse effects occurred from direct toxic effects or by interactions with other drugs.

Table 5.4 shows some of the potential side-effects of herbal medicines. These potential toxicities and potential interactions with medicines were reported by Chiu et al. (2009). They suggested developing a system of pharmacological surveillance, licensing and also the setting up of an international TCM toxicology database. Herbal products should be systematically labeled and monitored. These are very important initiatives if the development of TCM usage is to progress.

Table 5.4 Types of toxicity of traditional Chinese medicine

Toxicity	Manifestations
Hepatotoxicity	Transaminitis to fulminant liver failure
	Cholestasis
Nephrotoxicity	Acute tubular necrosis
	Interstitial nephritis
Haemopoietic	Anti-platelet activity
	Anti-coagulation
	Bone marrow suppression
Cardiovascular toxicity	Veno-occlusive disease
	Pulmonary hypertension
	Arrhythmia
Neuropsychiatric toxicity	Hearing impairment
	Neuropsychiatric drug interaction
	Opioid potentiation

5.7 Discussion on Current Evidence of Traditional Chinese Medicine

The practice of TCM is evolved from thousands of years of practical experience and has been valued by those who receive it over the ages. Through this evolution, some paradigms have shifted as well, open surgery was previously prohibited but now has become a focus of combining Western and Eastern methods.

The reasons for skepticism about its effectiveness lie in 4 major problems of the available data on this entity: lack of well designed studies, lack of standardization of treatment regimes, lack of reports of adverse effects and minimal available data in an easily accessible language.

Western medicine has progressed through hypothesis and experimentation with an understanding of the chemistry and biology of various phenomena. The practice of TCM on the other hand has always been considered an art more than a science over the ages with management methods passed down generations from teacher to student. Often some of these methods are considered secrets that should not be shared and thus many do not publish their results. This difference in philosophy has therefore impeded the scientific progress of TCM. It is however very encouraging that TCM is now slowly becoming a science with enthusiastic research now being performed in both Western and Eastern centres. Currently, however, results reported have been based on case series of a relatively small numbers of patients. Comparative studies available are also relatively small and the results reported lack properly defined outcome measures and end-points giving rise to questions on their reliability and validity.

The other problem with the current information on TCM is the lack of standardization of treatment regimes and combinations. The basic premise for treatment of the various aspects of cancer may be similar; for example some herbs are used for getting rid of toxins and some herbs are used for regulating qi; however there is a wide variation in prescription even for the same condition. Available literature has described innumerous permutations and combinations of the herbs at different doses with many claiming that their concoction gives rise to good results. These reported concoctions than beg the questions of whether each ingredient in the concoctions plays an important role or is it one or two of the ingredients that are the active ones? Are the effects of the ingredients additive in nature or is there a desirable interaction of the ingredients that gives rise to the required results. Unfortunately, there are inadequate well conducted basic and clinical studies that can answer these questions at the current moment. The rationales behind the use of the ingredients are sometimes abstract and physicians may differ in their opinion on their usage. In order to make these studies more reliable there is a need for consensus meetings among TCM physicians so that concepts and treatment regimes can be more standardized. These however have to be preceded by good basic and molecular translational research that is still lacking in the field of TCM. As such biological explanations to observed phenomena are often not available. To this end the expertise of Western trained physicians will be of tremendous help.

Reporting of exciting new therapeutic modalities have to go hand in hand with the reporting of potential adverse effects. Western medicine has developed strict criteria of reporting adverse events especially in prospective studies. Many studies on TCM however do not report any adverse effects in the series presented, nor are there clearly defined adverse effects for TCM. Similarly, there are seldomly reported about how adverse events are monitored. Combination with Western methods also seldom explores potential adverse interactions between the two. As such, this knowledge void makes it difficult for a Western practitioner to recommend TCM in the interest of not causing harm to the patient.

Professor RJ Nicholls, in a commentary of TCM emphasized the cultural scientific gulf between the Western system of medicine and TCM (Tan et al. 2008). The reason being that there has been no means of easy communication throughout history and believes that in reality the work by the Chinese will continue to be inaccessible due to the language problem. There is however, a growing number of Western physicians that are fluent in both English and Chinese and these physicians have to take the lead in bridging the East-West divide and promote cooperation.

5.8 Future Directions

While it is very easy for practitioners of Western medicine to be skeptical about TCM, we urge them to keep an open mind. The current enthusiasm in TCM in combination with Western practices has never been stronger before. There are an increasing number of studies and publications in these areas.

The main foci of these studies should be on the biological and molecular basis of TCM and these should then be translated to well-designed clinical trials with proper reporting of adverse events. Only through this can more light be cast on this ancient art with innumerous anecdotal good results. The most promising areas will be the areas where Western medicine continues to have inadequate solutions like the side-effects of surgery and medical treatment of cancer and also advanced cancers.

There is no better time for strong cooperation between practitioners of Western and Eastern medicine and doctors who are well versed in both the languages should take the lead in advancing this amalgamation.

Acknowledgements We thank Alexandra Hospital Nurse Clinician Phyllis Tan for her contribution towards the research for this chapter. Her input was valuable to the completion of the work.

References

Cai J, Xuan ZR, Wei YP et al. Effects of perioperative administration of rhubarb on acute inflammatory response in patients with gastric cancer. Zhong Xi Yi Jie He Xue Bao. 2005;3:195–8.

Chiu J, Yau T, Epstein RJ et al. Complications of traditional Chinese/herbal medicines (TCM)-a guide for perplexed oncologists and other cancer caregivers. Support Care Cancer. 2009;17:231–40.

Cho WC, Chen HY. Clinical efficacy of traditional Chinese medicine as a concomitant therapy for nasopharyngeal carcinoma: a systematic review and meta-analysis. Cancer Invest. 2009;27:334–44.

Dong WH, Zhan LY et al. The aetiology and management of acute urinary retention after rectal surgery. Xian Dai Zhong Xi Yi Jie He Zha Zhi. 2003;12:2082–3.

He YH. General survey of traditional Chinese medicine and Western medicine researches on tumor metastasis. Chin J Integr Med. 2006;12:75–80.

Hsu YL, Kuo PL, Tzeng TF et al. Huang-lian-Jie-du-Tang, a traditional Chinese medicine prescription, induces cell-cycle arrest and apoptosis in human liver cancer cells in vitro and in vivo. J Gastroenterol Hepatol. 2008;23:e290–e9.

Huangdi's Internal Classic (Huangdi Neijing).
Konkimalla VB, Efferth T. Evidence-based Chinese medicine for cancer therapy. J Ethnopharmacol. 2008;116:207–10.
Lee RT, Hlubocky FJ, Hu JJ et al. An international pilot study of oncology physicians' opinions and practices on Complementary and Alternative Medicine (CAM).. Integr Cancer Ther. 2008;7:70–75.
Liang C, Zhang SH, Cai ZD. Effects of early intestinal application of Sijunzi Decoction on immune function in post-operational patients of gastrointestinal tumor. Zhongguo Zhong Xi Yi Jie He Za Zhi. 2005;25:1070–3.
Liu W, Xu K. Clinical treatment of cancer with Chinese medicine. Beijing, China: Renming Weisheng Chubanshe; 2000.
Molassiotis A, Fernendez-Ortega P, Pud D et al. Use of complementary and alternative medicine in cancer patients: a European survey. Ann Oncol. 2005;16:655–63.
Ng TP, Tan CH, Kua EH et al. The use of Chinese herbal medicines and their correlates in Chinese older adults: the Singapore Chinese Longitudinal Aging Study. Age Ageing. 2004;33:135–42.
Peng B. Chinese medicine as intervention for acute cancerous colon obstruction. Beijing Zhong Yi. 2003;22:25.
Su F. Clinical observation of Taozhi Zhipo Fang used for preventing intestinal adhesion after surgical operation. Chin J Surg Integr Tradit Chin Med West Med. 2000;6:404–5.
Suehiro T, Matsumata T, Shikada Y et al. The effect of the herbal medicines Dai-kenchu-to and Keishi-bukuryo-gan on bowel movement after colorectal surgery. Hepatogastroenterology. 2005;52:97–100.
Sun Y. Cancer study. Beijing, China: Renming Weisheng Chubanshe; 2001.
Tan KY, Liu CB, Chen AH et al. The role of traditional Chinese medicine in colorectal cancer treatment. Tech Coloproctol. 2008;12:1–6.
Zhou YL. Colon cancer and acute intestinal obstruction. Treatment of 30 patients with Chinese medicine. Fujian Med J. 2004;26:158.
Zhou QM, Su SB. Review on experimental research of Chinese herbal medicine intervention for breast cancer. Zhongguo Zhong Yao Za Zhi. 2007;32:1947–50.

Chapter 6
Increasing Therapeutic Gain and Controlling Radiation-Induced Injuries with Asian Botanicals and Acupuncture

Stephen M. Sagar and Raimond K. Wong

Abstract Therapeutic gain by radiotherapy can be achieved through improved targeting, selectively sensitizing malignant cells, or protecting normal tissue. The majority of synthetic chemical radiation sensitizers and normal tissue protectors have proved too toxic at effective clinical doses. Asian botanicals (both from Chinese and Ayurvedic medicine) are being evaluated for their ability to improve therapeutic gain through various avenues that include the modulation of reactive oxygen species, increase in immunity, anti-inflammation, and anti-angiogenesis, as well as other molecular avenues. An increase in the efficacy of radiotherapy on tumour tissue allows a reduction in the applied dose to normal tissues. In addition, some botanicals can increase normal tissue repair following radiation therapy, and selective acupuncture may help in normal tissue cell repopulation.

6.1 Introduction

The concept of therapeutic gain in radiation oncology is to increase the degree of tumour damage whilst minimizing the acute and chronic damage to surrounding normal tissues. This is primarily achieved by physical techniques that target the tumour and restrict the dose to defined normal tissues. Outcome has improved since the development of high energy radiation, inverse planning systems, intensity modulated radiotherapy, and image guided radiotherapy applications. Localizing techniques and fractionated radiotherapy (which allow radiation damage repair and repopulation of new cells) have considerably improved the therapeutic gain. Fractionation also allows reoxygenation and can induce cell cycle synchronization, both of which can be further enhanced by sensitizers. The potential to improve

S.M. Sagar (✉)
Radiation Oncology, Juravinski Cancer Centre, Hamilton, ON, Canada
e-mail: stephen.sagar@jcc.hhsc.ca

W.C.S. Cho (ed.), *Supportive Cancer Care with Chinese Medicine*,
DOI 10.1007/978-90-481-3555-4_6, © Springer Science+Business Media B.V. 2010

therapeutic gain may be achieved through the development of selective radiosensitizers and protectors. The pharmacological properties of these compounds can enable them to be differentially distributed or activated between tumour and normal tissues and to have selective metabolic effects. Because of their toxicity, very few of the chemical compounds have established clinical indications. The most promising radioprotectors have been the sulfhydryls. Over 5,000 compounds were synthesized and screened by the Walter Reed Army Institute after World War II (Weiss and Simic 1988; Coleman et al. 2003). Only amifostine (WR-2721 or S-2-(3-aminopropyl-amino) ethyl phosphorothioic acid), a sulfhydryl pro-drug with reduced activation by malignant tissue, has been approved by the FDA for bone marrow and salivary gland protection, and it has some unacceptable toxicity too (Capizzi and Oster 1995).

Ionizing radiation is electromagnetic radiation that possesses sufficient energy to induce ionization. Low linear energy transfer (LET) radiation, such as x-irradiation, is sparsely ionizing and results in the formation of reactive oxygen species (ROS) and reactive nitrogen species (RNS) that can damage biological molecules that include DNA, lipids and proteins. This process enables opportunities for therapeutic gain by quenching these free radicals in normal tissues, and enhancing their effects in malignant tissue. Radiomodulators are agents that modify the radiation response and include both synthetic chemicals and compounds derived from botanicals. Radiosensitizers are compounds that when combined with radiation will achieve greater tumour inactivation than would have been expected from the additive effect of each modality (Urtasun 1998). They can also be defined as agents that do not have a therapeutic effect of their own, but act to enhance the therapeutic effect of radiation (Bump et al. 2003). Most synthetic radiosensitizers have proved too toxic to be used at effective clinical doses. Recent developments have focused on treatment with irradiation combined with chemotherapy drugs and targeted antibody or tyrosine kinase antagonists, an effective strategy that is often simply additive and does not necessarily spare normal tissues. Radioprotectors are compounds that protect against radiation damage to targeted normal cells, but do not provide similar protection to tumour cells (Urtasun 1998). Normally only agents administered pre-irradiation are considered radioprotectors. Those that are administered after irradiation to reduce toxicity are termed radiorecovery agents. Mitigators are agents that are administered both during and after irradiation, but before manifestation of radiation injury, whereas a radiation therapeutic is an agent administered after the emergence of clinical symptoms (Stone et al. 2004). The measurement of radiation damage can be through chemical, genetic, and biological assays that measure glutathione (GSH), glutathione-S-transferase (GST), glutathione peroxidase (GSHpx), superoxide dismutase (SOD), micronuclei, chromatid breaks, clastogenic factors (lipid peroxides), surviving cell colony forming units (CFU) of gastrointestinal epithelium (GI), bone marrow (MB), human peripheral blood lymphocytes (HPBLs), as well as symptoms of radiation sickness and death rates in animal studies. Evaluating relative damage between tumour and normal tissues in animal studies can follow these screening assays.

More recently, new avenues have been explored to improve therapeutic gain from radiotherapy. One approach is to use anti-angiogenic agents to improve tumour re-oxygenation without increasing normal tissue toxicity. Many botanicals display anti-angiogenic, as well as other multi-targeted effects that can reverse radiation-induced hypoxic factor and prevent metastases (Yance and Sagar 2006). New evidence suggests that radiation may expose tumour antigen and, together with immune-enhancing adjuvants, can function as a vaccine. Many Asian herbs display immune-enhancing activities (Sagar and Wong 2008) and could result in both a beneficial local as well as an abscopal effect when combined with radiotherapy (Demaria and Formenti 2007).

Unfortunately, our methodology for evaluating therapeutic gain in humans with cancer is limited, but new functional imaging techniques using SPECT and PET nuclear medicine scans or nuclear magnetic resonance (NMR) are promising. Minimal research has been done with botanicals (herb or plant-derived products) despite the fact that some manifest interesting radiosensitizing and radioprotecting properties when evaluated in the laboratory. Since both Chinese and Ayurvedic herbs have a common source and similar roots in traditional medicine, we will discuss preclinical properties of these compounds under the title of Asian herbs or botanicals. We will use their Western botanical categorization and describe their potential therapeutic use from a Western medicine approach, rather than through the challenging complexities of traditional medicine. We refer the reader to the original referenced reports for the details such as species categorization, plant parts, source, specific extracts, and exact assay methodology. These details can fundamentally change experimental and therapeutic outcome. Not surprisingly, there are very few quality randomized clinical trials using these botanicals or their derivatives. Although we can postulate possibilities from traditional experience, clearly they have not been utilized in the context of modern radiotherapy and chemotherapy until very recently. The challenge for utilizing Asian botanicals in Western oncology is to utilize quality assured products, verified by both chemical spectrographs (fingerprints) and biological assays, determine the advantages of single agent extraction *versus* complex mixtures, and to direct the promising agents though appropriate preclinical efficacy and toxicity studies, prior to phase I–III clinical trials. Since acupuncture is a fundamental part of Chinese medicine and there is emerging data for its ability to induce growth factors, we will complete this chapter with a short discussion of the potential role of acupuncture in stimulating neuro-chemicals and peptides that enhance the repopulation of normal tissue from progenitor and multipotent stem cells.

6.2 Botanical Radiosensitizers and Radioprotectors that Modulate Reactive Oxygen Intermediates (ROI's) and Associated Genes

Potential botanical radiosensitizers are listed in Table 6.1 and radioprotectors are listed in Table 6.2 (Arora et al. 2005; Garg et al. 2005; Jagetia 2007; Arora 2008). However, the differentiation between sensitizing and protecting may be dependent on administered dose, tissue type, local environmental factors (e.g. oxygenation status, pH, antioxidant to pro-oxidant ratio, etc), and fractionation of x-irradiation.

Table 6.1 Potential botanical radiosensitizers

Botanical name (Index constituent)	Potential mechanism	References
Alstonia scholaris (blackboard tree)	Decrease in glutathione	Jagetia and Baliga (2003a)
Azadirachta indica (neem)	Interacts with residual damage converting sub-lethal/ potentially-lethal damage into lethal damage; Inhibits double-strand break repair	Kumar et al. (2002)
Caffeine (caffeic acid or CAPE)	Depletes intracellular thiols; Inhibits NF-κB; Releases radiation-induced G2 block	Higuchi et al. (2000); Valenzuela et al. (2000); Chen et al. (2005)
Camptotheca acuminata (happy tree) (9-amino-camptothecin, 9-nitro-camptothecin)	Prevents topoisomerase 1 repair of DNA	Chen et al. 1997; Tamura et al. (1997); Kirichenko and Rich (1999); Sung et al. (2005)
Curcuma longa (common turmeric)	Potentiation of radiation-induced chromosome aberrations; Down-regulation of radiation-induced prosurvival factors	Araujo et al. (1999); Deeb et al. (2003)
Diospyros montana (diospyrin)	Regulates gene expression involved in cell cycle and apoptosis	Kumar et al. (2007)
Flavone derivatives (flavopyridol)	Inhibits cycline dependent kinases	Jung et al. (2003)
Glycine max (soya bean, genistein)	Down-regulation of apurinic/apyrimidinic endonuclease 1/redox factor 1 expression	Raffoul et al. (2007)
Gossypium (gossypol)	Inhibits DNA double-strand break repair	Xu et al. (2005); Kasten-Pisula et al. (2007)
Hypericum perforatum (St John's wort)	Inhibits protein kinase C	Zhang et al. (1996); Wessells et al. (2007)
Legumes (L-canavanine)	Preferentially sensitizes tumour at non-cytotoxic doses by altering pre-irradiation cell cycling	Bence et al. (2003)

Table 6.1 (continued)

Botanical name (Index constituent)	Potential mechanism	References
Nerium oleander (oleandrin)	Caspase-3 dependent apoptosis	Nasu et al. (2002)
Rabdosia rubescens (blushred rabdosia)	Supra-additive radiosensitization combined with misonidazole; More in hypoxic cells	Murayama et al. (1987)
Salvia miltiorrhiza (red sage root) (Tanshinone IIA)	Increased apoptosis and G2/M arrest	Dong et al. (2006)
Panax notoginseng (notoginseng) (Rb1)	Differential sensitization of tumour over normal tissue	Chen et al. (2001)
Tanacetum parthenium (parthenolide)	Inhibition of NF-κB pathway	Sun et al. (2007)
Taxus baccata (taxol)	Cell cycle arrest in most radiosensitive phase G2/M	–
Terminalia chebula (medicine terminalia fruit) (Ellagic acid)	Enhances radiation-mediated oxidative stress by decreasing antioxidant enzymes, e.g. SOD	Bhosle et al. (2005)
Tinospora cordifolia (berberine)	Decrease in cell glutathione	Rao et al. (2008)
Vitis vinifera (common grape vine) (resveratrol)	Down-regulates NF-κB and COX-2; Induces early S-phase cell-cycle checkpoint arrest	Subbaramaiah et al. (1998); Manna et al. (2000); Zoberi et al. (2002)
Withania somnifera (withaferin A)	Inhibits DNA repair; Cell cycle arrest; Reduces glutathione levels; Enhances apoptosis	Uma Devi (1996); Uma Devi et al. (2008) Kamath et al. (1999); Guruprasad (2009)

Table 6.2 Potential botanical radioprotectors

Botanical name (Index constituent)	Potential mechanism	References
Acanthopanax senticosus (Siberian ginseng)	Hematological, survival, and brain hemorrhage in mouse model	Yonezawa et al. (1989)
Aegle marmelos (bael)	HPBLs: reduce micronuclei and ROIs; Reduce radiation sickness, GI, BM deaths, lipid peroxidation, GSH, CFU; Increase villus height, crypt and goblet cells, in mouse model	Jagetia et al. 2003a, 2004a, b); Jagetia and Ventakesh (2005)
Ageratum conyzoides (billygoat-weed)	Radiation sickness, GI and BM deaths in mouse model	Jagetia et al. (2003b)
Aloe vera (aloes)	Scavenging hydroxyl radicals, SOD and glutathione peroxidase in mouse model	Sato (1990)
Amaranthus paniculatus (amaranth)	Survival, CFU, spleen weight, lipid peroxidation, GSH, in mouse model	Krishna and Kumar (2005)
Angelica sinensis (Chinese angelica root) (Polysaccharide: ferulic acid)	Survival and hematological in mouse model	Mei (1988); Mei et al. (1991)
Aphanamixis polystachya (meliaceae)	Aberrant nuclei, chromatid breaks, dicentrics, other aberrations in mouse model	Jagetia and Venkatesh (2006)
Archangelica officinalis (angelica)	Survival in mouse model	Narimanov (1993)
Centella asiatica (gotu kola)	Weight loss, taste aversion in rodent model	Shobi and Goel (2001); Sharma and Sharma (2002)
Curcuma longa (common turmeric)	Glyoxalase levels	Chaudhary et al. (1999)
Emblica officinalis (Indian gooseberry)	Survival, weight loss in mice model	Singh et al. (2005)
Ginkgo biloba (ginkgo seed)	Brain edema, clastogens, in humans	Hannequin et al. (1986); Emerit et al. 1995a, b)

Table 6.2 (continued)

Botanical name (Index constituent)	Potential mechanism	References
Glycyrrhiza uralensis (licorice root)	Lipid peroxidation microsomes, DNA strand breaks	Shetty et al. (2002)
Hippophae rhamnoides (sea buckthorn)	Increases survival in rats	Mizina and Sitnikova (1999)
Lycium barbarum (wolfberry fruit)	Hematological recovery in mouse model	Hsu et al. (1999)
Mentha haplocalyx (wild mint herb)	Radiation sickness, GI and BM deaths in mouse model	Jagetia and Baliga (2002)
Mentha piperita (peppermint)	BM, CFU, spleen weight, GI goblet cells/villus height, chromosomal damage, in mouse	Samarth et al. 2001, 2002); Samarth and Kumar (2003)
Moringa oleifera	Reduces % aberrant cells in metaphase chromosomes in mouse model	Rao et al. (2001)
Ocimum sanctum (holy basil)	Survival, CFU, chromosome damage, lipid peroxidation, glutathione, in mouse model	Uma Devi and Ganasoundari (1995); Ganasoundari et al. (1997)
Panax ginseng (ginseng) and *Panax quinquefolium* (American ginseng)	Survival, CFU, apoptosis, in mouse model; human lymphocytes, micronuclei assay	Takeda et al. (1982); Yonezawa et al. (1985); Zhang et al. (1987); Pande et al. (1998); Kim et al. 1993, 2001); Kumar et al. (2003); Lee et al. (2008)
Phyllanthus amarus	Hematological, ROI's (CAT, SOD, GST, GPx), chromosome aberrations, in mouse model	Kumar and Kuttan (2004)
Piper longum	Hematological, glutathione pyruvate transaminase, alkaline phosphatase, lipid peroxidation in mouse model	Sunila and Kuttan (2005)
Podophyllum hexandrum	GST, SOD, survival, BM and plasmid protection, apoptosis, in mouse model	Mittal et al. (2001); Sajikumar and Goel (2003); Kumar et al. 2005a, b) Chawla et al. (2006); Sagar et al. (2006); Goel et al. (2007); Lata et al. (2009)

Table 6.2 (continued)

Botanical name (Index constituent)	Potential mechanism	References
Salvia miltiorrhiza (red sage root) (Tanshinone IIA)	Antioxidant, protecting against lipid peroxidants; protects cochlea in guinea pig model	Yang et al. (1999)
Syzigium cumini	HPBLs micronuclei model	Jagetia and Baliga (2003b)
Tephrosia purpurea	Hemopoietic protection in mouse model	Taraphdar et al. (2002)
Tinospora cordifolia	Survival, CFU, hematological in mouse model	Pahadiya and Sharma (2003); Goel et al. (2004)
Zingiber officinale (ginger)	Protection of GI, BM; Reduction ROIs, GSH lipid peroxidation, in mouse model	Jagetia et al. 2003, 2004)

How do these botanicals interact with radiotherapy? Molecular biology research has shown that radiotherapy induces gene expression of NF-κB and tumour necrosis factor (TNF) (Jung and Dritschilo 2001). These are potent inducers of both pro-apoptotic and pro-survival pathways that contribute to both tumour cell death and to the development of resistance. The induction results from the generation of ROI's (Garg and Aggarwal 2002). In turn, NF-κB and TNF alter the membrane permeability of mitochondria, leading to cytochrome c release and caspase activation, resulting in apoptosis. In contrast, NF-κB also mediates prosurvival signaling (Garg et al. 2005) through regulation of genes involved in cellular survival (Bcl-2, COX-2, inhibitor of apoptosis protein or IAP, and superoxide dismutase). This polar effect is not clearly understood but may depend on other molecular and physiological conditions that differ between the tumour and normal tissue. A differential enhancement of the shift by administration of botanicals could result in increased cell survival in normal tissue (resistance to radiotherapy) compared to increased sensitivity in the tumour (sensitization to radiotherapy) (Fig. 6.1).

The final degree of damage between tumour and normal tissue depends on many complex variables (Camphausen et al. 2005). Approximately two thirds of DNA damage is caused by short-lived (nanoseconds to microseconds) high-energy primary and secondary free radicals. Most will be quenched rapidly outside of the high dose target. To act as a radioprotector by scavenging these free radicals, an antioxidant botanical or vitamin needs to be present in sufficient concentrations and have efficient radical scavenging capabilities in proximity to the target (DNA) during the radiation exposure. The free radical generation in tissues may continue after the radiation exposure as a consequence of an inflammatory response, with the generation of cytokines and sustained production of longer lived free radicals

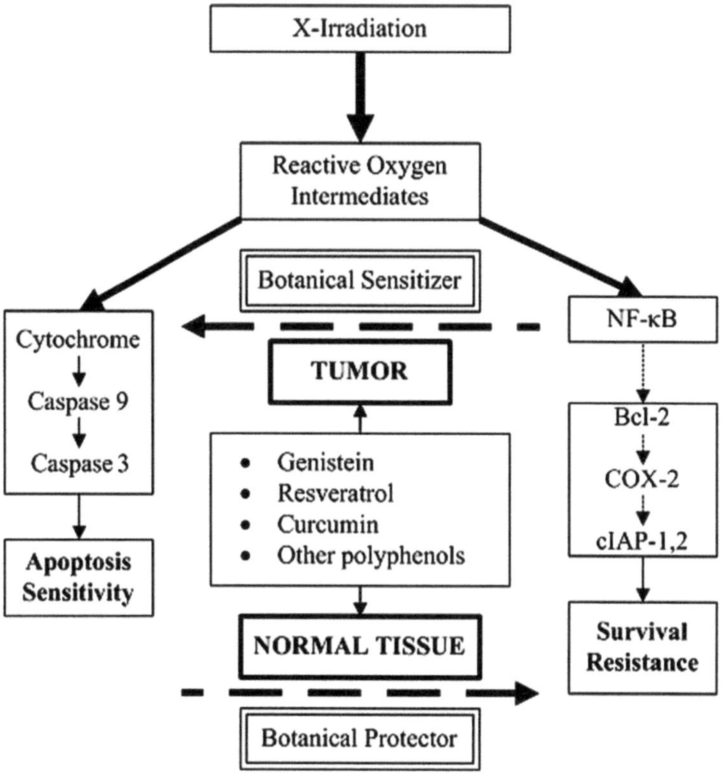

Fig. 6.1 Potential role of botanicals to improve therapeutic gain in tumour compared to normal tissue via differential polar outcomes from pro-apoptotic compared to anti-apoptotic signaling induced by radiation-generated reactive oxygen intermediates (ROI)

(Robbins and Zhao 2004). In this setting, particularly in normal tissues, antioxidant botanicals could be quite effective in protecting against sustained free-radical damage. As previously mentioned, free radicals can also serve as initiators for complex signal transduction and gene expression pathways governing pro- and anti-survival responses. Whether there is a differential inflammatory response in tumours is less clear, given their markedly different redox status. The situation of administering an antioxidant agent is further complicated by the level attained by the agent in the surrounding environment, and the effect it can have on altering the antioxidant effects of many molecules. For example, β-carotene is an antioxidant at low oxygen concentrations, but it acts as a pro-oxidant at high oxygen concentrations (Cook et al. 2004). The lack of reliable methods to predict the relative responses to irradiation of the tumour compared to normal tissue, in the presence of antioxidants, has led to caution in the administration of these agents until we have derived scientific methods to evaluate and predict response (Sagar et al. 2005; Lawenda et al. 2008).

Some interesting avenues are being explored to correlate oncogene activity and ROI generation, as well as the differential responses of tumour and normal tissue to antioxidants. There is a significant positive correlation between COX-2 expression and catalase activity in normal tissue and an inverse trend between p53 expression and superoxide dismutase and catalase activity in tumour tissue. In addition, patients with over expressed p53 protein levels have lower glutathione peroxidase enzyme levels in normal tissues and the converse in tumour tissue (Kaur et al. 2008). Administration of manganese superoxide dismutase-plasmid liposomes (MnSOD-PL) provides radiation protection mediated by MnSOD stabilization of the antioxidant pool including glutathione and total thiols in normal tissues. Animal experiments with orthotopic squamous cell tumours demonstrated paradoxical and beneficial tumour radiosensitization following intratracheal or intraoral MnSOD-PL, respectively. The mechanism of MnSOD-PL tumour radiosensitization may involve a difference in redox balance between tumours and normal tissues. Differences in handling radiation-induced oxidative stress between tumours and normal tissues can provide a fundamental basis to design new cancer therapeutic agents that can exploit differences between normal tissue and tumour mechanisms of handling the oxidative stress of ionizing radiation damage (Greenberger and Epperly 2007).

Agents that activate or support the antioxidant systems could enhance both tumour cell death and protect normal tissues. Clinical evaluation of this postulate is quite limited, mainly because of the fear that the efficacy of standard therapy would be reduced. Although we must be cautious, so far any adverse effect on tumour control has been in smokers in whom antioxidants seem to develop pro-oxidant characteristics that leave this unique population susceptible to second primary tumours (α-Tocopherol, β-Carotene Cancer Prevention Study Group 1994; Meyer et al. 2007). Treatment with antioxidant botanicals as an adjuvant therapy added to radiotherapy could protect the normal tissues against radiation-induced side effects, whereas other properties can increase tumour cell kill, either through conversion to pro-oxidant properties or via multiple targeting interactions with cell signaling pathways and modulation of genomic expression. Optimization of complex chemical mixtures would be a novel approach compared to the standard of isolating a single index chemical for therapy. Various cellular defense mechanisms such as the antioxidant vitamins and enzyme systems are normally induced in response to excessive ROIs, but they become overburdened during radiotherapy, potentially increasing late toxicity and suppressing mechanisms (such as the immune system) that reduce the spread of malignant cells. Some preliminary clinical studies with the Asian herbs, Naturin (Shen et al. 1996) and Vitexina (Hien et al. 2002) provide some limited support for reduced toxicity.

6.3 Antiangiogenic Botanicals

Botanicals that have a high degree of anti-angiogenic activity also display many other interactions that can inhibit tumour progression and reduce the risk of metastasis. They target various molecular pathways besides angiogenesis, including epidermal growth factor receptor (EGFR), the *HER-2/neu* gene, the COX-2 enzyme, the NF-κB transcription factor, the protein kinases, Bcl-2 protein and coagulation pathways. The following Asian herbs are traditionally used for anticancer treatment and are anti-angiogenic through multiple interdependent processes that include effects on gene expression, signal processing and enzyme activities: *Artemisia annua* (sweet wormwood herb), *Viscum album* (European mistletoe), *Curcuma longa* (common turmeric), *Scutellaria baicalensis* (baikal skullcap root), resveratrol and proanthocyanidin grape seed extract from *Vitis vinifera* (common grape vine), *Magnolia officinalis* (magnolia bark), *Camellia sinensis* (green tea), *Ginkgo biloba* (ginkgo seed), quercetin, *Poria cocus* (tuckahoe), *Zingiber officinale* (ginger), *Panax ginseng* (ginseng), *Rabdosia rubescens* (blushred rabdosia) and Chinese destagnation herbs. Asian botanicals with anti-angiogenic activity are listed in Table 6.3.

Some herbs and their derivatives that specifically inhibit VEGF and have direct activity against angiogenesis are listed below (Yance and Sagar 2006).

Table 6.3 Asian botanicals with potential direct and indirect antiangiogenic activity

Botanical name	References
Angelica sinensis (Chinese angelica root) (aqueous extracts)	Xu et al. (1989)
Artemisia annua (sweet wormwood herb) (artemisinin)	Chen et al. (2004a)
Camellia sinensis (green tea) (epigallocatechin)	Cao and Cao (1999); Pisters et al. (2001); Sartippour et al. (2002); Kojima-Yuasa et al. (2003); Tang et al. (2003); Fassina et al. (2004)
Chrysobalanus icaco (methanol extract)	Alves De Paulo and Teruszkin Balassiano (2000)
Curcuma longa (common turmeric)	Sreejayan (1997); Arbiser et al. (1998); Garcia-Cardena and Folkman (1998); Dorai et al. (2001); Gururaj et al. (2002); John et al. (2002); Kim et al. (2002); Shim et al. (2003); Chen et al. (2004c); Hahm et al. (2004)
Dysoxylum binectariferum (flavopiridol)	Melillo et al. (1999); Mohamed et al. (1999)
Magnolia biondii (magnolia flower) (magnosalin)	Bai et al. (2003); Chen et al. (2004b)
Ganoderma lucidum (lucid ganoderma) (triterpenoids)	Cao and Lin (2004); Stanley et al. (2005)

Table 6.3 (continued)

Botanical name	References
Ginkgo biloba (ginkgo seed) (ginkgolide B)	Zhang et al. (2002); Koltermann et al. (2008)
Glycyrrhiza uralensis (licorice root) (isoliquiritigenin, glabridin)	Sheela et al. (2006)
Hibiscus sabdariffa (roselle) (protocatechuic acid)	Huang et al. (2009)
Livistona chinensis (aqueous extract from seed)	Sartippour et al. (2001); Wang et al. (2008)
Matricaria chamomilla (flavonoids: apigenin, fisetin)	Liu et al. (2005); Fang et al. (2007)
Ocimum sanctum (carnosol, ursolic acid)	Das et al. (2005); Manikandan et al. (2007)
Magnolia obovata (honokiol)	Bai et al. (2003); Tse et al. (2005); Hahm et al. (2008); Li et al. (2009)
Panax ginseng (ginseng) (saponins: 20(R)- and 20(S)-ginsenoside-Rg3)	Sato et al. (1994); Sengupta et al. (2004); Xu et al. (2007)
Polypodium leucotomos (difur)	Gonzalez et al. (2000)
Polygonum cuspidatum (giant knotwood rhizome) (resveratrol)	Kimura and Okuda (2001)
Poria cocos (tuckahoe) (1-3-α-D-glucan)	Mizushina et al. (2005)
Rabdosia rubescens (blushred rabdosia) (ponicidin and oridonin)	Sartippour et al. (2005)
Rosmarinus officinalis (carnosol and ursolic acid)	Sohn et al. (1995); Cardenas et al. (2004)
Scutellaria baicalensis (baikal skullcap root) (baicalin and baicalein)	Liu et al. (2003); Wang et al. (2004)
Silybum marianum (milk thistle) (silymarin)	Jiang et al. (2000); Yang et al. (2003)
Tanacetum parthenium (parthenolide)	Curry et al. (2004); Kong et al. (2008)
Tabebuia avellanedae (β-lapachone)	Kung et al. (2007)
Taxus breviflora (taxoids)	Lau et al. (1999)
Viscum album (European mistletoe) (lectins)	Yoon et al. (1995)
Zingiber officinale (ginger) (6-gingerol)	Brown et al. (2009)

- Sweet wormwood herb
  [contains 95% Artemisinin, and other related terpenes and flavonoids]
- European mistletoe
  [contains mistletoe lectin III (ML3A)]
- Common turmeric
  [contains 95% Curcumin]
- Green tea
  [contains 95% phenols; 50% Epigallocatechin (EGCG)]
- Common grape vine
  [contains 95% proanthocyanidins]
- *Angelica sinensis* (Chinese angelica root)
  [contains 4-hydroxyderricin]
- *Taxus breviflora* (Pacific yew)
  [contains taxol]
- Baikal skullcap root
  [Contains 95% baicalin and flavonoids]
- *Polygonum cuspidatum* (giant knotwood rhizome)
  [contains 20% Resveratrol]
- *Silybum marianum* (milk thistle)
  [contains 80% Silymarin (Silibin)]
- Magnolia bark
  [contains 90% Honokiol]
- Ginger
  [contains 6-Gingerol]

Anti-angiogenic therapies may be combined with radiotherapy to improve local tumour control and to reduce the risk of metastases. During a course of radiotherapy, some tumours increase their angiogenic activity (Ansiaux et al. 2005). Radiation therapy in the form of x-rays is more effective at destroying tumour cells in tissue that reoxygenates well between fractions of treatment. Oxygen is necessary to generate ROIs. Tumours can become hypoxic from the poorly organized and chaotic vessels formed when the vascular endothelial growth factor (VEGF) to angiopoietin ratio is high. Combined-modality therapies with anti-angiogenic agents induce a normal microvascular bed out of the disorganized tumour vessels. There is a critical time during the anti-angiogenic treatment when the VEGF to angiopoietin ratio becomes balanced. At that point, pericytes are recruited, the vascular basement membrane adopts a thinner morphology and tumour oxygenation temporarily increases. This is a favorable time to apply ionizing radiation, since it is preferentially lethal to replicating and well-oxygenated cells. The combination of an anti-angiogenic agent and radiation therapy is optimally effective if this window of opportunity is exploited to increase local control and reduce the induction of metastases, without increasing normal tissue toxicity (Ergun et al. 2003; Koukourakis et al. 2001; Ma et al. 2003).

Various assays are used to screen botanicals for anti-angiogenic activity (Kruger et al. 2001; Miller et al. 2001). The assays used for screening include in vitro assays

Table 6.4 Anti-angiogenesis activity of Chinese medicinal herbal extracts (exhibiting more than 20% inhibition at 0.2 g herb/ml) (Wang et al. 2004)

Name	Used part	% Inhibition (CAM)	% Inhibition (BAEC)
Berberis paraspecta	Root	25	38
Catharanthus roseus	Leaf	27	30
Coptis chinensis (coptis root)	Rhizome	25	37
Scrophularia ningpoonsis (figwort root)	Root	20	34
Scutellaria baicalensis (baikal skullcap root)	Root	27	41
Polygonum cuspidatum (giant knotwood rhizome)	Whole plant	–	28
Taxus chinensis	Bark	–	26

Assays: chick embryo chorioallantoic membrane (CAM) and bovine aortic endothelial cells (BAEC) culture models

that are usually based on the use of endothelial cells (bovine aortic or human umbilical), such as the BAEC model, and the in vivo assays such as the chick embryo chorioallantoic membrane (CAM) model. Table 6.4 shows the results from Wang et al. (2004), which demonstrate quite clearly the potential for baikal skullcap root and other botanicals to be potential therapeutic agents.

In Chinese medicine, destagnation herbs are traditionally thought to overcome the blockage of qi and blood. Laboratory evidence now suggests that they may have anti-angiogenic and anti-coagulation properties (Huang et al. 2003; Samuels 2005). A randomized placebo-controlled trial from China showed that the addition of destagnation herbs, including *Salvia miltiorrhiza* (red sage root) and Chinese angelica root, to radiotherapy doubled both the local control and survival rates of patients with nasopharyngeal cancer (Xu et al. 1989). This sensitization to radiotherapy appears secondary to their anti-angiogenic activity, although other effects cannot be discounted.

6.4 Immunogenic Botanicals

Tumours inhibit the immune system, by suppressing the activation of anti-tumour T-cells and their differentiation into cytolytic T-cells (CTLs) that can recognize tumour antigen. Defective priming results from defective differentiation and maturation of antigen presenting cells (APCs) termed dendritic cells (DCs). Myeloid suppressor cells accumulate as a result of pathological cytokine production by the tumour. In addition to antigen, DCs require danger signals to induce maturation. Danger signals include pro-inflammatory cytokines that can be activated by interactions with toll like receptors (TLRs) on monocytes, such as DCs, and inflammatory agents such as radiotherapy. TLRs evolved to interact with the polysaccharides found in the walls of bacteria and are an essential part of developing and maintaining a competent immune system (Heine et al. 2005). The mature DC up-regulates the CD40 receptor to activate T-cells. Tumours can inhibit this process through gene activation that generates interleukin (IL)-10, VEGF, NF-κB, and the constitutive activation of signal transducer and activator of transcription (Stat)-3.

Regulatory T-cells (Treg) and myeloid suppressor cells inhibit the anti-cancer activity of NK and T-helper cells and are partly responsible for tumour progression, resistance to chemotherapy and ineffective anti-tumour vaccines. Enhancement of innate immunity seems to improve anti-cancer therapies. Treg are characterized by CD25 and FoxP3 expression. Their normal role is to control the adaptive immune response through cell contact-dependent mechanisms. The DCs modulate the interplay between Treg and antigen responsive T-cells. Immature myeloid precursors of DC suppress T-cell activation and induce Treg development. Mature monocytes (macrophages) override Treg mediated suppression. The mature DC-derived macrophages are activated through the TLR pattern recognition receptors found on monocytes in the mucosa-associated lymphoid tissue (MALT) of the GI tract. They then secrete IL-6, which renders T-helper and NK cells refractory to the suppressive effect of Tregs (Kabelitz et al. 2006). Other studies have shown that elimination of Tregs can significantly improve the outcome of cancer immunotherapy in preclinical models (Sutmuller et al. 2001). Myeloid suppressor cells may have additional properties that can compromise anti-cancer therapies, such as promotion of angiogenesis (Yang et al. 2004). Specific cytokines also play a role in immune suppression. IL-13 and IL-4 are cytokines that suppress NK cell immunosurveillance (Terabe et al. 2004).

Treg cells that suppress immune responses limit the efficiency of cancer immunotherapy. Recent findings indicate that TLRs directly regulate the suppressive activity of Treg cells. Linking TLR signaling to the functional control of Treg cells may offer new opportunities to improve the outcome of cancer immunotherapy by coadminstration of certain TLR ligands, including specific botanicals (Wang 2006). In inflamed tissue, TLR stimulation cause granulocyte/monocyte colony stimulating factor (GM-CSF) to divert progenitor cells from DCs to mature macrophage monocytes. In uninflamed tissues, TLR stimulation causes GM-CSF to induce the generation of immature DCs. Thus, TLR stimulation would guide the innate immune system to assure a sufficient supply of phagocytic cells in inflamed tissues. Garay reviewed the potential benefits of TLR agonists when added to chemotherapy. The TLR2/4 agonists induce a well-controlled tumour necrosis factor-alpha (TNF-α) secretion, at plasma levels known to permeabilize neoangiogenic tumour vessels to the passage of cytotoxic drugs (Garay et al. 2007). Moreover, TLR2/4 agonists induce inducible nitric oxide synthase (iNOS) expression, and nitric oxide is able to induce apoptosis of chemotherapy-resistant tumour cell clones. Finally, TLR2/4-stimulation activates dendritic cell traffic, macrophage production and cytotoxic T-cell responses.

Many Chinese herbs contain glycoproteins and polysaccharides (among them, constituents of *Coriolus versicolor* (multicolored polypore), *Ganoderma lucidum* (lucid ganoderma), *Grifola frondosa* (Maitake mushroom), *Astragalus membranaceus* (astragalus root), ginseng and various other medicinal mushrooms) that can modulate the innate immune system. Although these botanicals can have multiple anti-tumour activities in response to diverse phytochemicals (Cho and Leung 2007a, b), the polysaccharide components, in particular, can boost the innate immune system through interaction with the TLRs in MALT. This intervention may potentially improve the effectiveness of new anticancer vaccines and radiotherapy. Specific polysaccharides enhance the innate immune system through the stimulation of TLRs (Sen et al. 2005; Rezaei 2006; Tsan 2006). Polysaccharide extracts and complexes from Chinese medicinal herbs and mushrooms may have a potential role for enhancing innate immunity (Table 6.5). There is some evidence from clinical trials that they can improve survival (Chang 2002). Molecular mechanisms for the immuno-biological functions may be through various receptors on macrophages, monocytes and natural killer (NK) cells, which activate NF-κB and anti-tumour cytokine secretion. Interactions may include complement receptor type 3, CD14, mannose, and β-glucan receptors. There is evidence of interaction with TLRs, especially TLR4, with polysaccharides derived from astragalus root, *Acanthopanax senticosus* (Siberian ginseng), lucid ganoderma, *Platyloden grandiflorum* (platycodon root) and *Panax quinquefolium* (American ginseng) (Han et al. 2003, 2005; Schepetkin and Quinn 2006; Rosenthal et al. 2008).

This recent research on TLRs may have relevance for radiotherapy. Irradiation causes tissue inflammation and results in a physiological environment that may

Table 6.5 Botanicals containing polysaccharide complexes and extracts that enhance immunity

Botanical	Reference
Coriolus versicolor (multicolored polypore) (Krestin, PSK or PSP)	Mitomi et al. (1992); Nakazato et al. (1994); Ogoshi et al. (1995); Hayakawa et al. (1997); Munemoto et al. (2002); Koda et al. (2003); Tsang et al. (2003); Ito et al. (2004); Kanazawa et al. (2004); Ohwada et al. (2004); Wong et al. (2004); Wong et al. (2005); Zeng et al. (2005)
Ganoderma lucidum (lucid ganoderma)	Gao et al. (2003); Shao et al. (2004a); Lin (2005); Kuo et al. (2006)
Grifola frondosa (Maitake mushroom) (Maitake MD-fraction)	Atsuyuki et al. (2002); Kodama et al. (2002); Kodama et al. (2005)
Astragalus membranaceus (astragalus root)	Shao et al. (2004b)
Panax ginseng (ginseng)	Shin et al. (2002); Lim et al. (2004)
Other medicinal mushrooms	Ooi and Liu (2000); Lindequist et al. (2005); Zaidman et al. (2005)

allow synergy between TLR stimulated monocytes and DC assisted adaptive immunity. Recent findings indicate that irradiation of a tumour in vivo can sensitize the tumour stromal cells for killing by anti-tumour CTLs, and also that stromal elimination leads to tumour eradication (Zhang et al. 2007). Combining radiation therapy and TLR agonists may enhance the radiation therapy's ability to eradicate tumours, thus acting as an immunosensitizer (Demaria et al. 2005; Koski and Czerniecki 2005). Irradiation of the tumour can induce damage response signals required for an effective response of the immune system to the tumour. Cancer cells killed in vivo by radiation therapy can serve as a good source of antigens for APC to present to T-cells. In fact, it has been known for many years that irradiated syngeneic tumour cells can produce a protective anti-tumour response (Demaria et al. 2005; Obeid et al. 2007). The combination of botanical TLR agonists with radiotherapy can be viewed as a novel enhancement strategy or sensitizer that may increase systemic response through the abscopal effect, as well as increasing the local tumour response (Demaria et al. 2004; Mason et al. 2005).

6.5 Future Clinical Research

Most research is currently at the preclinical stage. Better quality assurance, safety, and validation of both chemical content and consistent biological activities are required prior to resource-intensive clinical trials (Fig. 6.2). Although many of these botanicals have been used traditionally in Chinese and Ayurvedic medicine, we require more validation in the context of modern therapies, such as radiotherapy, using current scientific standards.

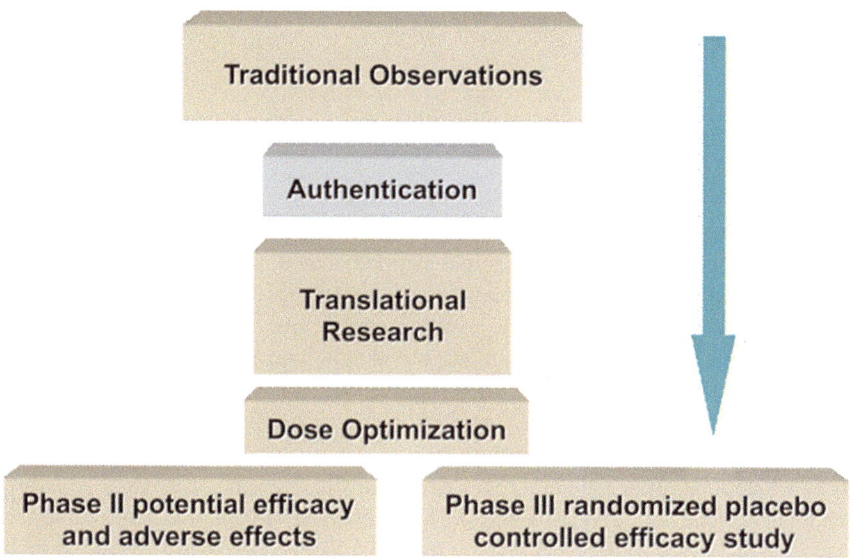

Fig. 6.2 Systematic botanical research

The lack of worldwide regulation of botanicals and their derivatives raises uncertainty with each product. There is wide variation in the composition of similar botanical agents. Even within the same species, biologic variation due to differences in soil conditions, moisture, temperature and harvesting conditions may lead to considerable variability in the concentrations of the bioactive constituents. Activity of the botanical may vary among the capsule, powder and suspension forms. The formulation used in both the preclinical experiments and the clinical trial needs to be precisely stated and should be a validated and verified identical preparation. Stability testing at regular intervals throughout the conduct of the studies is recommended to ensure that the product retains its potency. Quality testing to ensure minimally acceptable tolerances with regard to heavy metal content, bacterial and fungal counts, pesticide residues, and potential contamination with prescription pharmaceuticals is mandatory for clinical use. Chromatographic fingerprint analysis may be used for determining the identity, stability, and consistency of botanicals as well as the identification of adulterants (Blumenthal and Milot 2004).

Natural health products differ from pharmaceutical compounds in that they consist of complex mixtures of chemicals. The polypharmacy of complex botanicals may provide distinct advantages over single-ingredient drugs by containing a major chemical that acts synergistically with secondary compounds. In addition, the secondary compounds may mitigate the undesirable side effects caused by the predominant active ingredients. Multiple ingredients could act through multiple discrete pathways to therapeutically impact the host. Lower concentrations of each of the botanicals may therefore be more efficacious when used together than they would be individually. These theories could explain and justify complex botanical actions, but there is a dearth of studies done to demonstrate the mechanisms of action and authenticity of therapeutic usages of complex mixtures, and it is challenging to predict whether there is therapeutic gain or loss (Sagar 2007).

6.6 Acupuncture as a Biological Response Modifier of Cell Proliferation

There are some neuropeptides released in parotid gland saliva, including cholecystokinin, pentagastrin, vasointestinal peptide, calcitonin gene-related peptide, neuropeptide Y, Neurokinin A and peptide histidine methionine (Hauser-Kronberger et al. 1992; Dawidson et al. 1998, 1999). Acupuncture can stimulate the synthesis of neuropeptides that can modulate blood flow and increase or decrease cell proliferation (Table 6.6). Some neuropeptides release multipotent cells into the circulation after injury that can contribute to tissue repair (Gehron-Robey 2009). Acupuncture may play a role in the repair of normal tissue through repopulation from either progenitor or stem cells. Although the exact physiological pathways are unclear, its effect may be through stimulating the autonomic innervation that occurs in most tissues, including bone marrow. Evidence exists for regeneration of the parotid gland through neural electrical stimulation (Schneyer et al. 1993), and of

Table 6.6 Neuropeptides released in parotid gland saliva by electrostimulation or acupuncture

Neuropeptide	Function	Reference
Cholecystokinin	Stimulates digestive secretion; Induces cell proliferation	Thumwood et al. (1991)
Pentagastrin	Stimulates digestive secretion; Induces cell proliferation	Klingensmith et al. (1996); Szabo et al. (2000)
Vasointestinal peptide	Vasodilatation; Salivary secretion; Induces cell proliferation	Shimuzu and Taira (1979); Bengt et al. (1990); Koh et al. (1997); Guan et al. (2006)
Calcitonin gene-related peptide	Vasodilatation	Brain et al. (1985); Haegerstrand et al. (1990)
Neuropeptide Y	Neurone proliferation; Vascular muscle and endothelial cell proliferation	Zukowska-Grojek et al. (1998); Hansel et al. (2001)
Neurokinin and substance P	Hematopoiesis	Rameshwar et al. (2001)
Nerve growth factor	Parotid cell differentiation	Takeuchi et al. (2003)

the brain of rodents stimulated with acupuncture (Kim et al. 2002), as well as hematological recovery after anti-cancer therapy (Lu et al. 2007, 2009). Acupuncture reverses radiation-induced xerostomia partly through tissue recovery (Wong et al. 2003), and it may enhance neural regeneration leading to a promising role for chemotherapy-induced peripheral neuropathy (Wong and Sagar 2006).

6.7 Conclusion

Antioxidant, anti-angiogenic, and immunogenic Asian botanicals appear to be promising multi-targeting, anti-cancer agents that deserve further therapeutic exploration. Many preclinical screening studies, directed by the intuition and observation of traditional health systems, such as Chinese and Ayurvedic medicine, reveal that many plants exhibit a diverse array of biological activities that may be relevant to the mitigation of ionizing radiation-induced damage in normal tissues of humans. However, so far, only a fraction of these plants have been investigated. There is an urgent need to develop newer, more efficient and reliable bioassays for large scale rapid evaluation of both the radiosensitizing and radioprotective efficacy of plant extracts, and to systematically evaluate this efficacy using standardized extracts, and to identify the bioactive compounds responsible for their potential therapeutic effects. Isolation of the bioactive constituents and subsequent combination in appropriate proportions may further potentiate the effects of herbal preparations to protect normal tissues, and to enhance the tumouricidal effect of radiotherapy. Animal models show that there is usually a window of opportunity about 30 min–2 h prior to irradiation, when the administration of appropriate herbal preparations renders maximum therapeutic gain. There is a need to investigate formulations that can also be of use in the post-irradiation period. Recent evidence suggests a polar effect for some so-called radiosensitizers and radioprotectors in which their differential affects on tumours and normal tissues can result in a therapeutic gain. Other related interventions include anti-angiogenesis and immunomodulatory botanicals. Either additive, synergistic or adverse interactions could occur. Both reliable preclinical and clinical predictors of therapeutic gain are required. Clinical trials have not yet been undertaken with most herbal radiosensitizer, radioprotector and anti-angiogenic botanicals, but some of the clinical trials with immune-enhancers are promising. It is important to develop a scientific model based on sound pharmacological principles (Fig. 6.2).

References

Alpha-Tocopherol, Beta Carotene Cancer Prevention Study Group. The effects of vitamin E and beta carotene on the incidence of lung cancer and other cancers in male smokers. N Eng J Med. 1994;330:1029–35.

Alves De Paulo S, Teruszkin Balassiano I et al. *Chrysobalanus icaco* L. extract for antiangiogenic potential observation. Int J Mol Med. 2000;5:667–9.

Ansiaux R, Baudelet C, Jordan B et al. Thalidomide radiosensitizes tumors through early changes in the tumor microenvironment. Clin Cancer Res. 2005;11:743–50.

Araujo MC, Dias FL, Takahashi CS. Potentiation by turmeric and curcumin of gamma radiation-induced chromosome aberrations in Chinese hamster ovary cells. Teratog Carcinog Mutagen. 1999;19:9–18.

Arbiser JL, Klauber N, Rohan R et al. Curcumin is an in vivo inhibitor of angiogenesis. Mol Med. 1998;4:376–83.

Arora R. Herbal radiomodulators: applications in medicine, homeland defence and space. Wallingford, UK: CABI; 2008.

Arora R, Gupta D, Chawla R. Radioprotection by plant products: present status and future prospects. Phytother Res. 2005;19:1–22.

Atsuyuki I, Kodama N, Nanba H. Effect of maitake (*Grifola frondosa*) D-fraction on the control of the T lymph node Th-1/Th-2 proportion. Biol Pharm Bull. 2002;25:536–40.

Bai X, Cerimele F, Ushio-Fukai M et al. Honokiol, a small molecular weight natural product, inhibits angiogenesis in vitro and tumor growth in vivo. J Biol Chem. 2003;278:35501–7.

Bence AK, Damas VR, Crooks PA. L-canavanine as a radiosensitization agent for human pancreatic cancer cells. Mol Cell Biochem. 2003;244:37–43.

Bengt M, Bengt-Olof N, Jorgen E. Effects of repeated infusions of substance P and vasoactive intestinal peptide on the weights of salivary glands subjected to atrophying influence in rats. Br J Pharmacol. 1990;101:854–8.

Bhosle SM, Huilgol NG, Mishra KP. Enhancement of radiation-induced oxidative stress and cytotoxicity in tumour cells by ellagic acid. Clin Chim Acta. 2005;359:89–100.

Blumenthal M, Milot B. Bioassays for testing activity and bioavailability of botanical products. HerbalGram. 2004;63:48–51.

Brain SD, Williams TJ, Tippins JR et al. Calcitonin gene-related peptide is a potent vasodilator. Nature. 1985;313:54–6.

Brown AC, Shah C, Liu J et al. Ginger's (*Zingiber officinale* Roscoe) inhibition of rat colonic adenocarcinoma cells proliferation and angiogenesis in vitro. Phytother Res. 2009;23:640–5.

Bump EA, Hoffman SJ, Foye WO. Radiosensitizers and radioprotective agents. In: Abraham DA (ed). Burger's medicinal chemistry and drug discovery, vol 5: Chemotherapeutic drugs. USA: John Wiley and Sons Inc; 2003:151–211.

Camphausen K, Citrin D, Krishna CM et al. Implications for tumor control during protection of normal tissues with antioxidants. J Clin Oncol. 2005;23:5455–7.

Cao Y, Cao R. Angiogenesis inhibited by drinking tea. Nature. 1999;398:381.

Cao QZ, Lin ZB. Antitumor and anti-angiogenic activity of *Ganoderma lucidum* polysaccharides peptide. Acta Pharmacol Sin. 2004;25:833–8.

Capizzi RL, Oster W. Protection of normal tissue from the cytotoxic effects of chemotherapy and radiation by amifostine: clinical experiences. Eur J Cancer. 1995;31:8–13.

Cardenas C, Quesada AR, Medina MA. Effects of ursolic acid on different steps of the angiogenic process. Biochem Biophys Res Commun. 2004;320:402–8.

Chang R. Bioactive polysaccharides from traditional Chinese medicine herbs as anticancer adjuvants. J Altern Complement Med. 2002;8:559–65.

Chaudhary D, Chandra D, Kale RK. Modulation of radioresponse of glyoxalase system by curcumin. J Ethnopharmacol. 1999;64:1–7.

Chawla R, Arora R, Singh S et al. Variation in aryltetralin lignan content of *Podophyllum hexandrum* influences radioprotective efficacy. Evid Based Complement Alternat Med. 2006;3: 503–11.

Chen MF, Liao HF, Tsai TH et al. Caffeic acid phenethyl ester preferentially sensitizes CT26 colorectal adenocarcinoma to ionizing radiation without affecting bone marrow radioresponse. Int J Radiat Oncol Biol Phys. 2005;63:1252–61.

Chen AY, Okunieff P, Pommier Y et al. Mammalian DNA Topoisomerase 1 mediates the enhancement of radiation cytotoxicity by camptothecin derivatives. Cancer Res. 1997;57:1529–36.

Chen F, Wang T, Wu YF et al. Honokiol: a potent chemotherapy candidate for human colorectal carcinoma. World J Gastroenterol. 2004b;10:3459–63.

Chen FD, Wu MC, Wang HE et al. Sensitization of a tumour, but not normal tissue, to the cytotoxic effect of ionizing radiation using Panax notoginseng extract. Am J Chin Med. 2001;29: 517–24.

Chen HW, Yu SL, Chen JJ et al. Anti-invasive gene expression profile of curcumin in lung adenocarcinoma based on a high throughput microarray analysis. Mol Pharmacol. 2004c;65:99–110.

Chen HH, Zhou HJ, Wu GD et al. Inhibitory effects of artesunate on angiogenesis and on expressions of vascular endothelial growth factor and VEGF receptor KDR/flk-1. Pharmacology. 2004a;7:1–9.

Cho WC, Leung KN. In vitro and in vivo immunomodulating and immunorestorative effects of *Astragalus membranaceus*. J Ethnopharmacol. 2007a;113:132–41.

Cho WC, Leung KN. In vitro and in vivo anti-tumor effects of *Astragalus membranaceus*. Cancer Lett. 2007b;252:43–54.

Coleman NE, Blakely WF, Fike JR et al. Molecular and cellular biology of moderate dose (1–10 Gy) radiation and potential mechanisms of radiation protection. Radiat Res. 2003;159: 812–34.

Cook JA, Gius D, Wink DA et al. Oxidative stress, redox, and the tumor microenvironment. Semin Radiat Oncol. 2004;14:259–66.

Curry EA, Murry DJ, Yoder C et al. Phase I dose escalation trial of feverfew with standardized doses of parthenolide in patients with cancer. Invest New Drugs. 2004;22:299–305.
Das B, Yeger H, Tsuchida R et al. A hypoxia-driven vascular endothelial growth factor/flt1 autocrine loop interacts with hypoxia-inducible factor-1 through mitogen-activated protein kinase/extracellular signal-regulated kinase 1/2 pathway in neuroblastoma. Cancer Res. 2005;65:7267–75.
Dawidson I, Angmar-Månsson B, Blom M et al. Sensory stimulation (acupuncture) increases the release of vasoactive intestinal polypeptide in the saliva of xerostomia sufferers. Neuropeptides. 1998;32:543–8.
Dawidson I, Angmar-Månsson B, Blom M et al. Sensory stimulation (acupuncture) increases the release of calcitonin gene-related peptide in the saliva of xerostomia sufferers. Neuropeptides. 1999;33:244–50.
Deeb D, Yong X, Hao XU et al. Curcumin (diferuloyl-methane) enhances tumor necrosis factor-related apoptosis-inducing ligand-induced apoptosis in LNCaP prostate cancer cells. Mol Cancer Ther. 2003;2:95–103.
Demaria S, Formenti SC. Sensors of ionizing radiation effects on the immunological microenvironment of cancer. Int J Radiat Biol. 2007;83:819–25.
Demaria S, Kawashima N, Yang AM et al. Immune mediated inhibition of metastases following treatment with local radiation and CTLA-4 blockade in a mouse model of breast cancer. Clin Cancer Res. 2005;1:728–34.
Demaria S, Ng B, Devit M-L et al. Ionizing radiation inhibition of distant untreated tumors (abscopal effect) is immune mediated. Int J Radiat Oncol Biol Phys. 2004;58:862–70.
Dong X, Dong J, Wu G et al. Effects of tanshinone IIA on the radiotherapeutic sensitivities of MKN-45 cell line. Int J Radiat Oncol Biol Phys. 2006;66:S586.
Dorai T, Cao YC, Dorai B et al. Therapeutic potential of curcumin in prostate cancer-III: Curcumin inhibits proliferation, induces apoptosis and inhibits angiogenesis of LNCaP prostate cancer cells in vivo. Prostate. 2001;47:293–303.
Emerit I, Arutyunyan R, Oganesian N et al. Radiation-induced clastogenic factors: Anticlastogenic effects of *Ginkgo biloba* extract.. Free Rad Biol Med. 1995a;18:985–91.
Emerit I, Oganesian N, Sarkisian T et al. Clastogenic factors in the plasma of Chernobyl recovery workers: Anticlastogenic effects of *Ginkgo biloba* extract. Radiat Res. 1995b;144: 198–205.
Ergun A, Camphausen K, Wein LM. Optimal scheduling of radiotherapy and angiogenic inhibitors. Bull Math Biol. 2003;65:407–24.
Fang J, Zhou Q, Liu LZ et al. Apigenin inhibits tumor angiogenesis through decreasing HIF-1 and VEGF expression. Carcinogenesis. 2007;28:858–64.
Fassina G, Vene R, Morini M et al. Mechanisms of inhibition of tumor angiogenesis and vascular tumor growth by epigallocatechin-3-gallate. Clin Cancer Res. 2004;10:4865–73.
Ganasoundari A, Uma Devi P, Rao MN. Protection against radiation-induced chromosome damage in mouse bone marrow by *Ocimum sanctum*. Mutat Resh. 1997;373:271–6.
Gao Y, Zhou S, Jiang W et al. Effects of Ganopoly: A *Ganoderma lucidum* polysaccharide extract on the immune functions in advanced-stage cancer patients. Immunol Invest. 2003;32:201–15.
Garay RP, Viens P, Bauer J. Cancer relapse under chemotherapy: why TLR2/4 receptor agonists can help. Eur J Pharmacol. 2007;563:1–17.
Garcia-Cardena G, Folkman J. Is there a role for nitric oxide in tumor angiogenesis? J Natl Cancer Inst. 1998;90:560–1.
Garg A, Aggarwal BB. Reactive oxygen intermediates in TNF signaling. Mol Immunol. 2002;39:509–17.
Garg AK, Buchholz TA, Aggarwal BB. Chemosensitization and radiosensitization of tumors by plant polyphenols. Antioxid Redox Signal. 2005;7:1630–47.
Gehron-Robey P. Neuropeptide beckons cells that heal. Nat Med. 2009;15:367–9.
Goel HC, Prakash H, Ali A et al. *Podophyllum hexandrum* modulates gamma radiation-induced immunosuppression in Balb/c mice: implications in radioprotection. Mol Cell Biochem. 2007;295:93–103.

Goel HC, Prasad J, Singh S et al. Radioprotective potential of a herbal extract of *Tinaspora cordifolia*. J Radiat Res. 2004;45:61–8.

Gonzalez S, Alcaraz MV, Cuevas J et al. An extract of the Fern Polypodium leucotomos (Difur) modulates Thl/Th2 cytokines balance in vitro and appears to exhibit anti-angiogenic activities in vivo: Pathogenic relationships and therapeutic implications. Anticancer Res. 2000;20: 567–75.

Greenberger JS, Epperly MW. Antioxidant gene therapeutic approaches to normal tissue radioprotection and tumor radiosensitization. In Vivo. 2007;21:141–6.

Guan CX, Min Z, Qin XQ et al. Vasoactive intestinal peptide enhances wound healing and proliferation of human bronchial epithelial cells. Peptides. 2006;27:3107–14.

Guruprasad K. Effect of Withaferin A on the development and decay of thermotolerance in B16F1 melanoma: A preliminary study. Integr Cancer Ther. 2009;8:93–7.

Gururaj AE, Belakavadi M, Venkatesh DA et al. Molecular mechanisms of antiangiogenic effect of curcumin. Biochem Biophys Res Commun. 2002;297:934–42.

Haegerstrand A, Dalsgaard CJ, Jonzen B et al. Calcitonin gene-related peptide stimulates proliferation of human endothelial cells. Proc Natl Acad Sci USA. 1990;87:3299–303.

Hahm ER, Arlotti JA, Marynowski SW et al. Honokiol, a constituent of oriental medicinal herb *Magnolia officinalis*, inhibits growth of PC-3 xenografts in vivo in association with apoptosis induction. Clin Cancer Res. 2008;14:1248.

Hahm ER, Gho YS, Park S et al. Synthetic curcumin analogs inhibit activator protein-1 transcription and tumor-induced angiogenesis. Biochem Biophys Res Commun. 2004;321:337–44.

Han SK, Song JY, Yun YS et al. Ginsan improved Th-1 immune response inhibited by gamma radiation. Arch Pharm Res. 2005;28:343–50.

Han SB, Yoon YD, Ahn HJ. Toll-like receptor-mediated activation of B cells and macrophages by polysaccharide isolated from *Acanthopanax senticosus*. Int Immunopharmacol. 2003;3: 1301–12.

Hannequin D, Thibert A, Vaschalde Y. Development of a model to study the anti-oedema properties of *Ginkgo biloba* extract. Presse Med. 1986;15:1575–6.

Hansel DE, Eipper BA, Ronnett GV. Neuropeptide Y functions as a neuroproliferative factor. Nature. 2001;410:940–4.

Hauser-Kronberger C, Albergger K, Saria A et al. Neuropeptides in human salivary (submandibular and parotid) glands. Acta Oto-laryngologica. 1992;112:343–8.

Hayakawa K, Mitsuhashi N, Saito Y et al. Effect of Krestin as adjuvant treatment following radical radiotherapy in non-small cell lung cancer patients. Cancer Detect Prev. 1997;21:71–7.

Heine H, Almer AJ, Kabelitz D et al. Recognition of bacterial products by Toll-Like Receptors. Chem Immunol Allergy. 2005;86:99–119.

Hien VT, Huong BN, Hung PM et al. Radioprotective effects of Vitexina for breast cancer patients undergoing radiotherapy with Co^{60}. Integr Cancer Ther. 2002;1:38–43.

Higuchi K, Mitsuhashi N, Saitoh J et al. Caffeine enhanced radiosensitivity of rat tumour cells with a mutant type *p53* by inducing apoptosis in a *p53*-independemt manner. Cancer Lett. 2000;152:157–62.

Hsu HY, Yang JJ, Ho YJ et al. Difference in the effects of radioprotection between aerial and root parts of *Lycium chinese*. J Ethnopharmacol. 1999;64:101–8.

Huang CN, Chan KC, Lin WT. *Hibiscus sabdariffa* inhibits vascular smooth muscle cell proliferation and migration induced by high glucose a mechanism involves connective tissue growth factor signals. J Agric Food Chem. 2009;57:3073–9.

Huang GW, Xie CX, Kuang GQ. Treatment of 41 patients with advanced stage of nasopharyngeal cancer by combination therapy of radiation and Chinese herbal drugs for activating blood circulation to remove stasis as hirudo. Zhongguo Zhong Xi Yi Jie He Za Zhi. 2003;23: 777–8.

Ito K, Nakazato H, Koike A et al. Long-term effect of 5-fluorouracil enhanced by intermittent administration of polysaccharide K after curative resection of colon cancer. A randomized controlled trial for 7-year follow-up. Int J Colorectal Dis. 2004;19:157–64.

Jagetia GC. Radioprotective potential of plants and herbs against the effects of ionizing radiation. J Clin Biochem Nutr. 2007;40:74–81.

Jagetia GC, Baliga MS. Influence of the leaf extract of *Mentha arvensis* Linn (mint) on the survival of mice exposed to different doses of gamma radiation. Strahlentherapie und Onkologie. 2002;178:91–8.

Jagetia GC, Baliga MS. Treatment with *Alstonia scholaris* enhances Radiosensitivity in vitro and in vivo. Cancer Biother Pharm. 2003a;18:917–29.

Jagetia BC, Baliga MS. The evaluation of the radioprotective effect of the leaf extract of *Syzigium cumuni* (Jamun) in the mice exposed to lethal dose of gamma-radiation. Nahrung. 2003b;47: 181–5.

Jagetia BC, Baliga MS, Venkatesh P et al. Influence of ginger rhizome (*Zingiber officinale* Rosc) on survival, glutathione and lipid peroxidation in mice after whole-body exposure to gamma-irradiation. Radiat Res. 2003;160:584–92.

Jagetia BC, Baliga MS, Venkatesh P. Ginger (*Zingiber officinale* Rosc), a dietary supplement, protects mice against radiation-induced lethality: mechanism of action. Cancer Biother Pharm. 2004;19:422–35.

Jagetia GC, Shirwaikar A, Rau SK et al. Evaluation of the radioprotective effect of *Ageratum conyzoides* linn extract in mice exposed to different doses of gamma radiation. J Pharm Pharmacol. 2003a;55:1151–8.

Jagetia GC, Venkatesh P. Radioprotection by oral administration of *Aegle marmelos* (L) Correa in vivo. J Environ Pathol Toxicol Oncol. 2005;24:315–32.

Jagetia GC, Venkatesh VA. Treatment of mice with stem bark extract of *Aphanamixis polystachya* reduces radiation-induced chromosome damage. Int J Radiat Biol. 2006;82:197–209.

Jagetia GC, Venkatesh P, Baliga MS. Evaluation of radioprotective effect of *Aegle marmelos* (L.) Correa in the cultured human peripheral blood lymphocytes exposed to different doses of gamma-irradiation: a micronucleus study. Mutagenesis. 2003b;18:387–93.

Jagetia GC, Venkatesh P, Baliga MS. Evaluation of the radioprotective effect of bael leaf (*Aegle marmelos*) extract in mice. Int J Radiat Biol. 2004a;80:281–90.

Jagetia GC, Venkatesh P, Baliga MS. Fruit extract of *Aegle marmelos* protects mice against radiation-induced lethality. Integr Cancer Ther. 2004b;3:323–32.

Jiang C, Agarwal R, Lu J. Anti-angiogenic potential of a cancer chemopreventive flavonoid antioxidant, Silymarin: inhibition of key attributes of vascular endothelial cells and angiogenic cytokine secretion by cancer epithelial cells. Biochem Biophys Res Commun. 2000;276: 371–8.

John VD, Kuttan G, Krishnakutty K. Anti-tumour studies of metal chelates of synthetic curcuminoids. J Exp Clin Cancer Res. 2002;21:219–24.

Jung M, Dritschilo A. NF-kappa B signaling pathway as a target for human tumor radiosensitization. Sem Radiat Oncol. 2001;11:346–51.

Jung CP, Motwani MP, Kortmansky J et al. The cyclin-dependent kinase inhibitor flavopyridol potentiates gamma-irradiation-induced apoptosis in colon and gastric cancer cells. Clin Cancer Res. 2003;9:6052–61.

Kabelitz D, Wesch D, Oberg HH. Regulation of regulatory T cells: role of dendritic cells and toll-like receptors. Crit Rev Immunol. 2006;26:291–306.

Kamath R, Rao BSS, Uma Devi P. Response of a mouse fibrosarcoma to Withaferin A and radiation. Pharmacol Res Commun. 1999;5:287–91.

Kanazawa M, Mori Y, Yoshihara K et al. Effect of PSK on the maturation of dendritic cells derived from human peripheral blood monocytes. Immunol Lett. 2004;91:229–38.

Kasten-Pisula U, Windhorst S, Dahm-Dalphi J et al. Radiosensitization of tumour cell lines by the polyphenol Gossypol results from double-strand break repair and not from enhanced apoptosis. Radiother Oncol. 2007;5:1752–6.

Kaur T, Gupta R, Vaiphei K et al. Interplay between oncoproteins and antioxidant enzymes in esophageal carcinoma treated without and with chemoradiotherapy: A prospective study. Int J Radiat Oncol Biol Phys. 2008;70:563–71.

Kim SH, Cho CK, Yoo SY et al. In vivo radioprotective activity of *Panax ginseng* and diethyldithiocarbamate. In Vivo. 1993;7:467–70.

Kim EH, Jang MH, Shin MC et al. Acupuncture increases cell proliferation and neuropeptide Y expression in dentate gyrus of streptozotocin-induced diabetic rats. Neurosci Lett. 2002;327:33–6.

Kim SH, Son CH, Nah SY et al. Modification of radiation response in mice by *Panax ginseng* and diethyldithiocarbamate. In Vivo. 2001;15:407–11.

Kimura Y, Okuda H. Resveratrol isolated from *Polygonum cuspidatum* root prevents tumor growth and metastasis to lung and tumor-induced neovascularization in Lewis lung carcinoma-bearing mice. J Nutr. 2001;131:1844–9.

Kirichenko AV, Rich TA. Radiation enhancement by 9-aminocamptothecin: the effect of fractionation and timing of administration. Int J Radiat Oncol Biol Phys. 1999;44:659–64.

Klingensmith ME, Hallonquist H, McCoy PP et al. Pentagastrin selectivity modulates levels of mRNAs encoding apical H/K adenosine triphosphatase and basolateral Na-K-Cl cotransporter in rat gastric fundic mucosa. Surgery. 1996;120:242–7.

Koda K, Miyazaki M, Sarashina H et al. A randomized controlled trial of postoperative adjuvant immunochemotherapy for colorectal cancer with oral medicines. Int J Oncol. 2003;23: 165–72.

Kodama N, Komuta K, Nanba H. Can maitake MD-fraction aid cancer patients? Altern Med Rev. 2002;7:236–9.

Kodama N, Murata Y, Asakawa A. Maitake D-fraction enhances antitumor effects and reduces immunosuppression by mitomycin-C in tumor-bearing mice. Nutrition. 2005;21:624–9.

Koh SW, Yeh TH, Morris SM et al. Vasoactive intestinal peptide stimulation of human trabecular meshwork cell growth. Invest Ophthalmol Vis Sci. 1997;38:2781–9.

Kojima-Yuasa A, Hua JJ, Kennedy DO et al. Green tea extract inhibits angiogenesis of human umbilical vein endothelial cells through reduction of expression of VEGF receptors. Life Sci. 2003;73:1299–313.

Koltermann A, Liebl J, Fürst R et al. *Ginkgo biloba* extract EGb761 exerts anti-angiogenic effects via activation of tyrosine phosphatases. J Cell Mol Med. 2008;doi:10.1111/j.1582-4934.2008.00561.x.

Kong F, Chen Z, Li Q et al. Inhibitory effects of parthenolide on the angiogenesis induced by human multiple myeloma cells and the mechanism. J Huazhong Univ Sci Technol. 2008;28:525–30.

Koski GK, Czerniecki BJ. Combining innate immunity with radiation therapy for cancer treatment. Clin Cancer Res. 2005;11:7–11.

Koukourakis MI, Giatromanolaki A, Sivridis E et al. Squamous cell head and neck cancer: evidence of angiogenic regeneration during radiotherapy. Anticancer Res. 2001;21:4301–9.

Krishna A, Kumar A. Evaluation of radioprotective effects of rajgira (*Amaranthus paniculatus*) extract in Swiss albino mice. J Radiat Res. 2005;46:233–9.

Kruger EA, Duray PH, Price DK et al. Approaches to preclinical screening of antiangiogenic agents. Sem Oncol. 2001;28:570–6.

Kumar B, Joshi J, Kumar A et al. Radiosensitization by diospyrin diethylether in MCF-7 breast carcinoma cell line. Mol Cell Biochem. 2007;304:1–2.

Kumar KB, Kuttan R. Protective effect of an extract of *Phyllanthus amarus* against radiation-induced damage in mice. J Radiat Res. 2004;45:133–9.

Kumar A, Rao AR, Kimura H. Radiosensitizing effects of neem (Azadirachta indica) oil. Phytotherapy Res. 2002;16:74–7.

Kumar M, Sharma MK, Saxena PS et al. Radioprotective effect of Panax ginseng on the peroxidases and lipid peroxidation level in testes of Swiss albino mice. Biol Pharm Bull. 2003;26:308–12.

Kumar R, Singh PK, Arora R et al. Radioprotection by *Podophyllum hexandrum* in the liver of mice: A mechanistic approach. Environ Toxicol Pharmacol. 2005a;20:326–34.

Kumar R, Singh PK, Sharma A et al. *Podophyllum hexandrum* extract provides radioprotection by modulating the expression of proteins associated with apoptosis: role in radioprotection. Biotechnol Appl Biochem. 2005b;42:81–92.

Kung HN, Chien CL, Chau GY et al. Involvement of NO/cGMP signaling in the apoptotic and anti-angiogenic effects of beta-lapachone on endothelial cells in vitro. J Cell Physiol. 2007;211: 522–32.

Kuo MC, Weng CY, Ha CL et al. Ganoderma lucidum mycelia enhance innate immunity by activating NF-κB. J Ethnopharmacol. 2006;103:217–22.

Lata M, Prasad J, Singh S. Whole body protection against lethal ionizing radiation in mice by REC-2001: A semi-purified fraction of *Podophyllum hexandrum*. Phytomedicine. 2009;16: 47–55.

Lau DH, Xue L, Yond LJ et al. Paclitaxel (Taxol): an inhibitor of angiogenesis in a highly vascularized transgenic breast cancer. Cancer Biother Radiopharm. 1999;14:31–6.

Lawenda B, Kelly K, Ladas E et al. Should supplemental dietary antioxidant administration be avoided during chemotherapy and radiation therapy? J Nat Cancer Inst. 2008;100:773–83.

Lee TK, Wang W, O'Brien KF et al. Effect of north American ginseng on ^{137}Cs-induced micronuclei in human lymphocytes: a comparison with WR-1065. Phytother Res. 2008;22:1614–22.

Li Z, Liu Y, Zhao X et al. Honokiol, a natural therapeutic candidate, induces apoptosis and inhibits angiogenesis of ovarian tumor cells. Eur J Obstet Gynecol Reprod Biol. 2009;140:95–102.

Lim TS, Na K, Choi EM et al. Immunomodulating activities of polysaccharides isolated from *Panax ginseng*. J Med Food. 2004;7:1–6.

Lin ZB. Cellular and molecular mechanisms of immuno-modulation. *Ganoderma lucidum*. J Pharmacol Sci. 2005;99:144–53.

Lindequist U, Niedermeyer THJ, Julich WD. The pharmacological potential of mushrooms. Evid Based Complement Alternat Med. 2005;2:285–99.

Liu LZ, Fang J, Zhou Q et al. Apigenin inhibits expression of vascular endothelial growth factor and angiogenesis in human lung cancer cells: implication of chemoprevention of lung cancer. Mol Pharmacol. 2005;68:635–43.

Liu JJ, Huang TS, Cheng WF et al. Baicalein and baicalin are potent inhibitors of angiogenesis: Inhibition of endothelial cell proliferation, migration and differentiation. Int J Cancer. 2003;106:559–65.

Lu W, Hu D, Dean-Clower E et al. Acupuncture for chemotherapy-induced leukopenia: exploratory meta-analysis of randomized controlled trials. J Soc Integr Oncol. 2007;5:1–10.

Lu W, Matulonis U, Doherty Gilman A et al. Acupuncture for chemotherapy-induced neutropenia in patients with gynecologic malignancies: a pilot randomized, sham-controlled clinical trial. J Altern Complement Med. 2009;15:1–9.

Ma BB, Bristow RG, Kim J et al. Combined-modality treatment of solid tumors using radiotherapy and molecular targeted agents. J Clin Oncol. 2003;21:2760–76.

Manikandan P, Vidjaya Letchoumy P, Prathiba D et al. Proliferation, angiogenesis and apoptosis-associated proteins are molecular targets for chemoprevention of MNNG-induced gastric carcinogenesis by ethanolic Ocimum sanctum leaf extract. Singapore Med J. 2007;48: 645–51.

Manna SK, Mukhopadhyay A, Aggarwal BB. Resveratrol suppresses TNF-induced activation of nuclear transcription factors NF-kappa B, activator protein-1, and apoptosis: potential role of reactive oxygen intermediates and lipid peroxidation. J Immunol. 2000;164:6509–19.

Mason KA, Ariga H, Neal R et al. Targeting Toll-like receptor 9 with CpG oligodeoxynucleotides enhances tumor response to fractionated radiotherapy. Clin Cancer Res. 2005;11:361–9.

Mei QB. Effects of *Angelica sinensis* polysaccharides on hemopoietic stem cells in irradiated mice. Chung Kuo Yao Li Hsueh Pao. 1988;9:279–82.

Mei QB, Tao JY, Cui B. Advances in the pharmacological studies of *Radix Angelica Sinensis* (Oliv) diels (Chinese danggui. Chin Med J. 1991;104:776–81.

Melillo G, Sausville EA, Cloud K. Flavopiridol, a protein kinase inhibitor, down regulates hypoxic induction of vascular endothelial growth factor expression in human monocytes. Cancer Res. 1999;59:5433–7.

Meyer F, Bairati I, Fortin A et al. Interaction between antioxidant vitamin supplementation and cigarette smoking during radiation therapy in relation to long-term effects on recurrence and mortality: A randomized trial among head and neck cancer patients. Int J Cancer. 2007;122:1679–80.

Miller KD, Sweeney CJ, Sledge GW. Redefining the target: Chemotherapeutics as antiantiogenics. J Clin Oncol. 2001;19:1195–206.

Mitomi T, Tsuchiya S, Iijima N et al. Randomized, controlled study on adjuvant immunochemotherapy with PSK in curatively resected colorectal cancer. The Cooperative Study Group of Surgical Adjuvant Immunochemotherapy for Cancer of Colon and Rectum (Kanagawa). Dis Colon Rectum. 1992;35:123–30.

Mittal A, Pathania V, Agrawala PK et al. Influence of *Podophyllum hexandrum* on endogenous antioxidant defense system in mice; possible role in radioprotection. J Ethnopharmacol. 2001;76:253–62.

Mizina TY, Sitnikova SG. Antiradiation activity of juice concentrate from *Hippophae rhamnoides* L. fruits. Rastitel'nye Resursy. 1999;35:85–92.

Mizushina Y, Akihisa T, Ukiya M et al. A novel DNA topoisomerase inhibitor: dehydroebriconic acid; one of the lanostane-type triterpene acids from Poria cocos. Cancer Sci. 2004;95:354–60.

Mohamed EJ, Voss S, Devenny ME et al. Novel small molecule alpha-v integrinantagonists: comparative anticancer efficacy with known angiogenesis inhibitors. Anticancer Res. 1999;19:959–68.

Munemoto Y, Iida Y, Abe J et al. Significance of postoperative adjuvant immunochemotherapy after curative resection of colorectal cancers: Association between host or tumor factors and survival. Int J Oncol. 2002;20:403–11.

Murayama C, Nagano Y, Sano S et al. Effect of oridin, a Rabdosia diterpenoid, on radiosensitization with misonidazole. Experientia. 1987;43:1221–3.

Nakazato H, Hoike A, Saji S et al. Efficacy of immunochemotherapy as adjuvant treatment after curative resection of gastric cancer; Study Group of Immunochemotherapy with PSK for Gastric Cancer. Lancet. 1994;343:1122–6.

Narimanov AA. The antiradiation effectiveness of a mixture of *Archangelica officinalis* and *Ledum palustre* extracts in the fractionated gamma irradiation of mice. Radiobiologiia. 1993;33:280–4.

Nasu S, Milas L, Kawabe S et al. Enhancement of radiotherapy by oleandrin is a caspase-3 dependent process. Cancer Lett. 2002;185:145–51.

Obeid M, Tesniere A, Ghiringhelli F et al. Calreticulin exposure dictates the immunogenicity of cancer cell death. Nature Med. 2007;13:54–61.

Ogoshi K, Satou H, Isono K et al. Immunotherapy for esophageal cancer. A randomized trial in combination with radiotherapy and radiochemotherapy. Cooperative Study Group for Esophageal Cancer in Japan. Am J Clin Oncol. 1995;18:216–22.

Ohwada S, Ikeya T, Yokomori T et al. Adjuvant immunochemotherapy with oral Tegafur/Uracil plus PSK in patients with stage II or III colorectal cancer: a randomised controlled study. Br J Cancer. 2004;90:1003–10.

Ooi VE, Liu F. Immunomodulation and anti-cancer activity of polysaccharide-protein complexes. Curr Med Chem. 2000;**7**::715–29.

Pahadiya S, Sharma J. Alteration of lethal effects of gamma rays in Swiss albino mice by *Tinaspora cordifolia*. Phytother Res. 2003;17:552–4.

Pande S, Kumar M, Kumar A. Evaluation of radiomodifying effects of root extract of *Panax ginseng*. Phytother Res. 1998;12:13–7.

Pisters KM, Newman RA, Coldman B et al. Phase I trial of oral green tea extract in adult patients with solid tumors. J Clin Oncol. 2001;19:1830–8.

Raffoul JJ, Banerjee S, Singh-Gupta V et al. Down-regulation of apurinic/apyrimidinic endonuclease 1/redox factor 1 expression by soy isoflavones enhances prostate cancer radiotherapy in vitro and in vivo. Radiat Res. 2007;67:2141–9.

Rameshwar P, Zhu G, Donnelly RJ et al. The dynamics of bone marrow stromal cells in the proliferation of multipotent hematopoietic progenitors by substance P: an understanding of the effects of a neurotransmitter on the differentiating hematopoietic stem cell. J Neuroimmunol. 2001;121:22–31.

Rao SK, Rao PS, Rao BN. Preliminary investigation of the radiosensitizing activity of guduchi (*Tinospora cordifolia)* in tumor-bearing mice. Phytother Res. 2008;22:1482–9.

Rao AV, Uma Devi P, Kamath R. In vivo radioprotective effect of *Moringa oleifera* leaves. Indian J Exp Biol. 2001;39:858–63.

Rezaei N. Therapeutic targeting of pattern-recognition receptors. Int Immunopharmacol. 2006;6:863–9.

Robbins ME, Zhao W. Chronic oxidative stress and radiation-induced late normal tissue injury: A review. Int J Radiat Biol. 2004;80:251–9.

Rosenthal KL, Newton J, Patrick AJ. CVT-E002, a proprietary extract of North American ginseng, activates the vertebrate innate immune system to produce proinflammatory and anti-viral factors via MyD88 signaling. FASEB J. 2008;22:1b538.

Sagar S. Should patients take or avoid antioxidant supplements during anticancer therapy? An evidence-based review. Curr Oncol. 2005;12:44–54.

Sagar SM. Future directions for research on *Silybum marianum* for cancer patients. Integr Cancer Ther. 2007;6:166–73.

Sagar RK, Chawla R, Arora R et al. Protection of hematopoietic system by *Podophyllum hexandrum*. Planta Med. 2006;72:114–20.

Sagar SM, Wong RK. Chinese medicine and biomodulation in cancer patients (part two. Curr Oncol. 2008;15:8–30.

Sajikumar S, Goel HC. *Podophyllum hexandrum* prevents radiation-induced neuronal damage in postnatal rats exposed in utero. Phytother Res. 2003;17:761–6.

Samarth RM, Goyal PK, Kumar A. Modulatory effect of *Mentha piperita* (Linn.) on serum phosphatases activity in Swiss albino mice against gamma irradiation. Indian J Exp Biol. 2001;39:479–82.

Samarth RM, Goyal PK, Kumar A. Modulation of serum phosphatases activity in Swiss albino mice against gamma irradiation by *Mentha piperita* Linn. Phytother Res. 2002;16:586–9.

Samarth RM, Kumar A. *Mentha piperota* (Linn.) leaf extract provides protection against radiation-induced chromosomal damage in bone marrow of mice. Indian J Exp Biol. 2003;41:229–37.

Samuels N. Herbal remedies and anticoagulant therapy. Thromb Haemost. 2005;93:3–7.

Sartippour MR, Liu C, Shao ZM et al. Livistona extract inhibits angiogenesis and cancer growth. Oncol Rep. 2001;8:1355–7.

Sartippour MR, Seeram NP, Heber D et al. Rabdosia rubescens inhibits breast cancer growth and angiogenesis. Int J Oncol. 2005;26:121–7.

Sartippour MR, Shao ZM, Heber D et al. Green tea inhibits vascular endothelial growth factor (VEGF) induction in human breast cancer cells. J Nutr. 2002;132:2307–11.

Sato Y. Studies on chemical protectors against radiation. XXXI. Protection effects of *Aloe arborescens* on skininjury induced by x-irradiation. Yakugaku Zasshi. 1990;110:876–84.

Sato K, Mochizuki M, Saiki I et al. Inhibition of tumor angiogenesis and metastasis by a saponin of *Panax ginseng*, ginsenoside-Rb2. Biol Pharm Bull. 1994;17:634–9.

Schepetkin IA, Quinn MT. Botanical polysaccharides: Macrophage immunomodulation and therapeutic potential. Int Immunopharmacol. 2006;6:317–33.

Schneyer CA, Humphreys-Beher MG, Hall HD et al. Mitogenicactivity of rat salivary glands after electrical stimulation of parasympathetic nerves. Am J Physiol. 1993;264:935–8.

Sen G, Khan AQ, Chen Q et al. In vivo humoral immune responses to the isolated pneumococcal polysaccharides are dependent on the presence of associated TLR ligands. J Immunol. 2005;175:3084–91.

Sengupta S, Toh SA, Selers LA et al. Modulating angiogenesis-the Yin and the Yang in ginseng. Circulation. 2004;110:1219–25.

Shao BM, Dai H, Xu W et al. Immune receptors for polysaccharides. *Ganoderma lucidum*. Biochem Biophys Res Commun. 2004a;323:133–41.

Shao BM, Xu W, Dai H. A study on the immune receptors for polysaccharides from the roots of Astragalus membranaceus, a Chinese medicinal herb. Biochem Biophys Res Commun. 2004b;320:1103–11.

Sharma J, Sharma R. Radioprotection of Swiss albino mouse by *Centella asiatica* extract. Phytother Res. 2002;16:785–6.

Sheela ML, Ramakrishna MK, Salimath BP. Angiogenic and proliferative effects of the cytokine VEGF in Ehrlich ascites tumor cells is inhibited by Glycyrrhiza glabra. Int Immunopharmacol. 2006;6:494–98.

Shen RN, Lu L, Jia XQ et al. Naturin: a potent bio-immunomodifier in experimental studies and clinical trials. In Vivo. 1996;10:201–9.

Shetty TK, Satav JG, Nair CK. Protection of DNA and microsomal membranes in vitro by *Glycyrrhiza glabra* L. against gamma radiation. Phytother Res. 2002;16:576–8.

Shim JS, Kim JH, Cho HY et al. Irreversible inhibition of CD13/aminopeptidase-N by the antiangiogenic agent curcumin. Chem Biol. 2003;10:695–704.

Shimuzu T, Taira N. Assessment of the effects of vasoactive intestinal peptide (VIP) on blood flow through and salivation of the dog salivary gland in comparison with those of secretin, glucagon and acetylcholine. Br J Pharmacol. 1979;65:683–7.

Shin JY, Song JY, Yun YS. Immunostimulating effects of acidic polysaccharides extract of *Panax ginseng* on macrophage function. Immunopharmacol Immunotoxicol. 2002;24:469–82.

Shobi V, Goel HC. Protection against radiation-induced conditioned taste aversion by *Centella asiatica* extract. Physiol Behav. 2001;73:19–23.

Singh I, Sharma A, Nunia V et al. Radioprotection of Swiss albino mice by *Emblica officinalis*. Phytother Res. 2005;19:444–6.

Sohn KH, Lee HY, Chung HY et al. Anti-angiogenic activity of triterpene acids. Cancer Lett. 1995;94:213–8.

Sreejayan R. Nitric oxide scavenging by Curcuminoids. J Pharm Pharmacol. 1997;49:105–7.

Stanley G, Harvey K, Slivova V et al. *Ganoderma lucidum* suppresses angiogenesis through the inhibition of secretion of VEGF and TGF-beta1 from prostate cancer cells. Biochem Biophys Res Commun. 2005;330:46–52.

Stone HB, Moulder JE, Coleman CN et al. Models for evaluating agents intended for the prophylaxis, mitigation and treatment of radiation injuries. Radiat Res. 2004;162:711–28.

Subbaramaiah K, Chung WJ, Michaluart P et al. Resveratrol inhibits cyclooxygenase-2 transcription and activity in phorbol-ester treated human mammary epithelial cells. J Biol Chem. 1998;273:21875–82.

Sun Y, St Clair DK, Fang F et al. The radiosensitization effect of parthenolide in prostate cancer cells is mediated by nuclear factor-kB inhibition and enhanced by the presence of PTEN. Mol Cancer Ther. 2007;6:2477–86.

Sung H-K, Lee T-H, Yang D-C et al. ShiQuanDaBuTangJiaWeiBang inhibits tumor metastasis and angiogenesis via regulation of topoisomerase-1. J Ethnopharmacol. 2005;98:157–62.

Sunila ES, Kuttan G. Protective effect of *Piper longum* fruit ethanolic extract on radiation induced damage in mice: a preliminary study. Fitoteripia. 2005;76:649–55.

Sutmuller RP, van Duivenvoorde LM, van Elsas A. Synergism of cytotoxic T lymphocyte-associated antigen 4 blockade and depletion of CD25(+) regulatory T cells in antitumor therapy reveals alternative pathways for suppression of autoreactive cytotoxic T lymphocyte responses. J Exp Med. 2001;194:823–32.

Szabo I, Rumi G, Bodis B et al. Gastrin and pentagastrin enhance the tumour proliferation of human stable cultured gastric adenocarcinoma cells. J Physiol (Paris). 2000;94:71–4.

Takeda A, Katoh N, Yonezawa M. Restoration of radiation injury by ginseng III. Radioprotective effect of thermostable fraction of ginseng extract on mice, rats and guineapigs. J Radiat Res. 1982;23:150–67.

Takeuchi T, Aletta JM, Laychock SG et al. Role of nerve growth factor in the regulation of parotid cell differentiation induced by rat serum. Biochem Pharmacol. 2003;65:1507–13.

Tamura K, Takada M, Kawase I. Enhancement of tumor radio-response by irinotecan in human lung tumor xenografts. Jap J Cancer Res. 1997;88:218–23.

Tang FY, Nguyen N, Meydani M. Green tea catechins inhibit VEGF-induced angiogenesis in vitro through suppression of VE-cadherin phosphorylation and inactivation of Akt molecule. Int J Cancer. 2003;106:871–8.

Taraphdar AK, Shaw BP, Bhattacharya RK et al. Role of sharpunka (*Tephrosia purpurea*) in haemopoietic injury. Antiseptic. 2002;99:302–4.
Terabe M, Park JM, Berzofsky JA. Role of IL-13 in the regulation of anti-tumor immunity and tumor growth. Cancer Immunol Immunother. 2004;53:79–85.
Thumwood CM, Hong J, Baldwin GS. Inhibition of cell proliferation by the cholecystokinin antagonist L-364,718. Exp Cell Res. 1991;189:189–92.
Tsan MF. Toll-like receptors, inflammation and cancer. Sem Cancer Biol. 2006;16:32–7.
Tsang KW, Lam CL, Yan C et al. Coriolus versicolor polysaccharide peptide slows progression of advanced non-small cell lung cancer. Respir Med. 2003;97:618–24.
Tse KW, Wan CK, Shen XL et al. Honokiol inhibits TNF-alpha-stimulated NF-κB activation and NF-κB-regulated gene expression through suppression of IKK activation. Biochem Pharmacol. 2005;70:1443–57.
Uma Devi P. *Withania somnifera* Dunal (Ashwagandha): potential plant source of a promising drug for cancer chemotherapy and radiosensitization. Indian J Exp Biol. 1996;34:927–32.
Uma Devi P, Ganasoundari A. Radioprotective effect of leaf extract of Indian medicinal plant *Ocimum sanctum*. Indian J Exp Biol. 1995;33:205–9.
Uma Devi P, Utsumi H, Takata M et al. Enhancement of radiation-induced cell death in chicken B lymphocytes by Withaferin A. Indian J Exp Biol. 2008;46:437–42.
Urtasun RC. Chemical modifiers of radiation. In: Leibel SA and Phillips TL (eds). Text book of radiation oncology. Philadelphia, USA:WB Saunders Company; 1998. 42–52.
Valenzuela MT, Mateos S, Almmodoavar JMR et al. Variation in sensitizing effect of caffeine in human tumour cell lines after gamma-irradiation. Radiother Oncol. 2000;54:261–71.
Wang RF. Regulatory T cells and toll-like receptors in cancer therapy. Cancer Res. 2006;66: 4987–90.
Wang H, Li A, Dong XP et al. Screening of anti-tumor parts from the seeds of *Livistonia chinensis* and its anti-angiogenesis effect. J Chin Med Mater. 2008;31:718–22.
Wang S, Zheng Z, Weng Y et al. Angiogenesis and anti-angiogenesis activity of Chinese medicinal herbal extracts. Life Sci. 2004;74:2467–78.
Weiss JF, Simic MG. Perspectives in radioprotection. Pharmacol Ther. 1988;39:1–414.
Wessells J, Busse AC, Rave-Frank M et al. Photosensitizing and radiosensitizing effects of Hypericin on human renal carcinoma cells in vitro. Photochem Photobiol. 2007;84:228–35.
Wong CK, Bao YX, Wong EL et al. Immunomodulatory activities of Yunzhi and Danshen in post-treatment breast cancer patients. Am J Chin Med. 2005;33:381–95.
Wong RK, Jones GW, Sagar SM et al. A Phase I–II study in the use of acupuncture-like transcutaneous nerve stimulation in the treatment of radiation-induced xerostomia in head-and-neck cancer patients treated with radical radiotherapy. Int J Radiat Oncol Biol Phys. 2003;57:472–80.
Wong R, Sagar S. Acupuncture for chemotherapy-induced peripheral neuropathy: a case series. Acupunct Med. 2006;24:87–91.
Wong CK, Tse PS, Wong EL et al. Immunomodulatory effects of Yunzhi and Danshen Capsules in healthy subjects: a randomized, double-blind, placebo-controlled, crossover study. Int Immunopharmacol. 2004;4:201–11.
Xu GZ, Cai WM, Qin DX et al. Chinese herb "destagnation" series I: Combination of radiation with destagnation in the treatment of nasopharyngeal carcinoma: A prospective randomized trial on 188 cases. Int J Radiat Oncol Biol Phys. 1989;16:297–300.
Xu TM, Xin Y, Cui MH et al. Inhibitory effect of ginsenoside Rg3 combined with cyclophosphamide on growth and angiogenesis of ovarian cancer. Chin Med J. 2007;120:584–88.
Xu L, Yang D, Wang S et al. Gossypol enhances response to radiotherapy and results in tumour regression of human prostate cancer. Mol Cancer Ther. 2005;4:197–205.
Yance DR, Sagar SM. Targeting angiogenesis with integrative cancer therapies. Integr Cancer Ther. 2006;5:9–29.
Yang LM, DeBusk KF, Fingleton B. Expansion of myeloid immune suppressor Gr+CD11b+cells in tumor-bearing host directly promotes tumor angiogenesis. Cancer Cell. 2004;6:409–21.
Yang SH, Lin JK, Chen WS et al. Anti-angiogenic effect of silymarin on colon cancer LoVo cell line. J Surg Res. 2003;113:133–8.

Yang X, Lu Y, Xie D. Protective effect of *Radix salvia miltorrhizae* on radiation damage of the cochlea. Hunan Yi Ke Da Xue Bao. 1999;24:465–7.

Yonezawa M, Katoh N, Takeda A. Restoration of radiation injury by Ginseng IV. Stimulation of recoveries in CFU and megakaryocyte counts related to the prevention of occult blood appearance in x-irradiated mice. J Radiat Res. 1985;26:436–42.

Yonezawa M, Katoh N, Takeda A. Radiation protection by shigoka extract on split-dose in mice. J Radiat Res. 1989;30:247–54.

Yoon TJ, Yoo YC, Choi OB et al. Inhibitory effect of Korean mistletoe (Viscum album coloratum) extract on tumour angiogenesis and metastasis of haematogenous and non-haematogenous tumour cells in mice. Cancer Lett. 1995;97:83–91.

Zaidman BZ, Yassin M, Mahajna J et al. Medicinal mushroom modulators of molecular targets as cancer therapeutics. Appl Microbiol Biotechnol. 2005;67:453–8.

Zeng F, Hon CC, Sit WH et al. Molecular characterization of *Coriolus versicolor* PSP-induced apoptosis in human promyelotic leukemic HL-60 cells using cDNA microarray. Int J Oncol. 2005;27:513–23.

Zhang W, Anker L, Law RE et al. Enhancement of radiosensitivity in human malignant glioma cells by hypericin in vitro. Clin Cancer Res. 1996;2:843–6.

Zhang B, Bowerman NA, Salama JK et al. Induced sensitization of tumor stroma leads to eradication of established cancer by T cells. J Exp Med. 2007;204:49–55.

Zhang L, Rui YC, Yang PY et al. Inhibitory effects of *Ginkgo biloba* extract on vascular endothelial growth factor in rat aortic endothelial cells. Acta Pharmacol Sin. 2002;23:919–23.

Zhang JS, Sigdestad CP, Gemmell MA et al. Modification of radiation response in mice by fractionated extracts of *Panax ginseng*. Radiat Res. 1987;112:156–63.

Zoberi I, Bradberry CM, Curry HA et al. Radiosensitizing and anTiproliferative effects of resveratrol in two human cervical tumour cell lines. Cancer Lett. 2002;175:165–73.

Zukowska-Grojek Z, Karatowska-Prokopczuk E, Fisher TA et al. Mechanisms of vascular growth-promoting effects of neuropeptide Y: role of its inducible receptors. Regul Pept. 1998;75–76:231–8.

Chapter 7
Controlling Chemotherapy-Related Side Effects with Chinese Medicine

Shwu-Huey Liu, Yung-Chi Cheng, and Muhammad W. Saif

Abstract Chemotherapy remains a mainstream treatment for patients with advanced malignant tumours that are incurable by either local surgery or radiotherapy, but the success of chemotherapy is often limited by the occurrence of side effects. Some chemotherapy-induced side effects may be mitigated by conventional medicine, but a holistic approach cannot be accomplished. Realizing that Western medicine has limitations for the treatment of diseases such as cancer, diabetes and Alzheimer's disease, consumers and researchers in the US are paying more attention to complementary and alternative medicine (CAM), especially herbal medicine, as a way to counter such limitations. Traditional Chinese medicine (TCM) represents the well-documented type of herbal medicine. Traditional Chinese medicine is widely used by cancer patients in Asia as a way to reduce chemotherapy-induced side effects or control cancer progression, but TCM may also enhance the anticancer activity of chemotherapy. The major challenges facing acceptance of traditional Chinese medicine in non-Asian countries lie in the areas of manufacturing, preclinical and clinical studies, regulatory approval, education and legislation.

7.1 Introduction

Medical oncology has had a great impact in changing the practice of medicine in the past several decades as curative treatments for a variety of previously fatal malignancies have been identified. However, few categories of drugs in common use have a narrower therapeutic index and a greater potential for causing harmful side effects than do the antineoplastic drugs (Calabresi and Chabner 1996). Anticancer agents, like many other potent drugs with only moderate selectivity, may cause severe toxicity. This chapter presents information to support the premise that complementary and alternative medicine (CAM), particularly traditional Chinese medicine (TCM),

---

M.W. Saif (✉)
School of Medicine, Yale Cancer Center, Yale University, New Haven, CT, USA
e-mail: wasif.saif@yale.edu

W.C.S. Cho (ed.), *Supportive Cancer Care with Chinese Medicine*,
DOI 10.1007/978-90-481-3555-4_7,

may have a role in alleviating some of the side effects that occur with cancer chemotherapy and in enhancing the effectiveness of such chemotherapy.

7.1.1 Cancer

Many of us tend to think of cancer as a disease of our modern age, but people throughout history recognized the uniqueness of some tumours and sought to find treatments for them. Whether physicians in ancient times were able to distinguish malignant from benign tumours is uncertain, but as early as the first century AD there are references to treatment of what we know today as cancer or tumours. Modern chemotherapy has its roots deep in this past.

7.2 Cancer Chemotherapy

Chemotherapy, one facet of the armamentarium for the treatment of cancer, employs chemicals to destroy cancer cells. The drugs used for this purpose are varied in both their structure and in the way that they kill cancer cells. Table 7.1 lists some of the commonly used anticancer agents grouped according to type and/or site of action. Some of the drugs listed are available under more than one trade name, but for the sake of brevity, only one registered trade name is given.

Table 7.1 Cancer chemotherapeutic agents

Type and/or site of action	Drug name(s)
Alkylating agents	
Nitrogen mustard	Chlorambucil (Leukeran), cyclophosphamide (Cytoxan), isosfamide (IFEX), estramustine (Emcyt), mechlorethamine (Mustargen), melphalan (Megace)
Ethylenimine derivative	Thiotepa (triethylenethiophosphoramide, Thioplex)
Alkyl sulfonate	Busulfan (Myleran)
Nitrosourea	Carmustine (BiCNU), lomustine (CeeNU), semustine (methyl-CCNU)[a], streptozotocin (Zanosar)
Triazine	Dacarbazine (DTIC-Dome)
Metal salt	Cisplatin (Platinol), carboplatin (Paraplatin), oxaliplatin (Eloxatin)
Antimetabolites	
Folic acid analog	Methotrexate (Trexall)
Pyrimidine analog	Azacytidine (Vidaza), cytarabine (Cytosar), floxuridine (FUDR), fluorouracil (Efudex)

Table 7.1 (continued)

Type and/or site of action	Drug name(s)
Purine analog	Mercaptopurine (Purinethol), thioguanine (Tabloid), pentostatin (Nipent), cladribine (Leustatin), fludarabine (Fludara)
Natural products	
Mitiotic inhibitor	Vinblastine (Velban), vincristine (Oncovin), vindesine (Eldisine)[a], vinorelbine (Navelbine)
Microtubule polymer stabilizer	Paclitaxel (Taxol), docetaxel (Taxotere)
Podophyllum derivative	Etoposide (VP-16, Vepesid), teniposide (VM-26, Vumon)
Antibiotic	Bleomycin (Blenoxane), dactinomycin (Cosmegen), daunorubicin (DaunoXome), doxorubicin (Adriamycin), idarubicin (Idamycin), epirubicin (Ellence), plicamycin (Mithracin), mitomycin (Mutamycin), mitoxantrone (Novantrone), epirubicin (Ellence)
Enzyme	Asparaginase (Elspar)
Hormones and hormone antagonists	
Androgen	Fluoxymesterone (Halotestin) and others
Corticosteroid	Prednisone (Deltasone), dexamethasone (Decadron)
Estrogen	Diethylstilbestrol (DES)
Progestin	Megestrol acetate (Megace), medroxyprogesterone acetate (Provera)
Estrogen antagonist	Tamoxifen (Nolvadex)
Androgen antagonist	Flutamide (Eulexin), finasteride (Proscar), bicalutamide (Casodex)
Luteinzing hormone-releasing hormone (LHRH) agonist	Leuprolide (Lupron), goserelin (Zoladex)
Signal transduction inhibitors	
Tyrosine kinase inhibitors	Gefitinib (Iressa), imatinib (Gleevec), sorafenib (Nexavar), sunitinib (Sutent)
Monoclonal antibodies	
Epidermal growth factor receptor (EGFR) binder	Cetuximab (Erbitux)
HER-2 receptor binder	Trastuzumab (Herceptin)
B-cell inhibitors	Rituximab (Rituxan), alemtuzumab (Campath)
Antiangiogenesis agent [vascular endothelial growth factor (VEGF)-targeting monoclonal antibody]	Bevacizumab (Avastin)
Miscellaneous agents	
Substituted urea	Hydroxyurea (Hydrea)

Table 7.1 (continued)

Type and/or site of action	Drug name(s)
Methylhydrazine derivative	Procarbazine (Matulane)
Adrenocortical suppressant	Mitotane (Lysodren)
Steroid synthesis inhibitor	Aminoglutethimide (Cytadren)
Substituted melamine	Altretamine (hexamethylmelamine, Hexalen)
Acridine dye	Amascrine (Amsidine)[a]

[a]Investigational agents, not yet approved by the FDA for general use.

7.3 Side Effects of Cancer Chemotherapy

One of the characteristics that distinguish cancer chemotherapeutic agents from most other drugs is the frequency and severity of anticipated side effects at usual therapeutic doses. Most toxicity varies with specific agent, dose, schedule of administration, route of administration and predisposing factors in the patient, which may be known and predictive for toxicity or unknown and result in unexpected toxic effects. Such toxicities occur because the chemotherapy is very effective in killing cancer cells, but also deleteriously affects normal cells. Because of the severity of the side effects, it is critical to carefully monitor the patient for adverse reactions so therapy can be modified before the toxicity becomes life-threatening.

7.3.1 Types of Side Effects

Commonly-seen side effects of chemotherapy include gastrointestinal tract problems, hair loss, low blood cell counts, skin rashes, fatigue and infertility.

7.3.1.1 Gastrointestinal Side Effects

Gastrointestinal (GI) side effects are related to the esophagus, stomach, intestines, colon and bladder, and may include nausea, diarrhea, constipation, loss of appetite and mouth sores.

7.3.1.2 Myelosuppression

Chemotherapy affects the rapidly dividing cells of the bone marrow much like it affects cancer cells and many blood cells die, or is not produced, as a result. The decreased output of any of these cells can lead to anemia, neutropenia, and thrombocytopenia. As a result, many patients with these symptoms can exhibit fatigue, be subject to infection, or have blood-clotting difficulties.

7.3.1.3 Alopecia

Hair loss can occur because the chemotherapy causes hair follicles to stop reproducing, bringing hair growth to a halt. In addition to this, the weakened follicle is no longer able to support the hair strand coming out of it. The hair strand then either breaks off or falls out due to lack of support. The hair will grow back when the chemotherapy has stopped.

7.3.1.4 Sexual Side Effects

Chemotherapy may also cause low sperm counts or damage to the ovaries. In some cases, these effects are permanent.

7.3.1.5 Constitutional Side Effects

Fatigue, lack of energy, etc.

7.3.1.6 Delayed Organ Toxicities

Cardiac toxicity, pulmonary toxicity, nephrotoxicity, neurotoxicity, and hepatotoxicity may all be a consequence of cancer chemotherapy.

7.3.2 Drug-Specific Side Effects

Some chemotherapy-induced side effects are less common than others and are specific to individual drugs or classes of drugs. Examples of drugs and their related toxicities include the following.

- Vinca alkaloids: neurotoxicity
- Ifosamide and cyclophosphamide: hemorrhagic cystitis
- Anthracyclines: cardiomyopathy
- Bleomycin: pulmonary fibrosis
- Asparaginase: anaphylaxis (allergic reaction)
- Cisplatin: renal toxicity, neurotoxicity
- Ifosfamide: central nervous system toxicity
- Mitomycin: hemolytic-uremic syndrome
- Procarbazine: food and drug interactions

Anyone who administers chemotherapeutic agents must be familiar with the expected and the unusual toxicities of the chemotherapeutic agents the patient is receiving, and be prepared to avert severe toxicity when possible, and able to manage toxic complications when they cannot be avoided.

Cancer treatment can unleash a host of problems. Supportive medications have been developed to manage such toxicities. However, these medications carry their own toxicity profile.

7.3.3 Current Approaches to the Management of the Side Effects of Cancer Chemotherapy

As noted above, the side effects associated with the use of cancer chemotherapeutic drugs can often be severe enough that the chemotherapeutic treatment regimen must be modified (drug dosage reduced, treatment delayed) or they may even be life-threatening. Various drugs are employed to ameliorate chemotherapy-induced side effects as much as possible, so that the beneficial effects of such chemotherapy can be maximized. Some of these drugs are discussed below for the two most common classes of chemotherapy-induced side effects.

7.3.3.1 Gastrointestinal Side Effects

Nausea and vomiting are usually treated with antinauseants/antiemetics such as Aloxi (palonosetron HCl), Anzemet (dolasetron mesylate) Emend (aprepitant), Kytril (granisetron), Marinol (dronabinol) and Zofran (ondansetron). When acid reflux, ulcers and stomach pain are problems, drugs such as Aciphex (rabeprazole sodium), Nexium (esomeprazole magnesium), Prevacid (lansoprazole), Prilosec (omeprazole), Protonix (pantoprazole sodium), Zantac (ranitidine), Pepcid (famotidine) or Tagamet (cimetidine) can be given. In many cases, diarrhea can be treated with Imodium (loperamide) or Lomotil (diphenoxylate/atropine). Laxatives and stool softeners can usually successfully treat constipation; Examples include Colace (docusate), Dulcolax (bisacodyl), Kristalose (lactulose) and Senokot (senna).

7.3.3.2 Myelosuppression

Red blood cells or platelets can be replaced by transfusions, packed red blood cells, or platelets. Transfusions of white blood cells are ineffective and rarely given. Injections of growth factors are often used in cases of myelosuppression. These chemicals stimulate the bone marrow to make blood cells. Different growth factors are used to stimulate the different types of blood cells. Erythropoietin (EPO, Epogen) is used to stimulate red blood cell production, granulocyte colony-stimulating factor (G-CSF, filgastrim, Neupogen, Granocyte, Neulasta) and granulocyte-macrophage colony-stimulating factor (GM-CSF, sargramostim, Leukine) stimulate white blood cell production, and interleukin-11 (oprevelkin, Neumega) can increase platelet numbers. Erythropoietin injections can decrease the need for a transfusion and improve the quality of life. This drug has few side effects if the kidneys are healthy. G-CSF and GM-CSF can speed the return of neutrophils. Side effects seen with the use of G-CSF and GM-CSF include bone pain, fevers, rashes, muscle pains, and nausea. Interleukin-11 can increase platelet numbers. Use of interleukin-11 can result in fluid retention, a rapid heartbeat, red eyes, and difficulty breathing. Careful monitoring of possible neutropenia in cancer patients is important. If a cancer patient has a fever and other signs of possible infection, injected antibiotics may be employed, possibly for several days.

7.4 Historical Use of Chinese Medicine for Cancer Treatment

Realizing the limitations of Western medicine in the treatment of diseases with unmet needs, such as cancer and Alzheimer's disease, consumers and researchers alike in the US are giving more attention to CAM. According to recent studies, herbal therapies represent the most commonly used CAM; 18.6% of the population (over 38 million US adults) has used herbal medicines. In fact, these numbers may be higher since it is estimated that more than 50% of those who use herbal therapies did not disclose this information to a conventional medical professional (Eisenberg et al. 1998; Tindle et al. 2005).

Herbal medicine has been in use for centuries by peoples worldwide. In the United States, herbs have become commercially valuable in the dietary supplement industry and as such, they are monitored by the Food and Drug Administration (FDA) under the Dietary Supplement and Health Education Act (DSHEA) of 1994. According to a report by Gardiner et al. (2007), the top selling herbs were *Echinacea purpurea* (echinacea) (41%), *Panax ginseng* (ginseng) (25%), *Ginkgo biloba* (ginkgo seed) (22%) and *Allium satirum* (garlic) (20%); these are used to promote good health or improve quality of life (QoL). It was estimated that the global dietary supplement industry is projected to reach $187 billion by 2010 (Lersch et al. 1992; Tindle et al. 2005; Bar-Sela et al. 2007; Gardiner et al. 2007). Botanicals have also become a focal point for the identification of new active agents for the treatment of diseases. Active compounds, derived from plant extracts, are of continuing interest to the pharmaceutical industry. For example, taxol, an antineoplastic drug originally obtained from the bark of the Pacific yew tree, has been found to be widely useful in the treatment of different forms of cancer (Wani et al. 1971).

There are many types of herbal medicine around the world; these include Ayurveda, Unani, Sida and TCM. Of all herbal medicine types, experiences with TCM are the best documented. The first written Chinese medical document came from the Han dynasty (206 BC–AD 220) (Huang 1999). Western medicine generally uses purified compounds, either natural or synthetic, mostly directed towards a single physiological target. However, the compositions used in TCM are usually composed of multiple herbs and compounds which are aimed at multiple targets in the body based on unique and holistic concepts. Traditional Chinese medicine mainly uses processed crude natural products, in various combinations and formulations, to treat different maladies and the use of such formulations often results in few side effects based on conventional usage. The great potential of TCM has yet to be realized for the majority of the world's people.

The use of TCM is based on the interaction of multiple components acting synergistically and multifactorially to regulate functions of the body. The multiple components in a Chinese herbal formulation serve various functions; some provide efficacy while others decrease toxicity or enhance absorption of other phytochemical components in the same formula. Using a mixture of plant extracts instead of an isolated compound for the management of diseases is gaining greater appreciation in Western countries and represents the unique feature of Chinese herbal medicine. However, with reports of increasing incidences of herbal toxicities due to conventional used and the concern for herb-drug interactions when botanicals are used with Western medicines, tighter regulation on the use of botanicals will undoubtedly be forthcoming (Wong et al. 2001; Liu et al. 2004; Sagar and Wong 2008).

Traditional Chinese medicine has been claimed to relieve some of the symptoms that occur as side effects of the use of Western cancer chemotherapeutic agents. In addition, TCM has been reported to boost the immune system, and to help patients reduce stress through both herbal and physical interventions (Monro 2003; Shu et al. 2005; Wu et al. 2005; Quimby 2007; Armstrong and Gilbert 2008; Ito et al. 2008; Ragupathi et al. 2008; Wu et al. 2009).

Several commonly used TCM herbs, such as *Angelica sinensis* (Chinese angelica root), *Astragalus membranaceus* (astragalus root), *Coriolus versicolor* (multicolored polypore), *Panax ginseng* (ginseng) and *Ganoderma lucidum* (lucid ganoderma), have been claimed to have immunomodulatory activity in cancer patients and several traditional TCM formulas also have been claimed to have chemotherapeutic properties. Some of these TCM herbs or formulas are discussed in the following paragraphs.

7.4.1 Chinese Angelica Root

Chinese angelica root also known as Danggui, is used for strengthening the body organs and nourishing blood. It is also used to treat menstrual disorders as well as radiation-induced pneumonitis in humans (Xie et al. 2006). The latter effect is thought to be due to down-regulation, during the pneumonic phase, of tumor necrosis factor-α (TNF-α) and transforming growth factor-β1 (TGF-β1) in inflammatory cells of irradiated tissue. Recent preclinical studies indicated that the extract of Chinese angelica root also showed a dramatic anti-tumour effect, causing growth arresting and apoptosis of malignant brain tumours in vitro and in vivo; both p53-dependent and p53-independent pathways of apoptosis were involved in the cytotoxic mechanisms (Tsai et al. 2006; Kan et al. 2008). Chinese angelica root may also exert antiangiogenic effects. A case study by Armstrong suggested the potential use of Chinese angelica root for the treatment of brain tumours.

7.4.2 Astragalus Root

Astragalus root also known as Huangqi, is a Chinese medicinal plant commonly used to treat patients with deficiency in vitality which symptomatically presents with fatigue, diarrhea and lack of appetite. It has been reported that herbal formulations containing astragalus root can produce hepatoprotective (Cui et al. 2003), antiviral and antioxidative effects (Li et al. 2006). Recently, evidence from various animal and clinical studies has demonstrated that astragalus root may possess anticarcinogenic properties, which could attenuate the systemic side effects of some conventional antineoplastic drugs (Cho and Leung 2007). It has been shown to be capable of restoring impaired T-cell functions in cancer patients by activating the anti-tumour immune mechanism of the host. It has also been used to ameliorate the side effects of antineoplastic drugs because of its immunomodulatory nature. Recent studies demonstrated that total astragalus saponins (AST) possess anticarcinogenic and proapoptotic properties in human colon cancer cells and in tumour xenografts models (Auyeung et al. 2009).

Side effects, including nausea and vomiting, sore mouth, diarrhea, hepatotoxicity, myelosuppression and immunosuppression, are commonly encountered in patients with colorectal cancer who are treated with chemotherapy. A variety of Chinese herbal medicines have been used for managing these adverse effects. The results of a limited meta-analysis from four related randomized clinical trials were recently reported by Wu et al. (2005). These studies compared chemotherapy only or chemotherapy plus anti-emetics (tropisetron, sulpiride, etc) with chemotherapy plus Chinese herbs. All of the studies used a decoction containing astragalus compounds as the intervention with chemotherapy. Due to the methodological limitations of the studies, there is no robust demonstration of benefit. However, no evidence of harm arising from the use of Chinese herbs was found. The authors suggested that high quality randomized controlled studies investigating the effects of decoctions of Chinese herbs, particularly astragalus root, upon chemotherapy-related side effects should be conducted.

7.4.3 Ginseng

Ginseng has been viewed as a panacea and a promoter for longevity in Asia since the Han dynasty. The efficacy of ginseng has been known in the West since the eighteenth century. Ginseng's pharmacological effects have included cardiovascular, neurologic, hematologic, immunologic and antineoplastic effects (Forman 1994; Attele et al. 1999; Konkimalla and Efferth 2008; Yang et al. 2008; Barton et al. 2009; Fishbein et al. 2009). Seven major species of ginseng are distributed in East Asia, Central Asia and North America. Three common species: *Panax ginseng* (Asian ginseng), *Panax quinquefolium* (American ginseng) and *Panax japonicus* (Japanese ginseng) have been studied extensively. In vitro studies, animal models, case studies and cohort studies suggested that ginseng may prevent or ameliorate various cancers.

Ginsenosides are being considered as the active ingredients of ginseng for most of its pharmacological actions (Ota et al.1987; Yun and Choi 1995; Gillis 1997). More than 20 ginsenosides have been identified; several of these, such as Rh2, have been shown to have direct cytotoxic and growth inhibitory activities against tumour cells. In vitro studies indicated that Rh2 arrested cell cycle progression at the G1 stage in B16-BL6 melanoma cells. Intravenously or orally administered ginsenoside Rg3 led to a decrease in lung metastasis of B16-BL6 melanoma cells. Choi et al. (1995) showed that total ginseng extracts enhance the proofreading activity of eukaryotic DNA polymerase. Preclinical studies suggested that ginseng may have a non-organ-specific anticarcinogenic effect. Kim et al. (1998) suggested that ginseng possesses some immunomodulatory properties, primarily associated with NK cell activity. However, a large-scale double-blind, randomized, placebo-controlled clinical study is needed to validate these hypotheses.

The results of a cross-sectional survey among 160 patients with cancer receiving outpatient chemotherapy at a medical center in northern Taiwan have been reported by Yang et al. (2008). A majority of the participants reported CAM use ($n = 157$, 98.1%). Over fifteen percent (15.3%) of patients took grape seed and ginseng while over fourteen percent (14.4%) of patients did not know the name of the herbs they took. The most commonly reported reasons for CAM use were to boost the immune system (55.4%) and relieve stress (53.5%).

A randomized, double-blind, dose-finding evaluation of American ginseng was conducted at the Mayo Clinic (Barton et al. 2009). This pilot trial sought to investigate whether any of three doses of American ginseng might help cancer-related fatigue. A secondary aim was to evaluate toxicity. Two hundred and ninety patients were accrued to this trial. Non-significant trends for all outcomes were seen in favor of the 1,000 and 2,000 mg/day doses of American ginseng. More than twice as many patients on American ginseng perceived a benefit and were satisfied with treatment as compared to those on placebo. There were no significant differences in any measured toxicities between any of the arms. It was concluded that there appeared to be some beneficial effects on cancer-related fatigue at the 1,000–2,000 mg/day doses of American ginseng; toxicity at these dose levels was tolerable.

Although previous studies showed that ginseng may help cancer and/or cancer supportive care, there is limited data exploring the use of ginseng as an adjuvant to chemotherapy, and minimal mechanistic studies related to possible synergism between ginseng and the chemotherapeutic agent. Further studies of ginseng in well designed clinical studies are necessary.

7.4.4 Ganoderma

Ganoderma is the most popular and intensely investigated genus among the medically active mushrooms. It is also well known as Lingzhi (Chinese) or Reishi (Japanese). Ganoderma has been used in China for longevity and health promotion since ancient times. Within the genus ganoderma, over 250 taxonomic names have been reported worldwide including *Ganoderma lucidum*, *Ganoderma sinense* and *Ganoderma tsugae* (Boh et al. 2007). The most popular species is *Ganoderma lucidum* (lucid ganoderma), a polypore mushroom that grows on the lower trunks of deciduous trees. Dried powder of lucid ganoderma was popular as a cancer chemotherapy agent in ancient China. Among the many bioactive molecules isolated from ganoderma extracts, the most striking are triterpenes and polysaccharides. The major use of ganoderma extracts in controlled clinical settings has been as an immune stimulant (Zhuang et al. 2009). Ganoderma is widely used in traditional treatments of cancer (Yuen and Gohel 2005; Mahajna et al. 2009), and lucid ganoderma has been extensively studied in vitro in cancer cells and in vivo animal models (Zhou et al. 2007; Weng et al. 2008). Lucid ganoderma extracts exhibited anticancer activity in the in vitro systems against a variety of cancer cells including leukemia, lymphoma, breast, prostate, liver, lung and myeloma cell lines. The anticancer activity of lucid ganoderma includes the inhibition of proliferation, induction of apoptosis, induction of cell cycle arrest, inhibition of invasive behavior, and suppression tumour angiogenesis in many experimental systems including prostate cancer. Pharmacological studies indicated that the mechanism of action of lucid ganoderma includes its inhibition of the function of androgen receptors and interference with the PI3K/Akt/NF-κB pathway (Weng et al. 2008). It also has been shown that lucid ganoderma extracts exhibit diverse pharmacologic functions (Zhou et al. 2007).

Lucid ganoderma has been reported to be associated with suppressed motility, invasion and metastasis of several types of cancers, but its exact mechanism of action still remains unclear. Its preclinical anticancer activities have been used to support its use for cancer treatment and prevention. It remains debatable as to whether ganoderma is a food supplement for health maintenance or actually a therapeutic drug for medical proposes. Thus far there has been no report of human trials using ganoderma as a direct anticancer agent, despite some evidence showing the usage of ganoderma as a potential supplement to cancer patients.

A number of clinical trials have shown promising efficacies of lucid ganoderma extracts or powders in cancer treatment as well as in other indications. However, some of the clinical trials were not well designed and lacked appropriate controls. It is strongly believed that there is a need to explore the full potential of lucid ganoderma to assess its safety and efficacy in well-designed, double-blind, randomized, placebo-controlled clinical trials as a stand-alone treatment or in combination with other treatments.

7.5 Recent Developments in the Clinical Use of Chinese Medicines for Cancer Treatment in the United States

Although there are no FDA approvals to date for an oral botanical drug, the FDA has taken the first steps by creating a blueprint for botanical drug approval in a document entitled "Guidance for Industry: Botanical Drug Products" published in June of 2004 and by approving the first botanical drug, Veregen, as a topical lotion to treat genital and perianal warts in October 2006 (Mayeaux and Dunton 2008). Several botanical products have been reported to be under study in the US for the treatment of cancer or for cancer supportive care.

7.5.1 PC-SPES

PC-SPES was commercially available from November 1996 until 2002. PC-SPES was a combination of eight different herbs: *Chrysanthemum morifolium* (chrysanthemum flower), *Ganoderma lucidum* (lucid ganoderma), *Glycyrrhiza uralensis*

Table 7.2 Constituent herbs in PC-SPES

Scientific name	Common name	Chinese pinyin
Chrysanthemum morifolium	Chrysanthemum flower	Juhua
Isatis tinctoria	Indigowoad root	Banlangen
Glycyrrhiza uralensis	Licorice root	Gancao
Ganoderma lucidum	Lucid ganoderma	Lingzhi
Panax notoginseng	Notoginseng	Sanqi
Rabdosia rubescens	Blushred rabdosia	Donglingcao
Serenoa repens	Saw palmetto	Juzonglu
Scutellaria baicalensis	Baikal skullcap root	Huangqin

(licorice root), *Isatis tinctoria* (indigowoad root), *Panax notoginseng* (notoginseng), *Rabdosia rubescens* (blushred rabdosia), baikal skullcap root and *Serenoa repens* (saw palmetto) (Table 7.2). PC-SPES was marketed for its effects in reducing prostate specific antigen (PSA) levels, improving pain, and enhancing the QoL of those with hormone-refractory prostate cancer (DiPaola et al. 1998; De la Taille et al. 1999, 2000; Small et al. 2000; Meyer and Gillatt 2002). There have been 119 clinical and preclinical studies of PC-SPES published to date, but there have been no randomized controlled trials conducted.

Small et al. (2000) conducted the largest PC-SPES clinical study in 70 patients. Thirty-three men with androgen-dependent prostate cancer and 37 men with androgen-independent prostate cancer were enrolled in the study. Each patient received up to 9 capsules of PC-SPES per day (each capsule contained 320 mg). The most beneficial dose was not determined in the study. It was reported that all 33 of the androgen-dependent group experienced a reduction in prostate specific antigen (PSA) of >80% and that 19 of the 37 with androgen-independent prostate cancer experienced a >50% decrease in their PSA. Although this report indicated that further study was needed, it was concluded that PC-SPES seemed to have activity in the treatment of both androgen-dependent and -independent prostate cancer. It was claimed that the toxicity of PC-SPES was tolerable. However, the claim of acceptable toxicity should be questioned as three out of 70 patients developed a pulmonary embolus, two developed left ventricular dysfunction and four developed hypertriglyceridemia.

There are differences in the frequency of side effects between different studies with PC-SPES. However, the De la Teille et al. (1999, 2000) trial, along with others, contained no placebo arm and involved only small numbers of patients (Kellis and Vickery 1984; Small et al. 2000). As such, these trials are limited in the conclusive evidence that can be provided to support the use of PC-SPES in the treatment of hormone-refractory prostate cancer. All other studies so far conducted only contain small numbers of patients, thus, only limited conclusions can be drawn from them.

Attempts to identify the active compounds in PC-SPES have yielded incongruous results. Moreover, warfarin was identified in the serum of a patient taking PC-SPES who experienced a bleeding disorder. Sovak et al. (2002) analyzed PC-SPES lots manufactured from 1996 through mid-2001 and found that PC-SPES lots manufactured from 1996 through mid-1999 contained the synthetic compounds indomethacin (range = 1.07–13.19 mg/g) and diethylstilbestrol (range = 107.28–159.27 μg/g). They also found that batches of PC-SPES manufactured from 1996 through mid-1999 had two to six times more antineoplastic and up to 50 times more estrogenic activity than lots manufactured after the spring of 1999. In lots manufactured after mid-1999, gradual declines in the concentrations of indomethacin (from 1.56 to 0.70 mg/g), diethylstilbestrol (from 46.36 to 0.00 μg/g), and total phytosterols (from 0.586 to 0.085 mg/g) were observed. Warfarin was identified for the first time in lots manufactured after July 1998 (range = 341–560 μg/g). In the August 2001 lot, increases were found in concentrations of the natural products licochalcone A (from 27.6 to 289.2 μg/g) and baicalin (from 12.5 to 38.8 mg/g). The phytochemical composition of PC-SPES varied by lot, and chemical analyses detected various amounts of the synthetic drugs diethylstilbestrol, indomethacin, warfarin and several natural products.

To qualify for clinical pharmacologic exploration, nutritional supplements including herbal mixtures should meet standards of quality control under the Good Manufacturing Practice (GMP) system, and the manufacturers of such supplements should provide reliable analytical quality assurance. Although PC-SPES had shown some promising clinical results in patients with prostate cancer, the fatal flaw with PC-SPES was in the more fundamental issue of product integrity (Marcus and Grollman 2002; White 2002; Larimore and O'Mathuna 2003). The California Department of Health Services issued a warning about the product and its manufacturer, BotanicLab in February 2002. Simultaneously, the manufacturer voluntarily recalled PC-SPES nationwide. The FDA published a medical product safety alert, and Canada and Ireland also announced recalls of the product. A multicenter clinical trial comparing PC-SPES and diethylstilbestrol was stopped. BotanicLab went out of business in June 2002 and PC-SPES is no longer available.

7.5.2 Selected Vegetables and Herb Mix

Lung carcinoma is the leading cause of cancer related deaths in North America. Non-small cell lung cancer (NSCLC) causes the death of more than 400,000 patients annually in the US and Western Europe. The benefit of conventional therapies, such as chemotherapy and radiotherapy, for unresectable stage IIIB and IV NSCLC patients is marginal; the generally accepted median survival time of late stage patients has remained 4–6 months in the supportive care group and 6–9 months in the chemotherapy treatment group; the one-year survival is about 20%. The NCI, in a recent publication, concluded that more effective treatments for NSCLC are urgently needed (Sun et al. 1999).

To achieve the goals of (1) prolonged patient survival, (2) minimal toxicity, (3) improvement in the patient's QoL, and (4) reduction of the expense of current chemotherapy for advanced NSCLC, Selected Vegetables and Herb Mix, also called Sun's Soup, which consists of 19 botanicals, has been promoted as a treatment for NSCLC cancer. There have been several formulas of the soup, two of which are marketed in the United States as dietary supplements. One type called Selected Vegetables (SV) consists of 19 freeze-dried vegetable and herb ingredients, including *Glycine max* (soya bean), *Lentinus edodes* (Shiitake mushroom), *Ziziphus jujuba* (red date), *Allium ascalonicum* (scallion), *Allium satirum* (garlic), *Lens culinaris* (lentils), *Allium tuberosum* (leek), *Phaseolus radiatus* (mung bean), *Crataegus cuneata* (hawthorn fruit), *Allium cepa* (onion), American ginseng, *Angelica dahurica* (angelica root), licorice root, *Taraxacum officinale* (dandelion root), *Polygala senega* (senegal root), *Zingiber officinale* (ginger), *Olea europaea* (olive), *Sesamum indicum* (sesame seed) and *Petroselinum crispum* (parsley). The second formula is called Frozen Selected Vegetables (FSV). Either type of Selected Vegetables soup is taken as part of the diet.

In 1999, the results of a phase I/II study in which SV was used in patients with NSCLC, was published (Sun et al. 1999). All patients were treated with conventional therapies (surgery, chemotherapy and radiation therapy). Selected Vegetables was added to the daily diet of 5 stage I patients in the toxicity study group (TG) and 6 stage III and IV patients in the treatment group (SVG), but not to the diet of 13 stage III and IV patients in the control group (CG). The study was not randomized or blinded. It was found that Karnofsky performance status declined in the CG patients (79 ± 8 to 55 ± 11) but improved in the SVG patients (75 ± 8 to 80 ± 13) one to three months after treatment. The median survival time and mean survival of the CG patients were 4 and 4.8 months, respectively, but in the SVG patients these values were 15.5 and 15 months ($P < 0.01$). No clinical signs of toxicity were found in the TG patients in the 24-month study period. Adding SV to the daily diet of NSCLC patients was found to be nontoxic and associated with improvement in weight maintenance and survival of patients with advanced NSCLC.

In another clinical study published in 2001, of a total of 16 patients with NSCLC enrolled, 12 patients took FSV while undergoing standard medical treatment (Sun et al. 2001). The study was not randomized or blinded. Patients who received FSV were compared with historical controls, referring to a group of patients treated in the past. Because historical controls often differ in relevant characteristics from the experimental group, studies using this design are not considered as reliable as randomized controlled clinical trials. According to comments from the American Cancer Society, the available scientific evidence does not support claims that the SV soup can help treat cancer.

A large randomized, blinded, placebo-controlled, clinical trial to validate the use of SV in patients with advanced small cell lung cancer has been enrolling patients since mid-2007 at Mount Sinai School of Medicine (www.clinicaltrials.gov). Two patient populations have been involved: (Study 1) patients who will be receiving a standard chemotherapy regimen and (Study 2) patients who refuse standard chemotherapy but will receive best supportive care. The primary end point is survival time while the secondary end points are tumour response, QoL and toxicity of SV.

7.5.3 PHY906

PHY906, a traditional Chinese herbal formulation composed of parts of four distinct herbs: the roots of baikal skullcap, licorice and *Paeonia lactiflora* (white peony), and the fruit of black date, has been used for thousands of years to treat various gastrointestinal ailments such as abdominal cramps, fever, headache, vomiting, thirst and diarrhea. In 1999, Liu et al. (2000) at Yale University School of Medicine discovered that PHY906 decreased toxicities and enhanced the anti-tumour activity of a broad spectrum of chemotherapeutic agents in various types of cancers in mouse xenograft model systems; the chemotherapeutic agents tested included capecitabine, irinotecan (Camptosar, CPT-11), 5-fluorouracil, VP-16, oxaliplatin, thalidomide, taxol, gemcitabine and sorafenib in colon 38 and a murine pancreatic cancer line (PAN-2) in BDF-1 mice, and a human HCC tumour line (HepG2) and a human pancreatic cancer line (PAN-1) in nude mice (Liu et al. 2002).

Initial in-depth studies with PHY906 were centered on the ability of this formulation to reduce the severity of the gastrointestinal toxicity seen with the chemotherapeutic agent irinotecan. Irinotecan, an active agent in the treatment of colorectal cancer, has severe late-onset diarrhea as its dose-limiting toxicity (Saltz et al. 2000). In pre-clinical studies, PHY906 was shown to reduce the severity of irinotecan-induced toxicity without compromising antitumour efficacy in an in vivo animal model. Given the promising preclinical activity of PHY906 and the historically documented safety of the product, one proposed development path for PHY906 was for the short-term treatment of late-onset National Cancer Institute-Common Toxicity Criteria (NCI-CTC) toxicity grade 3 or 4 diarrhea that accompanies irinotecan-based chemotherapy (Farrell and Kummar 2003).

The primary goal for the first clinical trial in the first path for PHY906 was to evaluate the safety, tolerability and efficacy of PHY906 in alleviating diarrhea in patients with advanced colorectal cancer receiving irinotecan/5-fluorouracil/leucovorin (IFL) combination chemotherapy. Patients would act as their own controls in this placebo-controlled, cross-over phase I/IIa clinical trial. The effect of PHY906 on the pharmacokinetics of 5-fluorouracil and irinotecan was investigated to ensure that this herbal medicine did not alter their metabolism.

Kummar et al. (2009) conducted the phase I/IIa trial in 17 patients with advanced, metastatic colorectal cancer. Thirteen patients were enrolled into low dose (1.2 g/day) of PHY906 in cohort 1, and 4 patients into medium dose (2.4 g/day) of PHY906 in cohort 2. No patients experienced treatment-related, life-threatening (grade 4) toxicity during treatment with PHY906 plus IFL chemotherapy. In contrast, 2 of 16 patients (6.3%) experienced treatment-related, life-threatening (grade 4) adverse events (neutropenia and GI hemorrhage) during treatment with placebo plus IFL chemotherapy. The study showed that fewer patients required anti-diarrheals to control their loose stools while receiving PHY906 as compared to placebo and that there was indeed a reduction in the overall incidence of grade 3 or 4 diarrhea. In addition, there was also a trend towards lower frequency and severity of vomiting for cycles in which patients received PHY906 as opposed to placebo. Interestingly, during the conduct of this study, it was readily apparent to the patients, their family members, and the staff supporting this clinical trial that there was a difference in the overall qualitative function and QoL between treatment with PHY906 and placebo.

Unfortunately, the study was closed prematurely due to slow accrual as a result of changes in the standard care of treatment of patients with advanced colorectal cancer. Therefore, it is difficult to make firm conclusions regarding the potential effect of PHY906 on the clinical efficacy of the IFL regimen. However, while the patient numbers enrolled on to this study are small, the preliminary results suggest that PHY906 may not compromise the clinical activity of irinotecan-based chemotherapy as 14 of the 16 patients showed either a partial response or stable disease when evaluated after two cycles of therapy. A formal randomized trial is certainly needed to further evaluate the effect of PHY906 on the clinical activity and safety profile of irinotecan-based chemotherapy, whether it be irinotecan in combination with the infusional 5FU/LV regimen (FOLFIRI), or irinotecan in combination with the oral fluoropyrimidine capecitabine (XELIRI), or irinotecan monotherapy (Kummar et al. 2009).

The second developmental path for PHY906 was based on the positive results from a preclinical study conducted by Liu et al. (2003), as well as a pilot clinical trial (Yen et al. 2008, 2009). In preclinical studies, PHY906 combined with capecitabine (Xeloda) in HepG2 xenografted NCr athymic nude mice was found to enhance the antitumour activity of capecitabine. Capecitabine had been used off-label for the treatment of patients with hepatocellular carcinoma (HCC) prior to the FDA approval of the first drug, sorafenib (Nexavar), for the treatment of HCC in November 2007 (Sandhu et al. 2008). The first clinical study conducted with PHY906/capecitabine combination by Yen et al. (2008) was a multicenter, open-label, dose escalation phase I/II safety and efficacy clinical trial of PHY906 given concomitantly with capecitabine to patients with advanced HCC. Phase I was designed to determine a safe and tolerable dosing regimen of PHY906 plus capecitabine, and phase II was designed to determine whether PHY906 enhanced the response rate of capecitabine, time to disease progression (TTP), and overall survival time (OS). The QoL of patients undergoing treatment was monitored.

Forty-two patients with HCC were enrolled: 18 patients in phase I and 24 patients in phase II (Yen et al. 2009). Twenty-five patients (59.5%) were classified Child-Pugh A and 17 (40.5%) Child-Pugh B. All patients were eligible for safety evaluation; two who received the cohort 1 treatment regimen and 27 who received the cohort 2 or cohort 3 regimens were evaluable for efficacy. Among 27 efficacy-evaluable patients, 13 (48%) received prior chemoembolization, 4 (15%) other prior treatments, and previous treatment information was unavailable for 4 (15%). Three cohorts were involved in this study: (1) capecitabine 1,000 mg/m^2 BID and PHY906 1,000 mg BID; (2) capecitabine 750 mg/m^2 BID and PHY906 600 mg BID; and (3) capecitabine 750 mg/m^2 BID and PHY906 800 mg BID.

Of the first three patients recruited into cohort 1, two developed drug-related grade 3 dose-limiting toxicity (DLT): one with colitis, hyperbillirubinemia and stomatitis, and one with hand-foot skin reaction. Enrollment of further patients into this cohort was therefore terminated and both capecitabine and PHY906 doses were adjusted downward. The combination of PHY906 (600 mg or 800 mg BID) and capecitabine (750 mg/m^2 BID) was well tolerated ($n = 39$). Twenty-eight of 39 patients (71.8%) reported adverse events (AEs). The most frequently experienced grade 3 drug-related AEs were mucositis/stomatis (7.7%), dehydration (5.1%), neutropenia (2.6%), hyperbilirubinemia (2.6%) and hand-foot skin reaction (2.6%). No patients experienced drug-related grade 4 or 5 toxicities. Among 27 efficacy-evaluable patients, 5 patients each had one drug-related grade 3 toxicity: neutropenia, dehydration, ALP elevation, hyperglycemia or hand-foot skin reaction. One patient experienced two drug-related grade 3 toxicities (poor appetite and AST elevation). Among 20 efficacy-evaluable Child-Pugh A patients, 4 patients each experienced one drug-related grade 3 toxicity: neutropenia, dehydration, ALP elevation or hyperglycemia. No correlation was observed between grade-3 drug-related toxicity and ethnicity, Child-Pugh status, hepatitis or previous treatment.

Among four patients treated with capecitabine 750 mg/m^2/PHY906 600 mg, two patients had minor response (MR) (tumour reduced 33.5 and 34%, respectively), one had stable disease (SD), and one had progressive disease (PD) after two cycles of treatment. At the capecitabine 750 mg/m^2/PHY906 800 mg dose level ($n = 23$), no complete (CR) or partial (PR) responses were seen; 8.7% ($N = 2$) had an MR (39.7 and 44% tumour reduction, respectively), 56.5% ($N = 13$) exhibited SD, and 34.8% ($N = 8$) had PD. Median time to progression was 3.4 months and median OS was 9.2 months. The 12-month survival rate was 44.5%. Seventy-four percent ($N = 20$) of the 27 efficacy-evaluable patients were classified as Child-Pugh A. Median OS values for Child-Pugh A and Child-Pugh B patients were 10.9 and 6.5 months, respectively. No difference in the 6-month survival rate was observed between Child-Pugh A and Child-Pugh B patients. However, the 12-month survival rate was 51% for Child-Pugh A patients and 29% for Child-Pugh B patients.

Median OS values for Asian and non-Asian subgroups were 16.5 and 6.2 months, respectively ($P = 0.03$). Median OS values for Asian and non-Asian Child-Pugh A patients were 16.5 and 6.7 months, respectively ($P = 0.05$). No significant correlation was observed for either nuclear grade or degree of differentiation of tumour. The results suggest that the PHY906/capecitabine combination provides a survival benefit and a tolerable safety profile in advanced HCC patients and that the combination has promise as a treatment for this disease. Use of the PHY906/capecitabine combination may prove to be particularly efficacious for Asian Child-Pugh A HCC patients. In light of the very poor prognosis of HCC patients and the 100% tumour progression rate seen with sorafenib therapy, the PHY906/capecitabine combination provides an additional opportunity to stabilize the disease for relatively longer periods of time.

The data illustrate that a widely-used TCM formulation, PHY906, can be used in combination with a widely-used Western cancer chemotherapeutic agent, capecitabine, to successfully treat patients with advanced HCC (Yen et al. 2009). The results with Asian patients are particularly noteworthy. A follow-up phase II study is currently conducted in Taiwan. An additional large size, randomized, double-blind, controlled study of capecitabine/PHY906 in HCC patients is required to validate these findings.

Use of the PHY906/capecitabine combination may not be limited to HCC. A single institution, open-label, phase I study of PHY906 800 mg BID in combination with escalating doses of capecitabine (1,000, 1,250, 1,500 and 1,750 mg/m^2) orally twice daily on days 1–7 of a 14-day cycle (7/7 schedule) was conducted in patients with advance pancreatic cancer or other gastrointestinal malignancies at the Yale Cancer Center by Saif et al. (Hoimes et al. 2008, Sandhu et al. 2008; Saif et al. 2009a, b). A total of 24 patients were enrolled and received a total of 116 cycles. There were no DLTs at the maximum capecitabine dose level of 1,750 mg/m^2, however, the delivered dose-intensity of capecitabine was similar at the 1,750 mg/m^2 dose level and the 1,500 mg/m^2 dose level. Therefore, the MTD was defined as 1,500 mg/m^2 of capecitabine in this 7/7 schedule with PHY906 800 mg BID on days 1–4. Hematologic toxicity was uncommon with no grade 3–4 toxicities observed. Two patients experienced grade 1–2 neutropenia (dose levels 3 and 4), and 8 patients experienced grade 1–2 thrombocytopenia. There were no dose reductions due to hematologic toxicity. One patient achieved a partial response and 13 patients had stable disease greater than six weeks. This combination was well tolerated and warrants further study. A phase II clinical trial in patients with advanced and recurrent pancreatic cancer refractory to capecitabine is currently ongoing at the Yale Cancer by Saif et al. (Saif 2008; Saif et al. 2009a, b).

The mechanisms of PHY906 drug action are multi-factorial. In preclinical studies, PHY906 has been shown to have inhibitory activity on multi-drug resistant protein (MDR) and CYP450; the presence of these inhibitions can facilitate the oral uptake of chemotherapeutic agents (Ye et al. 2007). Examination of the tumour tissues and compounds involved suggest that the integrity of blood vessels and the pathways of HIF-α and Fos/Juk transcription are affected by PHY906. In vitro studies also reveal that PHY906 has inhibitory activities against NF-κB and matrix metalloproteases (MMPs), which are possible contributors to the enhancement of the antitumour action of chemotherapeutic agents. Possible mechanisms of action for the reduction of gastrointestinal toxicity by PHY906 are the inhibition of Tachykinin NK-1, and/or opiate δ receptors, and may be acetylcholinesterase-based. The structures for 64 bioactive compounds, including flavonoids, triterpene saponins and monoterpene glycosides, were proposed based on the LC/MS analysis.

7.5.4 Clinical Studies in the United States with Other Botanical Preparations

In addition to the formulations mentioned above, several herbal regimens have been or are being studied in US for cancer or cancer-supportive care (as listed at www.clinicaltrials.gov). These include:

A randomized, double-blind, placebo-controlled study to assess the feasibility, toxicity and efficacy (phase I/II) of a Chinese herbal therapy for symptom management in women undergoing chemotherapy for stage I/II/III breast cancer is being conducted at the University of California – San Francisco Helen Diller Family Comprehensive Cancer Center (ClinicalTrials.gov Identifier: NCT00028964). The goal of this study is to determine the toxic effects and safety of Chinese herbal therapy when administered for toxicity attenuation in combination with adjuvant doxorubicin and cyclophosphamide in women with stage I, II, or early stage III breast cancer.

A non-randomized, open label, single group phase I/II clinical trial assessing safety and efficacy of BZL101 for metastatic breast cancer is under way (ClinicalTrials.gov Identifier: NCT00454532). BZL101 is an aqueous extract from *Scutellaria barbata* (barbat skullcap) of the Lamiaceae family. Preclinical studies suggest that this herb has antitumour activity for breast cancer and preliminary clinical data suggest that it is tolerable in patients with metastatic breast cancer.

A randomized dose-escalation, safety and exploratory efficacy study of Kanglaite (KLT) plus gemcitabine (G+K) *versus* gemcitabine alone in patients with advanced pancreatic cancer has been conducted at several study sites in the US (ClinicalTrials.gov Identifier: NCT00733850). Kanglaite is a novel broad-spectrum anti-cancer drug produced from the TCM herb, *Coix lachryma-jobi* (coix seed). It was approved in China in 1995 and has become one of the popular anti-cancer drugs in that country. In June 2001, a phase I study of KLT commenced at the Huntsman Cancer Institute in Salt Lake City, Utah. The objectives of this study were: (a) to determine the maximum tolerated dose (MTD) and the safety profile of KLT in patients with refractory solid tumours; (b) to determine the pharmacokinetics of KLT in patients with refractory solid tumours; and (c) to gather preliminary efficacy data.

A pilot safety, feasibility, efficacy and correlative (phase I/II) study assessing barbat skullcap for the treatment of metastatic breast cancer is ongoing (ClinicalTrials.gov Identifier: NCT00028977). The study was conducted based on the hypothesis that the Chinese herb barbat skullcap may contain ingredients that slow cancer growth and that may be an effective treatment for metastatic breast cancer.

Although several Western anti-nausea drugs, e.g. dolasetron (Anzemet), granisetron (Kytril), ondansetron (Zofran), palonosetron (Aloxi), dexamethasone (Decadron) and aprepitant (Emend), prescribed for people taking chemotherapy are effective at reducing nausea and vomiting in many cases, these drugs often do not totally eliminate all nausea. A randomized, double-blind, placebo-controlled, multicenter study to determine the safety and efficacy of ginger in reducing the prevalence and severity of chemotherapy-induced nausea and vomiting has been conducted by the National Center for Complementary and Alternative Medicine (NCCAM) (ClinicalTrials.gov Identifier: NCT00040742). Patients were randomized to 1 of 3 treatment arms. Patients were stratified according to concurrent antiemetic type ($5HT_3$ antagonist versus NK1 antagonist). This was a 3-arm study: (a) patients received lower-dose oral ginger twice daily; (b) patients received higher-dose oral ginger twice daily; (c) patients received oral placebo twice daily. In all arms, treatment began immediately after the chemotherapy treatment and continued for 3 days.

The results for 644 patients from 23 nationwide private oncology practices affiliated with the University of Rochester Cancer Center Community Clinical Oncology Program were presented by J Ryan at the 2009 annual meeting of the American Society of Clinical Oncology. All doses of ginger significantly ($P = 0.003$) reduced nausea compared with placebo. However, ginger had a relatively minimal effect on vomiting, largely because antiemetic drugs are already so effective at eliminating that chemotherapy-related side effect (Rhode et al. 2007).

Hematologic toxicity is a major side effect of many chemotherapy treatments and sometimes can be life-threatening. The standard treatment for neutropenia and chemotherapy-associated anemia is administration of G-CSF and erythropoietin. However, both GCSF and erythropoietin can cause substantial side effects and may not be deemed to be cost effective. Treatments designed to reduce myelotoxicity without additional side effects and at reasonable cost may be much more acceptable than the currently available treatments. Herbal medicines may prove to play an important role in this regard.

7.6 Procedures and Challenges for the Development and Acceptance of Traditional Chinese Medicine in Non-Asian Countries: Development of PHY906 in the United States as an Example

7.6.1 Procedures for Traditional Chinese Medicine Development

Traditional Chinese medicine is known to rely on testimonials to prove its effectiveness and consequently, it has been prone to broad therapeutic claims for a given herbal formula. These practices must be substituted with more rigorous clinical and scientific studies that provide robust statistical analyses before TCM is widely accepted into mainstream Western medicine. The material presented below represents how the necessary rigor and robustness may become part of TCM development. The development of PHY906 is used as an example.

7.6.1.1 Food and Drug Administration Guidance for Developing Botanical Drugs

The draft "Guidance for Industry: Botanical Drug Products" published by the FDA in June, 2004 forms the basis for development of botanical drugs in the United States. This guidance describes regulatory approaches that must be followed. A botanical product is defined as a drug under section 201(g)(1)(B) of the FD&C Act, 21 USC 321(g)(1)(B), if it is intended for use in diagnosing, mitigating, treating curing or preventing disease. Such a drug product must be marketed under an approved NDA or FDA's OTC drug monograph system.

There are three main approval criteria raised in the FDA guidance for botanical medicines: (1) safety in human use; (2) efficacy in the indicated disease; and (3) consistency in batch-to-batch drug quality. Botanical drugs that can prove their safety and efficacy through historical usage will be able to move quickly to the clinical trial stage of development following acceptance of an Investigational New Drug (IND) application. The regulatory policies for the development of botanical drug products differ somewhat from those for conventional chemical entities. These differences include: (1) no preclinical animal studies are required for botanicals prior to the IND application; and (2) botanicals with historical documentation of safe use do not require human clinical phase I trials and therefore can undergo directly human clinical phase II trials. As for conventional drugs, an IND approval by the FDA is required for botanicals prior to the initiation of clinical trials.

7.6.1.2 Historical Usage and Preclinical Information

At the outset, the focus of the development of PHY906 as an FDA-approvable drug was on treating the documented severe and often life-threatening side effects of prevailing cancer chemotherapies. As a first step, a literature search of Chinese medicine formulas that have been used for the treatment of gastrointestinal symptoms similar to those observed in the use of many cancer chemotherapeutic agents used in Western medicine was prepared. Among the many formulas examined, focus was placed on those that: (1) were well established formulas, used for hundreds of years to successfully treat a variety of ailments including diarrhea, abdominal spasms, fever, headache, vomiting, nausea and loss of appetite; (2) had documented prior human use, and so could be fast-tracked into a relevant human clinical trials using the recently established guidelines for botanical drugs outlined by the FDA; and (3) had a well-defined botanical composition of individual herbs that had been well documented and that could be manufactured under GMP conditions. Of the several candidates selected and studied, a botanical formulation, named PHY906, was found to be superior to all others.

Given the historical usage of PHY906 for the treatment of gastrointestinal distress, initial clinical efforts were directed towards the evaluation of PHY906 as a potential chemotherapeutic modulator that could specifically alleviate chemotherapy-induced toxicities thereby resulting in improved QoL for cancer patients.

7.6.1.3 Chemistry, Manufacturing and Control

To comply with the FDA draft guidance on botanicals, batch-to-batch consistency and good quality of botanical product are essential. This requires not only appropriate quality control of final product testing, but also control of the botanical raw materials, in-process controls during manufacturing, and final process validation, especially for the drug substance. To sustain initial clinical trials, sufficient quantities of the botanical drug product must be prepared in a single batch from a single source of the botanical drug substance and/or raw materials.

The manufacturing procedure for PHY906 adheres to TCM methods. The process involves the extraction of a mixture of the herbal raw materials at the proper ratio with boiling water followed by filtration. The decoctions are concentrated by evaporation under reduced pressure and spray-dried to yield dry powder. To ensure that the quality of the botanical drug substance and product meets release specifications, appropriate control and analytical procedures are in place, and are implemented throughout the entire manufacturing process. To ensure the uniformity and integrity of the botanical drug substances, adequate in-process controls include checking the volume of the process liquor and HPLC determinations to establish chemical fingerprints to identify marker substances presented in the intermediates produced in each unit operation and final product etc; these are implemented according to Standard Operation Processes (SOPs). Purified marker substances are used for identification and quality control of the raw materials, as well as the botanical drug substances and product. Batch records are prepared and kept ready for inspection.

7.6.1.4 Clinical Studies

Clinical evaluation of botanical drug products for safety and efficacy does not differ significantly from the evaluation of any synthetic or highly purified drugs. For example, a phase I/IIA double-blind placebo-controlled dose escalation clinical study of PHY906 under an IND with the FDA was initiated in 2002 to evaluate PHY906's efficacy in modulating the Saltz regimen- and/or irinotecan-induced late onset diarrhea in advanced colorectal cancer patients. Another phase I/II open label dose escalation clinical trial under existing IND has been done to evaluate PHY906 as an adjuvant for capecitabine in the treatment of hepatocellular carcinoma. Finally, because of recent encouraging results obtained in a PAN01 xenograft animal pancreatic cancer model, a clinical study that uses PHY906 as an adjuvant for capecitabine in the treatment of pancreatic cancer is under way. These clinical trials are typically conducted at teaching hospitals in the US.

7.6.2 Challenges to Traditional Chinese Medicine Development

7.6.2.1 Quality Control

Quality control is a major challenge in bringing TCM into the mainstream medicine of the twenty-first century. Quality control of TCM should adopt a holistic approach that includes: (1) raw material produced by Good Agriculture Practices (GAP); (2) manufacturing batches of clinical samples with GMP; and (3) selecting parameters for in-process controls with both chemical and biological markers.

The first step of TCM quality control should start with herbs grown under GAP. The herbs used in formula preparation should be carefully monitored in terms of their growth, levels of inorganic contamination, contamination by herbicides, fungicides, pesticides, and fertilizers, and harvest conditions that ensure the highest levels of consistency in the raw herbs. Good Agriculture Practices for botanical cultivation, which has been initiated recently in China, represents one of the most important steps toward gaining FDA approval of a botanical drug.

Good Manufacture Practice is the system used to enforce the consistency and quality of the manufacturing process of botanical products. Current manufacturing quality control for consistency relies on the measurement of marker compounds contained in single herbs. In addition to GMP applied during production, good quality control should include not only chemical fingerprints but also biological fingerprints of botanicals. Some advanced analytic technologies such as LC-MS and LC-NMR should be developed as chemical quality control for TCM development, in addition to traditional analytical instrumentation, such as HPLC and GC. Without attempting to employ such techniques, the development of proper and standard methods that will allow TCM to be brought into the mainstream of Western medicine will be difficult to achieve.

Parameters for in-process controls, such as chemical and biological markers, must be developed and selected. Currently, the contents of marker compounds in botanicals are determined using one or more chemical analyses in botanical industries. In most cases, it is not clear whether the marker compounds are responsible for the biological activity of the formulation. Thus, the value of the determination of the content of those marker compounds for quality control of herbal formulations is questionable. The significance of each chemical in a botanical product as well as their combined synergy could be deduced eventually through bioassays. Bioassays, including in vivo and in vitro assays, relevant animal models, and a panel of surrogate pharmacological assays are being evaluated. In addition, several newly developed technologies such as genomics, proteomics and metabolomics that monitor multiple parameters including gene expression, protein expression and alterations of metabolizing enzymes should be combined with bioinformatics as a future approach for developing TCM. This kind of holistic approach is not only good for the quality control of such medicines, but also useful for the discovery of new indications or the development of new formulations.

7.6.2.2 Combination Drug Regulations

In the FDA's non-binding document "Guidance for Industry: Botanical Drug Products" issued in June 2004, the applicability of combination drug regulations to botanical drugs is considered. In essence, these regulations state that when drugs are used in combination, each component or active ingredient must be shown to contribute to the claimed effects of the combination before marketing approval will be granted. Botanical drug products that are derived from a single part (stem, leaves, roots, etc) of a plant, or from a single species of alga or macroscopic fungus, are not considered to be fixed-combination drugs within the meaning of the combination drug regulations. Currently, however, botanical drugs composed of parts of different species of plants, algae, or macroscopic fungi or even composed of multiple parts of a single species of plant, algae, or macroscopic fungi, are subject to the combination drug requirements.

For multi-herbal formulations such as PHY906, it is as yet unclear whether the FDA will require only that the contribution of each individual herb to the claimed effects of the overall formulation be documented or whether the agency will require that the contributions of all active moieties in the formulation be documented. For TCM such as PHY906, the latter requirement would be extremely problematic.

As noted previously, TCM is based often on the use of multiple herbs, or parts of different herbs, in combination; particular active substances are not extracted from the herbs, purified, and then used as individual drugs as is the case in Western medicine (e.g. taxol originally purified from the bark of the Pacific yew tree). In the case of PHY906, parts from four different herbs are employed. Analytical methods have revealed that the PHY906 formulation contains more than 100 different phytochemicals. Some of these phytochemicals have been definitively identified, some tentatively identified, and others are of unknown chemical structure, even after rigorous attempts to identify them over several years of investigation. In addition, which of these phytochemicals would be considered active according to the FDA is unknown. Therefore, if the FDA were to implement stringent combination drug regulations that require that all active substances in a particular formulation be documented, the approval of multi-herbal TCM formulations, such as PHY906, for marketing purposes would be difficult, if not impossible.

In the 2004 guidance document referred to above, it is stated that the FDA is considering revising its regulations to allow for the exemption of botanical drugs such as PHY906 that are composed of parts of different species of plants, algae, macroscopic fungi, or composed of multiple parts of a single species of plant, algae, or macroscopic fungi, from application of the combination drug requirements under certain circumstances. To date, however, no such revision has taken place.

Acknowledgments The authors wish to acknowledge Dr Gerald Crabtree for his critical reading of this chapter.

References

A phase I/II clinical trial assessing safety and efficacy of BZL101 for metastatic breast cancer. Clinical Trials Gov Identifier: NCT00454532.

Armstrong TS, Gilbert MR. Use of complementary and alternative medical therapy by patients with primary brain tumors. Curr Neurol Neurosci Rep. 2008;8:264–8.

Attele AS, Wu JA, Yuan CS. Ginseng pharmacology: multiple constituents and multiple actions. Biochem Pharmacol. 1999;58:1685–93.

Auyeung KK, Cho CH, Ko JK. A novel anticancer effect of astragalus saponins: transcriptional activation of NSAID-activated gene. Int J Cancer. 2009;125:1082–91.

Bar-Sela G, Tsalic M, Fried G et al. Wheat grass juice may improve hematological toxicity related to chemotherapy in breast cancer patients: a pilot study. Nutr Cancer. 2007;58:43–8.

Barton DL, Soori GS, Bauer BA et al. Pilot study of *Panax quinquefolius* (American ginseng) to improve cancer-related fatigue: a randomized, double-blind, dose-finding evaluation: NCCTG trial N03CA. Support Care Cancer. 2009. doi:10.1007/s00520-009-0642-2.

Boh B, Berovic M, Zhang J. *Ganoderma lucidum* and its pharmaceutically active compounds. Biotechnol Annu Rev. 2007;13:265–301.

Calabresi P, Chabner BA. Chemotherapy of neoplastic diseases. In: Goodman and Gilman, editors.

The pharmacological basis of therapeutics, 9th ed. Section X. New York: McGraw-Hill; 1996. pp. 1225–32.

Choi SW, Cho EH, Chi SY. Ginsenosides activate DNA polymerase from bovine placenta. Life Sci. 1995;57:1359–65.

Cho WC, Leung KN. In vitro and in vivo anti-tumor effects of *Astragalus membranaceus*. Cancer Lett. 2007;252:43–54.

Combination chemotherapy after surgery with or without Chinese herbal therapy to treat symptoms in women with breast cancer. Clinical Trials Gov Identifier: NCT00028964.

Cui R, He J, Wang B et al. Suppressive effect of *Astragalus membranaceus* Bunge on chemical hepatocarcinogenesis in rats. Cancer Chemother Pharmacol. 2003;51:75–80.

De la Taille A, Hayek OR, Burchardt M et al. Role of herbal compounds (PC-SPES) in hormone-refractory prostate cancer: two case reports. J Altern Complement Med. 2000;6:449–51.

De la Taille A, Hayek OR, Buttyan R et al. Effects of a phytherapeutic agent, PC-SPES, on prostate cancer: a preliminary investigation on human cell lines and patients. BJU Int. 1999;84: 845–50.

DiPaola RS, Zhang H, Lambert GH et al. Clinical and biologic activity of an estrogenic herbal combination (PC-SPES) in prostate cancer. N Engl J Med. 1998;339:785–91.

Eisenberg DM, Davis RB, Ettner SL et al. Trends in alternative medicine use in the United States, 1990–1997: results of a follow-up national survey. JAMA. 1998;280:1569–75.

Farrell MP, Kummar S. Phase I/IIA randomized study of PHY906, a novel herbal agent, as a modulator of chemotherapy in patients with advanced colorectal cancer. Clin Colorectal Cancer. 2003;2:253–6.

Fishbein AB, Wang CZ, Li XL et al. Asian ginseng enhances the anti-proliferative effect of 5-fluorouracil on human colorectal cancer: comparison between white and red ginseng. Arch Pharm Res. 2009;32:505–13.

Forman WB. The role of chemotherapy and adjuvant therapy in the management of colorectal cancer. Cancer. 1994;74:2151–3.

Gardiner P, Graham R, Legedza AT et al. Factors associated with herbal therapy use by adults in the United States. Altern Ther Health Med. 2007;13:22–9.

Gillis NC. *Panax ginseng* pharmacology: a nitric oxide link? Biochem Pharmacol. 1997;54:1–8.

Ginger in treating nausea in patients receiving chemotherapy for cancer. Clinical Trials Gov Identifier: NCT00040742.

Herbal therapy in treating women with metastatic breast cancer. Clinical Trials Gov Identifier: NCT00028977.

Hoimes CJ, Lamb L, Ruta S et al. A phase I/II study of PHY906 plus capecitabine (CAP) in patients (pts) with advanced pancreatic cancer. J Clin Oncol. 2008;20:15538.

Huang KC. The pharmacology of Chinese herbs. Boca Raton, FL: CRC Press; 1999.

Ito I, Mukai M, Ninomiya H et al. Comparison between intravenous and oral postoperative adjuvant immunochemotherapy in patients with stage III colorectal cancer. Oncol Rep. 2008;20:1521–6.

Kan WL, Cho CH, Rudd JA et al. Study of the anti-proliferative effects and synergy of phthalides from *Angelica sinensis* on colon cancer cells. J Ethnopharmacol. 2008;120:36–43.

Kellis JT, Vickery LE. Inhibition of human oestrogen synthetase (aromatase) by flavones. Science. 1984;225:1032–4.

Kim YS, Kim DS, Kim SI. Ginsenoside Rh2 and Rh3 induce differentiation of HL-60 cells into granulocytes: modulation of protein kinase C isoforms during differentiation by ginsenoside Rh2. Int J Biochem Cell Biol. 1998;30:327–38.

Konkimalla VB, Efferth T. Evidence-based Chinese medicine for cancer therapy. J Ethnopharmacol. 2008;116:207–10.

Kummar S, Copur MS, Rose M et al. A phase I study of the Chinese herbal medicine PHY906 as a modulator of irinotecan-based chemotherapy in patients with advanced colorectal cancer. 2009;submitted.

Larimore WL, O'Mathuna DP. Quality assessment programs for dietary supplements. Ann Pharmacother. 2003;37:893–8.

Lersch C, Zeuner M, Bauer A et al. Nonspecific immunostimulation with low doses of cyclophosphamide (LDCY), thymostimulin, and Echinacea purpurea extracts (echinacin) in patients with far advanced colorectal cancers: preliminary results. Cancer Invest. 1992;10:343–8.
Li X, He D, Zhang L et al. A novel antioxidant agent, astragalosides, prevents shock wave-induced renal oxidative injury in rabbits. Urol Res. 2006;34:277–82.
Liu SH, Jiang Z, Cheng YC. Botanical activity relationship in traditional Chinese medicine: studies of PHY906 as an adjuvant therapy with cancer chemotherapeutic agents. Proc Am Assoc Cancer Res. 2002;43:961, 4758.
Liu SH, Jiang Z, Gao W et al. PHY906, a Chinese herbal formulation enhances the therapeutic effect of cancer chemotherapy in human colorectal and liver cancer. Proc Am Soc Clin Oncol. 2003;864.
Liu SH, Jiang Z, Liddil J et al. Prevention of CPT-11 induced toxicity by a Chinese medicinal formulation, PHY-906. Proc Am Assoc Cancer Res. 2000;41:410, 2608.
Liu SH, Su T, Jiang Z et al. Developing TCM as FDA approved botanical drugs. Proceedings of 2004 SATEC meeting.
Mahajna J, Dotan N, Zaidman BZ et al. Pharmacological values of medicinal mushrooms for prostate cancer therapy: the case of Ganoderma lucidum. Nutr Cancer. 2009;61:16–26.
Marcus DM, Grollman AP. Botanical medicines – the need for new regulations. N Engl J Med. 2002;347:2073–6.
Mayeaux EJ, Jr, Dunton C. Modern management of external genital warts. J Low Genit Tract Dis. 2008;12:185–92.
Meyer JP, Gillatt DA. PC-SPES: a herbal therapy for the treatment of hormone refractory prostate cancer. Prostate Cancer Prostatic Dis. 2002;5:13–5.
Monro JA. Treatment of cancer with mushroom products. Arch Environ Health. 2003;58:533–7.
Ota T, Fujikawa-Yamamoto K, Zong ZP et al. Plant-glycoside modulation of cell surface related to control of differentiation in cultured B16 melanoma cells. Cancer Res. 1987;47:3863–7.
Quimby EL. The use of herbal therapies in pediatric oncology patients: treating symptoms of cancer and side effects of standard therapies. J Pediatr Oncol Nurs. 2007;24:35–40.
Ragupathi G, Yeung KS, Leung PC et al. Evaluation of widely consumed botanicals as immunological adjuvants. Vaccine. 2008;26:4860–5.
Rhode J, Fogoros S, Zick S et al. Ginger inhibits cell growth and modulates angiogenic factors in ovarian cancer cells. BMC Complement Altern Med. 2007;7:44.
Safety and exploratory efficacy of Kanglaite injection in pancreatic cancer. Clinical Trials Gov Identifier: NCT00733850.
Sagar SM, Wong RK. Chinese medicine and biomodulation in cancer patients – part one. Curr Oncol. 2008;15:42–8.
Saif MW. Is there a standard of care for the management of advanced pancreatic cancer? Highlights from the Gastrointestinal Cancers Symposium, Orlando, FL, USA, January 25–27, 2008. JOP 2008;9:91–8.
Saif MW, Lansigan F, Ruta S et al. Phase I study of the botanical formulation PHY906 with capecitabine in advanced pancreatic and gastrointestinal malignancies. Phytomedicine. 2009a. in press.
Saif MW, Li J, Lamb L et al. A phase II study of capecitabine (CAP) plus PHY906 in pts with advanced pancreatic cancer (APC) proc. Proc Am Soc Clin Oncol. 2009b; e15508.
Saltz LB, Cox JV, Blanke C et al. Irinotecan plus fluorouracil and leucovorin for metastatic colorectal cancer. N Engl J Med. 2000;343:905–14.
Sandhu DS, Tharayil VS, Lai JP et al. Treatment options for hepatocellular carcinoma. Expert Rev Gastroenterol Hepatol. 2008;2:81–92.
Shu X, McCulloch M, Xiao H et al. Chinese herbal medicine and chemotherapy in the treatment of hepatocellular carcinoma: a meta-analysis of randomized controlled trials. Integr Cancer Ther. 2005;4:219–29.
Small EJ, Frohlich MW, Bok R et al. Prospective trial of the herbal supplement PC-SPES in patients with progressive prostate cancer. J Clin Oncol. 2000;18:3595–603.

Sovak M, Seligson AL, Konas M et al. Herbal composition PC-SPES for management of prostate cancer: identification of active principles. J Natl Cancer Inst. 2002;94:1275–81.

Sun AS, Ostadal O, Ryznar V et al. Phase I/II study of stage III and IV non-small cell lung cancer patients taking a specific dietary supplement. Nutr Cancer. 1999;34:62–9.

Sun AS, Yeh HC, Wang LH et al. Pilot study of a specific dietary supplement in tumor-bearing mice and in stage IIIB and IV non-small cell lung cancer patients. Nutr Cancer. 2001;39:85–95.

Tindle HA, Davis RB, Phillips RS et al. Trends in use of complementary and alternative medicine by US adults: 1997–2002. Altern Ther Health Med. 2005;11:42–9.

Tsai NM, Chen YL, Lee CC et al. The natural compound n-butylidenephthalide derived from *Angelica sinensis* inhibits malignant brain tumor growth in vitro and in vivo. J Neurochem. 2006;99(4):1251–62.

Wani MC, Taylor HL, Wall ME et al. Plant antitumor agents. VI. The isolation and structure of taxol, a novel antileukemic and antitumor agent from *Taxus brevifolia*. J Am Chem Soc. 1971;93:2325–7.

Weng CJ, Chau CF, Hsieh YS et al. Lucidenic acid inhibits PMA-induced invasion of human hepatoma cells through inactivating MAPK/ERK signal transduction pathway and reducing binding activities of NF-kappaB and AP-1. Carcinogenesis. 2008;29:147–56.

White J. PC-SPES-A lesson for future dietary supplement research. J Natl Cancer Inst. 2002;94:1261–2.

Wong R, Sagar CM, Sagar SM. Integration of Chinese medicine into supportive cancer care: a modern role for an ancient tradition. Cancer Treat Rev. 2001;27:235–46.

Wu T, Munro AJ, Guanjian L et al. Chinese medical herbs for chemotherapy side effects in colorectal cancer patients. In: The cochrane collaboration. New York: John Wiley and Sons Ltd; 2009.

Wu T, Munro AJ, Liu G. Chinese medical herbs for chemotherapy side effects in colorectal cancer patients. Cochrane Database Syst Rev. 2005;1:CD004540.

Xie CH, Zhang MS, Zhou YF et al. Chinese medicine *Angelica sinensis* suppresses radiation-induced expression of TNF-alpha and TGF-beta1 in mice. Oncol Rep. 2006;15:1429–36.

Yang C, Chien LY, Tai CJ. Use of complementary and alternative medicine among patients with cancer receiving outpatient chemotherapy in Taiwan. J Altern Complement Med. 2008;14:413–6.

Ye M, Liu SH, Jiang Z et al. Liquid chromatography/mass spectrometry analysis of PHY906, a Chinese medicine formulation for cancer therapy. Rapid Commun Mass Spectrom. 2007;21:3593–607.

Yen Y, So S, Rose M et al. Phase I/II study of capecitabine and PHY906 in hepatocellular carcinoma. Proc Am Soc Clin Oncol. 2008;4610.

Yen Y, So S, Rose M et al. Phase I/II study of PHY906/capecitabine in advanced hepatocellular carcinoma. Anticancer Res. 2009;29:4083–92.

Yuen JW, Gohel MD. Anticancer effects of *Ganoderma lucidum*: a review of scientific evidence. Nutr Cancer. 2005;53:11–7.

Yun TK, Choi SY. Preventive effect of ginseng intake against various human cancers: a case study on 1987 pairs. Cancer Epidemiol Biomarkers Prev. 1995;4:401–8.

Zhou X, Lin J, Yin Y. Ganodermataceae: natural products and their related pharmacological functions. Am J Chin Med. 2007;35:559–74.

Zhuang SR, Chen SL, Tsai JH et al. Effect of citronellol and the Chinese medical herb complex on cellular immunity of cancer patients receiving chemotherapy/radiotherapy. Phytother Res. 2009;23:785–90.

Chapter 8
Cancer Pain Control with Traditional Chinese Medicine

Ting Bao, Lixing Lao, and Aditya Bardia

Abstract Cancer pain is the most common and one of the most distressing and feared symptoms among cancer patients. This chapter focuses on summarizing and evaluating the current clinical evidence on using different modalities of traditional Chinese medicine (TCM) to control cancer pain. Traditional Chinese medicine includes multiple modalities such as herbal medicine, acupuncture, dietary therapy, massage, and qigong therapy. Clinical trials of acupuncture for cancer pain suggest that acupuncture might be efficacious in reducing cancer related pain, particularly short term and in the post-operative setting. Similarly, massage is a promising therapy for control of cancer related pain, particularly short term benefit. While few Chinese herbal regimens appear promising as therapies for cancer related pain, based on the current scientific evidence, it cannot be recommended for routine clinical practice yet. The idea of qigong reducing cancer pain is quite stimulating as this is an intervention with minimal risk but research in this area is quite limited. Overall, TCM has the potential to provide effective complementary therapy to decrease cancer pain. However, the current research for TCM modalities in treating cancer pain are limited by methodological weaknesses such as small sample size, lack of standard outcome measurement, and lack of effective randomization and blinding method. Further studies on TCM for cancer pain with rigorous study design are warranted.

8.1 Introduction

Cancer pain is the most common and one of the most distressing and feared symptoms among cancer patients. It is estimated that up to two thirds of patients with metastatic cancer suffered from cancer related pain (Cleeland et al. 1994). More than 75% of hospitalized oncology patients experienced cancer related pain (Brescia

A. Bardia (✉)
School of Medicine, The Sidney Kimmel Comprehensive Cancer Center, Johns Hopkins University, Baltimore, MD, USA
e-mail: adityabardia@gmail.com

W.C.S. Cho (ed.), *Supportive Cancer Care with Chinese Medicine*,
DOI 10.1007/978-90-481-3555-4_8,

et al. 1992; McMillan et al. 2000; Wells 2000). Due to its importance, pain is often referred to as the fifth vital sign of oncology patients. Cancer pain varies both by types of malignancy and sites of cancer involvement (Foley 1979). The majority of cancer pain is caused by direct effect of cancer as a result of visceral involvement, bony metastasis, soft tissue invasion, or infiltration to the nerve or nerve plexus (Banning et al. 1991). Cancer treatments such as chemotherapy, radiation and surgery may also cause treatment-induced cancer pain (Coyle et al. 1990; Zech et al. 1995).

Based on etiology, pain can be divided into three categories: somatic pain, visceral pain and neuropathic pain. Somatic pain is caused by injury to skin, bones or muscles causing constant localized tenderness. In cancer patients, bony metastasis is the most common cause of somatic pain (Foley 1985). Somatic pain results from nociceptors being triggered by mechanical, thermal or chemical stimuli. In contrast, visceral pain is a poorly localized pain that is dull, colicky and usually associates with nausea and diaphoresis. It is experienced often by patients with pancreatic cancer. Its mechanism is not well understood but was thought to be caused through activation of visceral autonomic afferent nerves by stimuli such as ischemia, inflammation, and torsion (McMahon 1994). Neuropathic pain is a prolonged, severe, burning type of pain. It may associate with focal neurologic deficits and is usually constant but may be interrupted by sudden crescendo of pain. It is usually resistant to opioids and therefore the most challenging to treat (Portenoy et al. 1990).

Cancer pain has traditionally been treated with opioids and interventional anesthetic or neurosurgical procedures. Despite maximal use of pain medications and application of interventional procedures, a significant portion of cancer patients still suffer from pain. In addition, the undesired side effects of long term usage of opioid pain medication, particularly change of mental status, constipation, nausea, fear of dependence, could be an issue. As a result, cancer patients often seek help in complementary alternative medicine (CAM), including Traditional Chinese medicine (TCM) parting an attempt to control their pain.

Complementary alternative medicine therapies, although used widely by patients, have been the subject of debate. They have been criticized for their soft science. Critics note that some therapies are no more effective than placebo, and may be associated with adverse effects and negative interactions like conventional medicines. Thus, it has been suggested that these therapies, like conventional medicine, should be used in an evidence-based fashion.

This chapter provides an overview of the TCM for control of cancer related pain, with focus on the scientific evidence behind the interventions.

8.2 Traditional Chinese Medicine

Traditional Chinese medicine originated in China thousands of years ago and has been widely practiced in Asia. In the US, it has been widely used among cancer patients (Richardson et al. 2000). Traditional Chinese medicine's philosophy stems from Taoism, which believes that human being's health is the result of harmony among different parts of the body, and between the body and nature. Illness occurs when such harmony fails to be achieved. Traditional Chinese medicine believed that a vital energy, qi, travels along energy channels and meridians in the body to guarantee harmony. When there is qi blockage or qi deficiency, harmony is disturbed and pain occurs. The TCM treatment for cancer pain is therefore to use different TCM modalities to either unblock the qi stagnation or replete qi (Lao 1999).

Traditional Chinese medicine includes multiple modalities such as herbal medicine, acupuncture, dietary therapy, massage and qigong therapy. Among these modalities, herbal medicine and acupuncture are most frequently practiced by TCM practitioners, and would be discussed in details in this chapter. Each section is divided into overview of therapy, potential scientific basis for analgesic effect, review of clinical studies, adverse effects and conclusion. Deliberate emphasis has been made on the scientific evidence for reasons outlined above.

8.2.1 Acupuncture

8.2.1.1 Overview

Acupuncture is an ancient TCM technique that has been widely used as a complementary therapy to treat wide range of illnesses by many patients, especially oncology patients.

8.2.1.2 Scientific Basis for Analgesic Effect

The Western medicine basis of analgesic potential of acupuncture is based on the Gate control theory of pain (GCT). According to GCT, pain is considered a noxious stimuli that maybe increased or decreased by modulations within the gating mechanisms, either intensifying the pain by allowing the pain pathways to be open or decreasing the pain by closing the pain pathways. Most of the analgesic effects of acupuncture are mediated by opioid peptides, which act on various regions of the nervous system including the anterolateral tract in the spinal cord, the reticulogigantocellular nucleus, the raphe magnus, the dorsal part of the periaqueductal central gray, the posterior and anterior hypothalamus, and the medial part of the centromedian nucleus of the thalamus (Alimi et al. 2000). Other substances, including serotonin, catecholamines, inorganic chemicals, and amino acids such as glutamate and α-aminobutyric acid (GABA), are proposed to mediate certain analgesic effects of acupuncture, but at present their role is poorly understood. The benefit of acupuncture is of particular value in neuropathic pain where traditional pharmacological therapies are of, at best, modest value but acupuncture is believed to help by activating certain brain pathways and reflexes that contribute to the neuropathic pain.

8.2.1.3 Review of Clinical Studies

Even though acupuncture has been widely used among cancer patients to control cancer pain, the role of acupuncture in controlling cancer pain has not been clearly established through well designed clinical trials (Bardia et al. 2006). A number of randomized controlled trials (RCTs) have been conducted to study the role of acupuncture in treating cancer pain and are summarized in Table 8.1.

Among them, three recent RCTs studied the efficacy of different types of acupuncture in controlling postoperative pain and presented mixed results. Deng et al. (2008) published a randomized, sham acupuncture controlled clinical trial on 162 cancer patients experiencing post-thoracotomy pain. One hundred and six patients were evaluable with 52 patients received small intradermal needles in bilateral BL12 to BL19, ST36 and Shenmen points, and 54 patients received sham needle (ring without needle) at non-acupuncture points for 1 month. The patient's pain at the 30-day follow-up was measured by Brief Pain Inventory and showed no statistical difference between the real versus sham acupuncture groups. No statistical difference between the two groups in terms of 60 and 90 days follow-up pain scores, in-patient pain and medication usage. This is a well designed study with large sample size and strong statistic consideration. The efficacy of the unique intradermal needles used in this study is questionable though.

Wong et al. (2006) published a randomized sham acupuncture controlled clinical trial on the effect of electroacupuncture in post-thoracotomy pain. Twenty-seven lung cancer patients were enrolled in the study, with 25 patients deemed evaluable. Thirteen patients were randomized to electroacupuncture group and 12 to sham acupuncture group. Sham acupuncture was designed to use blunt-Tip needles on the same acupuncture points as the real electroacupuncture did. All patients received twice daily electro or sham acupuncture, for the first 7 postoperative days and their pain levels were measured by visual analog scale each day. Their usage of patient-controlled analgesia was also recorded for the first 3 postoperative days. This study showed a trend of lower VAS pain scores in patients receiving electroacupuncture when compared to patients receiving sham acupuncture on postop days 2 and 6; and a statistically significant lower cumulative dose of patient controlled analgesia on postop day 2 ($P < 0.05$). This study is limited by its small sample size and the sham acupuncture design as it used the same acupuncture points as the real acupuncture group.

Mehling et al. (2007) published a RCT on comparing acupuncture plus massage with usual care in controlling postoperative pain, nausea, vomiting and depressive moods. Ninety-three patients were randomized to acupuncture plus massage group and 45 patients to the usual care group. Patients received acupuncture and massage on postop days 1 and 2, and filled out questionnaires evaluating their postop symptoms on postop days 1, 2 and 3. The patients who received acupuncture plus massage had a significantly larger decrease of pain score from baseline to postop day 3 (1.4) when compared to the patients in the control group (0.4) with $P = 0.038$. In addition, among patients who reported baseline pain greater than 3/10, the patients in the intervention group had a 1.8 point decrease of pain score at postop day 3 whereas the usual care group had a 0.3 point decrease ($P = 0.001$). This study suggested that postop acupuncture and massage in addition to usual care significantly improved pain control when compared to usual care alone. However, with no sham therapy group in the study, it is difficult to tease out the placebo effect, and leave the question that if the professionally trained acupuncturists and massage therapists and real acupuncture needles are required in the intervention remained unanswered.

Table 8.1 Summary of randomized controlled trials on acupuncture for cancer pain relief

References	Sample size	Treatment groups	Treatment duration	Evaluation method	Results	Limitations
Li et al. (1994)	16	1. Chinese herbs ± ear-acupuncture ± epidural morphine 2. Placebo group	5 days	VAS	Combined treatments were superior to placebo control group	Small sample size; Questionable study design
Dang and Yang (1998)	48	1. Acupuncture 2. Acupuncture point injection 3. Western analgesics	2 months	WHO pain scale	No difference among the 3 groups in long-term effective rate of analgesia, 81% in all groups	Small sample size; Limited statistical Discussion
He et al. (1999)	80	1. Acupuncture 2. No acupuncture	Postop days 3, 5, 7 and day of discharge	VAS and range of movement	The acupuncture group had an improved postop pain ($P \leq 0.01$) and range of movement ($P = 0.001$)	Lack of placebo control arm
Wong et al. (2006)	27	1. Electroacupuncture 2. Sham acupuncture	7 days	VAS and medication quantification	Lower cumulative dose of patient controlled analgesic morphine used on postop day 2 in EA group ($P < 0.05$)	Small sample size; Sham acupuncture design; Short duration of acupuncture treatment and follow up

Table 8.1 (continued)

References	Sample size	Treatment groups	Treatment duration	Evaluation method	Results	Limitations
Mehling et al. (2007)	138	1. Acupuncture and massage 2. Usual care	2 days	Pain numeric rating scale	The treatment group has less pain ($P = 0.038$), being less depressed ($P = 0.003$)	No sham acupuncture control
Alimi et al. (2003)	90	1. Auricular acupuncture 2. Sham control 3. Control	2 month	VAS	The acupuncture group had a significant decrease ($P < 0.01$) in pain intensity after 2 months (35% decrease) compared with the control groups	Single acupuncturist
Deng et al. (2008)	162	1. Intradermal acupuncture 2. Sham acupuncture	1 month	Brief pain inventory, analgesic medication quantification	No difference between the two groups	Unique acupuncture device (intradermal acupuncture)

Four other trials have studied the effect of acupuncture in controlling cancer pain. Among them, Alimi et al.'s RCT is the most relevant and best designed trial (Alimi et al. 2003). This is a randomized, blinded, controlled trial conducted on 90 cancer patients with peripheral or central neuropathic pain arising after cancer treatment. The patients were randomized into one of three arms: one arm receive real auricular acupuncture at real ear acupuncture points that is defined as points where electro-dermal signal being detected; the other two arms were placebo arms with one arm received real auricular acupuncture at the placebo points, and the third arm receiving sham acupuncture through an auricular seeds at the placebo points. Different from any other acupuncture RCT so far, this study provided individualized auricular acupuncture to patients randomized to real acupuncture as the number of points and location of the points were selected individually for each patient. All patients received two courses of real or placebo auricular acupuncture in 2 months, 1 month apart. Their pain intensity measured by VAS at the end of the second month was used to measure the treatment efficacy. This study showed that in the group received real acupuncture, pain intensity decreased by 36% at the end of 2 months when compared with baseline, whereas it only decreased by 2% in the placebo groups ($P < 0.0001$).

The other three acupuncture-for-cancer-pain trials were less convincing with small sample size and incomplete statistical discussions (Li et al. 1994; Dang and Yang 1998; He et al. 1999). Li et al. (1994) evaluated the effect of various combinations of auricular acupuncture, Chinese herbs and epidural morphine to relieve postoperative pain in 16 patients with liver cancer. The study design was rather complicated and had very small sample size ($n = 2$ per group). Based on the visual analog scale (VAS) 0–100 mm, all the combination groups experienced better analgesia than placebo control group did. Dang and Yang (1998) published a study using the WHO pain scale to compare the effects of classical Chinese acupuncture (acupuncture point injection with freeze-dried human transfer factor) with conventional Western analgesia on patients with stomach cancer pain. After 2 months of treatment, researchers observed equivalent long-term effect of analgesia in the three groups. The authors reported that patients in both acupuncture treatment groups experienced improved quality of life and a decrease in the side effects of chemotherapy in addition to analgesia.

Another non-randomized study conducted by He et al. (1999) reported on the effect of acupuncture in postoperative pain management and movement in 80 breast cancer patients after surgical excision of the cancer and axillary lymphadenectomy. Forty-eight patients were given acupuncture on the postoperative days 3, 5 and 7 after surgery and on the day of discharge. Pain was measured by VAS. Compared to the control group of 32, who were not treated with acupuncture, the treatment group reported significant pain relief during arm movement on discharge and postoperative days 5 and 7. Range of motion also significantly increased in the treatment group compared to the control group during the same time period ($P < 0.001$). The authors also stressed that acupuncture point selection based on the state of the patient and obtaining a needling qi (de qi) sensation were important to achieving an effective acupuncture treatment.

8.2.1.4 Adverse Effects

Acupuncture is an invasive procedure, and adverse effects include minor side effects, such as transient hypotension and minor bruising, which are relatively common and self-limited. More serious effects, such as pneumothorax, hemopericardium, nerve damage and organ puncture are rare. Serious complications including life-threatening ones have also been reported but are extremely rare (Lao et al. 2003).

8.2.1.5 Conclusion

Overall, while there is a lack of definitive evidence, small studies do suggest that acupuncture might be efficacious in reducing cancer related pain, particularly in the short term and post-operative pain. Acupuncture might be a reasonable option to employ for pain relief especially in patients with other symptoms such as nausea (as acupuncture helps these symptoms as outline below), and those with neuropathic pain. For the latter, conventional medications are less efficacious and acupuncture might help such pain by activating certain brain pathways that contribute to the neuropathic pain.

8.2.2 Chinese Herbal Medicine for Cancer Pain Control

8.2.2.1 Introduction

An herb is any plant or plant product used for its scent, flavor and/or therapeutic properties. Herbal therapy refers to the use of preparations that contain herbs, either singly or in mixtures. They are generally used orally and come under the classification of dietary supplements. There are hundreds different types of Chinese herbal medicines, which may be applied to patients in different ways to decrease cancer pain, including transdermal, oral, intravenous, spray, inhalation or clysma.

8.2.2.2 Scientific Mechanism for Pain Relief

The scientific mechanism varies by the type of herbal supplement. For example, herbs containing salicylates like willow extracts may work primarily by activating slow pain pathways via interfering with the production of bradykinin and cytokines released during tissue destruction, while herbs like devils claw contain various anti-inflammatory and analgesic iridoid glycosides that could account for its analgesic effect. In general, the herbal drugs modulate the release of various central neurokines and endorphins in the central nervous system. The exact pathway depends on the particular herbal agent, and for many it is actually unknown, and that further studies should be conducted to elucidate the mechanism(s).

8.2.2.3 Review of Clinical Studies

Assessing the efficacy and safety of herbal medications is complex given the multitude of herbal therapies. In addition, these Chinese herbal medicines may be put together into different formula when used in patients.

Xu et al. (2007) published a thorough review of the current clinical research in China on using Chinese herbal medicine to treat cancer pain. A total of 115 studies were identified and 41 were identified as RCTs. None of the studies used the same formula of Chinese herbal medicines and the results were mixed. In addition, even though the studies have been labeled as RCTs, they often were not randomized or controlled. The results from various randomized trials are summarized in Table 8.2. The formula of various herbal medications is summarized in Table 8.3.

Among those trials, Kangfu Zhitong Adhesive Plaster was compared with morphine in treating 250 patients with cancer pain (Chen et al. 2001). The analgesic effects were found to be equivalent between the two groups after three days of treatment. Similar results were reported in a few other RCTs comparing the effect of other external Chinese herbal medicine such as Shebin Zhitong Gao (Ji et al. 2005), Chanshu Powder (Chen et al. 2004) and Zhongyao Tubu Ji (Yang and Yu 2003) were compared with conventional analgesics in reducing cancer pain. One trial did show topical herbal remedy Ai-tong-lin spray was superior to Western pain medicine lidocaine plus cholrhexine acetate aerosol with greater pain relieve in the herbal medicine group $P < 0.01$ (Zhou 1995). All the above studies were conducted in China and published in Chinese.

Cao and Xu (2006) published a RCT on evaluating the additional analgesic effect of Zhuang-gu-zhi-tong-san when added to cancer pain medication such as aspirin, tramal and pethidine on 82 patients experiencing cancer related bone pain. It was found that Zhuang-gu-zhi-tong-san prolonged analgesic duration by 2 h when compared with Western analgesic medicine alone ($P < 0.01$). However, the study is limited by its lack of effective blinding procedure, small sample size and lack of statistical analysis. The choice of Western analgesic medicine is also unique and difficult to interpret in the modern setting where opioids are used on cancer patients for cancer pain.

Another RCT evaluated the analgesic effect of a special type of nourishing yin and unblocking meridians Recipe in relieving caner pain in 84 patients suggested a trend of additive analgesic effect of Chinese herbal remedy (Zhang et al. 2006). The study showed that adding nourishing yin and unblocking meridians Recipe to morphine for 14 days caused pain reduction in 92% patients whereas the morphine along group only has 83% reduction, with the inter-group P-value more than 0.05. Chen et al. (2005) also published a RCT showing that adding Zhongyao-Zhitong Capsule to Western analgesic regimen comprised of indomethacin, tramal and morphine significantly increased pain relief from 52 to 80% ($P < 0.05$). However, the study results should be interpreted with caution given its small sample size (50 patients), lack of randomization and effective blinding mechanism.

Table 8.2 Summary of clinical trials on herbal therapies for cancer pain (Xu et al. 2007)

References	Study type	Type of cancer	Number of patients	Evaluation methods and pain assessment	Benefit reported	Administration methods	Adverse effects (number of patients)
A. Externally applied Chinese medicine for cancer pain							
Chen et al. (2001)	RCT	Liver, lung, gastric, colon, pancreatic cancer, gastro-metastasis	$N = 250$ Tx: $n = 182$ Ctr: $n = 68$	VRS Tx: I:10, II:114, III:58 Ctr: I:5, II:35, III:28	Total pain relief rate ($P > 0.05$): Tx: CR-90, PR-84 Ctr: CR-22, PR-40 Initiation time of analgesic action (min) ($P < 0.01$): Tx: 47.81 ± 33.12, Ctr: 13.05 ± 5.95 Analgesic duration (h) ($P < 0.01$): Tx:23.91 ± 12.31, Ctr: 15.97 ± 8.55	Tx: Kang-fu-zhi-tong adhesive plaster for 3 days; Ctr: Morphine 10 mg p.o. every 6 h for 3 days	Tx: Erubescence (178); Ctr: Not reported

Table 8.2 (continued)

References	Study type	Type of cancer	Number of patients	Evaluation methods and pain assessment	Benefit reported	Administration methods	Adverse effects (number of patients)
Jia et al. (2002)	RCT	Lung, liver, breast gastric, esophageal cancer, pancreatic, colorectal cancer	$N = 156$ Tx: $n = 80$ Ctr: $n = 76$	VRS, NRS Tx: 5.48 ± 1.29 Ctr: 5.27 ± 1.34	Total pain relief rate ($P < 0.05$): Tx: 92.5%, Ctr: 90.8% Pre-treatment pain intensity: Tx: 5.48 ± 1.29, Ctr: 5.27 ± 1.34 Post-treatment pain intensity: Tx: 1.16 ± 0.89, Ctr: 1.25 ± 0.93 Initiation time of analgesic action (t/h) ($P > 0.05$): Tx: 0.51 ± 0.17, Ctr: 0.52 ± 0.19 Analgesic duration (t/min) ($P > 0.05$): Tx: 7.32 ± 2.36, Ctr: 6.93 ± 2.17	Tx: Hua-jian-ba-du-mo external application 60 ml/m2, 2–3 times daily for 7 days; Ctr: Tramal 100–200 mg, 3–4 times daily for 7 days	Tx: Erythra (3); Ctr: Nausea and vomiting (30), dizziness (25), somnolence (25), constipation (23)

Table 8.2 (continued)

References	Study type	Type of cancer	Number of patients	Evaluation methods and pain assessment	Benefit reported	Administration methods	Adverse effects (number of patients)
Kou et al. (2003)	RCT	Thyroid, prostatic carcinoma, esophageal, breast, liver, lung, bone metastasis	$N = 58$ Tx: $n = 38$ Ctr: $n = 20$	VAS Tx: I:8, II:23, III:7 Ctr: I:5, II:12, III:3	Total pain relief rate ($P < 0.05$): Tx: 86.84%, Ctr: 65% Tx: CR-3, PR-30 Ctr: CR-0, PR-13 Initiation of analgesic action (t/min) ($P < 0.01$): Tx: 0.43 ± 0.5, Ctr: 1.39 ± 0.26	Tx: Yuan-she-zhi-tong physic liquor transdermal application several times a day for 7 days; Ctr: 1% Voltaren emulsion transdermal application several times a day for 7 days	Not reported

Table 8.2 (continued)

References	Study type	Type of cancer	Number of patients	Evaluation methods and pain assessment	Benefit reported	Administration methods	Adverse effects (number of patients)
Yang and Yu (2003)	RCT	Lung, liver, breast gastric, esophageal cancer, pancreatic cancer	$N = 135$ Tx: $n = 68$ Ctr: $n = 67$	NRS Tx: I:6, II:16, III:21 Ctr: I:5, II:43, III:19	Total pain relief rate ($P < 0.05$): Tx: CR-18, PR-28, MR-14 Ctr: CR-11, PR-24, MR-13 Initiation time of analgesic action (t/min) ($P < 0.01$): Tx: 21.23 ± 7.96, Ctr: 35.70 ± 12.16 Analgesic duration (t/min) ($P < 0.05$): Tx: 16.30 ± 8.75, Ctr: 12.42 ± 5.67	Tx: Zhong-yao-tu-bu-ji transdermal plaster, 2 times a day for 7 days; Ctr: Chan-su plaster once a day for 7 days	Tx: Erubescence (3); Ctr: Erubescence (1)

Table 8.2 (continued)

References	Study type	Type of cancer	Number of patients	Evaluation methods and pain assessment	Benefit reported	Administration methods	Adverse effects (number of patients)
Chen et al. (2004)	RCT single blind	Lung, liver, breast gastric, esophageal cancer, gastrointestinal cancer	$N = 90$ Tx: $n = 60$ Ctr: $n = 30$	NRS Tx: I:7, II:22, III:31 Ctr: I:4, II:12, III:14	Total pain relief rate ($P < 0.05$): Tx: 93.3%, Ctr: 80.0% Initiation time of analgesic action (t/min) ($P < 0.05$): Tx: 29.36 ± 8.41, Ctr: 30.46 ± 6.86 Analgesic duration (t/min) ($P < 0.05$): Tx: 16.50 ± 4.20, Ctr: 12.40 ± 5.30	Tx: Compound Chansu powder external application, once 24 h for 5 days; Ctr: Chan-su plaster (herbal preparation) external application, once 24 h for 5 days	Tx: Pruritus and roseola (3): Ctr: Pruritus and roseola (2)
Li (2004)	RCT	Liver	$N = 87$ Tx: $n = 43$ Ctr: $n = 44$	VRS Tx: I:17, II:20, III:6 Ctr: I:18, II:20, III:6	Total pain relief rate ($P > 0.05$): Tx: CR-8, PR-30 Ctr: CR-5, PR-32	Tx: Shuang-bai-san power, 150–300 g/6 h for 7 days; Ctr: Conventional analgesic treatment for 7 days (NSAIDs and opioids)	Tx: Erubescence & pruritus (1); Ctr: Dizziness (5), constipation (5), vomiting (4), abdominal distension (4)

Table 8.2 (continued)

References	Study type	Type of cancer	Number of patients	Evaluation methods and pain assessment	Benefit reported	Administration methods	Adverse effects (number of patients)
Tian et al. (2004)	RCT	Liver, lung, breast cancer, bone metastasis	$N = 60$ Tx: $n = 40$ Ctr: $n = 20$	VAS	Pain lessen ($P <$ 0.05): Tx: 26/40, Ctr: 7/20 Analgesic primary time (2 h after treatment): Tx: 14/40, Ctr: 6/20	Tx: Ai-li-tong transdermal plaster + Indometacin or Paracetamol + Dihydrocodeine for 10 days; Ctr: Placebo + Indometacin or Paracetamol + Dihydrocodeine for 10 days	Tx: Skin stimulation (6), hypersensitivity reaction of drug (3); Ctr: Skin stimulation (2), hypersensitivity reaction of drug (1)
He (2005)	RCT	Lung, breast, rectal, prostatic carcinoma, gastric, endometrial carcinoma, liver cancer with bone metastasis	$N = 66$ Tx: $n = 33$ Ctr: $n = 33$	VRS	Pain relief after 1 week ($P < 0.001$): Tx: CR-7, PR-10, MR-14 Ctr: CR-0, PR-0, MR-15 Pain relief after 4 weeks ($P < 0.05$): Tx: CR-24, PR-4, MR-5 Ctr: CR-18, PR-3, MR-8	Tx: Radiotherapy + Chinese medicine plaster; Ctr: Radiotherapy, 350 Gy, 3/week, 4 weeks, total 42 Gy/12 times	Not reported

Table 8.2 (continued)

References	Study type	Type of cancer	Number of patients	Evaluation methods and pain assessment	Benefit reported	Administration methods	Adverse effects (number of patients)
Ji et al. (2005)	RCT	Liver	$N = 46$ Tx: $n = 26$ Ctr: $n = 20$	VRS	Total pain relief rate ($P < 0.05$): Tx: 88.5%, Ctr: 90.0% Tx: CR-5, AR-9, MR-9 Ctr: CR-4, AR-7, MR-7 Initiation time of analgesic action (t/h) ($P < 0.01$): Tx: 0.43 ± 0.51, Ctr: 1.39 ± 0.26	Tx: She-bin-zhi-tong transdermal plaster, every 8 h for 7 days; Ctr: Tramal, 100 mg every 12 h for 7 days	Tx: Cutaneous reaction (4), nausea and vomiting (1); Ctr: Dizziness (2), nausea & vomiting (4), cutaneous reaction (1)
Sun et al. (2005)	RCT	Liver, lung, gastric cancer, colon, pancreatic cancer, malignant lymphoma	$N = 60$ Tx: $n = 45$ Ctr: $n = 15$	VRS, VAS Tx: I:4, II:30, III:11 Ctr: I:1, II:10, III:4	Pain relief rate ($P < 0.05$): Tx:100%, Ctr: 80%	Tx: Ai-tong-ning transdermal plaster, every 6–10 h for 7 days; Ctr: Duragesic, 25 mg every 3 days	Not reported

Table 8.2 (continued)

References	Study type	Type of cancer	Number of patients	Evaluation methods and pain assessment	Benefit reported	Administration methods	Adverse effects (number of patients)
Wan and Li (2005)	RCT	Liver, breast, lung, gastric, colon, pancreatic, prostatic, endometrial, malignant lymphoma, rhab-domyosar-coma, all stage IV	$N = 65$ Tx: $n = 32$ Ctr: $n = 33$	VRS, NRS Tx: II:18, III:14 Ctr: II:19, III:14	Total pain relief rate ($P < 0.05$): Tx: 90.7%, Ctr: 84.8% Tx: CR-9, PR-14, MR-6 Ctr: CR-4, PR-13, MR-11 Initiation time of analgesic action (t/min) ($P < 0.05$): Tx: 32.83 ± 14.42, Ctr: 27.42 ± 11.40 Analgesic duration (t/h) ($P < 0.05$): Tx: 18.10 ± 5.93, Ctr: 4.67 ± 1.57	Tx: Tong-kuai-xiao transdermal cataplasma, every 24 h for 7 days; Ctr: Bucinperazine, 100 mg intramuscular 3 times a day for 7 days	Not reported

Table 8.2 (continued)

References	Study type	Type of cancer	Number of patients	Evaluation methods and pain assessment	Benefit reported	Administration methods	Adverse effects (number of patients)
Yuan et al. (2005)	RCT	Liver cancer	$N = 91$ Tx: $n = 62$ Ctr: $n = 29$	VRS Tx: I:18, II:34, III:10 Ctr: I:6, II:18, III:5	Total pain relief rate ($P < 0.05$): Tx: 95.16%, Ctr: 79.30%	Tx: Ai-tong waistcloth external application on waist once 10 days; Ctr: Bucinnazine, 100 mg i.v. twice a day	Not reported
Liu et al. (2006)	RCT	Bone metastasis	$N = 40$ Tx: $n = 20$ Ctr: $n = 20$	VRS	Pain relief after 1 week ($P < 0.01$): Tx: CR-4, PR-8, MR-6 Ctr: PR-2, MR-8	Tx: Radiotherapy + Chinese medicine tincture; Ctr: Radiotherapy, 350 Gy, 5/week, 4 weeks, total 42 Gy/12 times	Not reported

Table 8.2 (continued)

References	Study type	Type of cancer	Number of patients	Evaluation methods and pain assessment	Benefit reported	Administration methods	Adverse effects (number of patients)
Sun et al. (2006)	RCT	Liver, lung, breast, large intestinal cancer	$N = 79$ Tx: $n = 41$ Ctr: $n = 38$	VRS Tx: I:13, II:16, III:12 Ctr: I:11, II:14, III:13	Total pain relief rate ($P < 0.05$): Tx: 92.68%, Ctr: 76.32% Tx: CR-15, PR-17, MR-6 Ctr: CR-10, PR-12, MR-7	Tx: Tong-shu-gao twice a week + Morphine 10 mg every 12 h for 2 months; Ctr: Morphine 10 mg every 12 h for 2 months	Tx: constipation (5), dysuresia (5); Ctr: constipation (12), dysuresia (12)
B. Oral administration of Chinese herbal medicine for cancer pain							
Gao et al. (1998)	RCT	Lung cancer, non-Hodgkin's lymphoma	$N = 66$ Tx: $n = 26$ Ctr: $n = 40$	VRS	The total pain relief rate: Tx: 88.5%, Ctr: 97.5% Mean analgesic duration (t/h) ($P <$ 0.05): Tx: 6, Ctr: 8	Tx: Kangsaide Zhitong-tang 60–120 ml p.o. 3 times a day for 7–10 days; Ctr: Morphine sulfate modified release tables 10–60 mg p.o. once 12 h for 7–10 days	Tx: Nausea (15), vomiting (6), constipation (2), diarrhea (2), headache (1), dry mouth (1); Ctr: Nausea (11), vomiting (8), constipation (22), dizziness (3), fatigue (5), flustered (2), hidrosis (5), somnolence (1), short of breath (1)

Table 8.2 (continued)

References	Study type	Type of cancer	Number of patients	Evaluation methods and pain assessment	Benefit reported	Administration methods	Adverse effects (number of patients)
Chen et al. (2000)	RCT multi-center	Liver, lung, breast, gastric, pancreatic	Tx: $n = 214$ Ctr: $n = 114$ Op: $n = 100$	NRS mean pain score: Tx: 6.09, Ctr: 5.78 ($P < 0.05$)	Pain relief: Tx: 73.53%, Ctr: 69.30%, Op: 71.00% Initiation of analgesic action in hours ($P > 0.05$): Tx: 1.087 ± 0.808, Ctr: 1.405 ± 0.899 Analgesic duration in hours ($P > 0.05$): Tx: 5.94 ± 1.78, Ctr: 5.71 ± 1.76	Tx: Gui-shen analgesic mixture 50 ml, placebo drug 2 tablets, every 8 h for 7 days; Ctr: Placebo herbs 50 ml, Bucinperazine 60 mg, every 8 h for 7 days; Open: Gui-shen analgesic mixture 50 ml, every 8 h for 7 days	Drowsiness: Tx: 22.67%, Ctr: 16.46%; Dizziness: Tx: 14%, Ctr: 13%; Nausea: Tx: 18%, Ctr: 13.93%; Vomiting: Tx: 4%, Ctr: 3.8%

Table 8.2 (continued)

References	Study type	Type of cancer	Number of patients	Evaluation methods and pain assessment	Benefit reported	Administration methods	Adverse effects (number of patients)
Wang et al. (2000a)	NRCT	Breast cancer with bone metastasis	$N = 97$ Tx: $n = 53$ Ctr: $n = 44$	VRS Tx: I:24, II:21, III:8 Ctr: I:19,II:20, III:5	Pain relief ($P < 0.05$): I:CR+PR: Tx: 24, Ctr: 19 II:CR+PR: Tx: 20,Ctr: 13 III:CR+PR: Tx: 4,Ctr: 1	Tx: Vinorelbine + Cisplatin regimen + Chinese medicinal decoction; Ctr: Vinorelbine + Cisplatin regimen + standard practice pain management (below) for 2 months: I: Indometacin 25 mg,3 times daily; II: Tramal, 50 mg, 3 times daily; III: Controlled release Morphine 30 mg, twice daily	Not reported

Table 8.2 (continued)

References	Study type	Type of cancer	Number of patients	Evaluation methods and pain assessment	Benefit reported	Administration methods	Adverse effects (number of patients)
Wang et al. (2000b)	NRCT	Lung, liver, breast gastric, rectal, esophageal	$N = 84$ Tx: $n = 41$ Ctr: $n = 43$	VRS Tx: I:15, II:18, III:8 Ctr: I:14, II:20, III:9	After discontinuing any medicine for 4 weeks, the recurrence or increasing rate of pain ($P < 0.05$): Tx: I:7.7%, II:20.0%, III:25.0% Ctr: I:49.2%, II:60.0%, III:77.8%	Tx: Chemotherapy regimen + Chinese medicinal broth 2 times daily for 2 months; Ctr: Chemotherapy regimen for 2 months (chemotherapy regimen determined by primary cancer)	Not reported

Table 8.2 (continued)

References	Study type	Type of cancer	Number of patients	Evaluation methods and pain assessment	Benefit reported	Administration methods	Adverse effects (number of patients)
Lin et al. (2001)	RCT	Esophageal, gastric liver, lung, breast, rectal	$N = 60$ Tx: $n = 30$ Ctr: $n = 30$	VRS Tx: I:9, II:15, III:6 Ctr: I:10, II:14, III:6	Pain relief: Tx: CR-14, PR-9, MR-6, NR-1 Ctr: CR-5, PR-12, MR-11, NR-2 Total rate of pain relief ($P < 0.05$): Tx: 96.67%, Ctr: 93.33%	Tx: I: Jia-wei-nian-tong capsule 4 pills; II: Jia-wei-nian-tong capsule 4 pills + Tramadol tablet 50 mg; III: Jia-wei-nian-tong capsule 4 pills + Pethidine 50 mg; 4 times daily: Ctr: I: Aspirin 0.5 g; II: Tramal tablet 50 mg; III: Pethidine 50 mg; 4 times daily	Tx: I: Slight diarrhea (few); II & III: Nausea (7), dizziness (6), constipation (3), slight diarrhea (2); Ctr: I: Nausea (many); II & III: Nausea (13), vomiting (8), dizziness (6), constipation (18)

Table 8.2 (continued)

References	Study type	Type of cancer	Number of patients	Evaluation methods and pain assessment	Benefit reported	Administration methods	Adverse effects (number of patients)
Zhang (2001)	RCT	Stomach, liver, lung, breast, colon, pancreatic and submaxillary gland (most metastasis)	$N = 110$ Tx: $n = 82$ Ctr: $n = 28$	VRS Tx: I:0, II:52, III:30 Ctr: I:0, II:16, III:12	Pain relief: Tx: CR-24, PR-28, MR-16; Ctr: CR-8, PR-10, MR-6 Total rate of pain relief ($P > 0.05$): Tx: 82.9%, Ctr: 85.7% Total dose of pethidine: Tx: 50 mg × 139, Ctr: 50 mg × 83	Tx: Compound Strychnos capsule p.o. 0.25 g, 3 times a day for 3 weeks; Ctr: Indomethacin suppos 50 mg, twice daily for 3 weeks; After 1 week, if patients still felt Grade II or III pain, Pethidine (50 mg) until pain became mild, average Pethidine: Tx: 2.21/case/week, Ctr: 3.61/case/week	Tx: Muscle twitching of oral area and numbness of tongue (1), slight numbness of tongue (4); Ctr: Liver and renal functional lesion (3), nausea, dyspepsia and loose stool (7)

Table 8.2 (continued)

References	Study type	Type of cancer	Number of patients	Evaluation methods and pain assessment	Benefit reported	Administration methods	Adverse effects (number of patients)
Li et al. (2002)	RCT	Liver, colon, head pancreas, prostate, stomach, ovarian gallbladder, renal bladder	$N = 84$ Tx: $n = 46$ Ctr: $n = 38$	VAS I:22.6%, II:61.9%, III:15.5%	Pain relief ($P >$ 0.05): Tx: CR+PR–23, MR–14 Ctr: CR+PR–19, MR–11	Tx: Lamiophlomis rotata Kudo capsule 3 pills, 3 times daily for 3 days; Ctr: Indomethacin 25 mg, 3 times daily for 3 days	Tx: Nausea and stomach discomfort (2); Ctr: Gastrointestinal tract discomfort (14), stomach discomfort, nausea, abdominal pain, headache and dizziness (2)
Ma et al. (2003)	RCT	Gastric	$N = 62$ Tx: $n = 31$ Ctr: $n = 31$	VRS Tx: 65.02 ± 5.26 Ctr: 67.45 ± 4.71	Tx: CR–8, AR–15, PR–6; Ctr: CR–8, AR–15, PR–5 Total rate of pain relief ($P > 0.05$): Tx: 93.55%, Ctr: 90.32%; Average initiation of analgesia ($P >$ 0.05): Tx: 17.26 min, Ctr: 16.57 min	Tx: Jia-wei-bao-an-ke-li 9 g, 3 times daily for 15 days: Ctr: Daning (analgesic drug) 1 pill, 2 times daily for 15 days	Not reported

Table 8.2 (continued)

References	Study type	Type of cancer	Number of patients	Evaluation methods and pain assessment	Benefit reported	Administration methods	Adverse effects (number of patients)
Wei et al. (2003)	RCT	Lung, liver, gastric cancer	$N = 200$ Tx: $n = 100$ Ctr: $n = 100$	VRS	Rate of moderate pain relief ($P > 0.05$): Tx: 83%, Ctr: 85%; Initiation of analgesic action (for moderate pain) in hours: Tx: 2.80, Ctr: 2.13	Tx: Tian-chan capsule, 3 capsules, plus placebo drug 1 tablet, 3 times a day for 5 days; Ctr: Paracetamol codeine phosphate, 1 tablet, plus placebo drug 3 tablets, 3 times a day for 5 days	Tx: Nausea and vomiting (3), calor mordax on back (1)
Chen et al. (2004)	RCT	Gastro-intestinal cancer	$N = 124$ Tx: $n = 73$ Ctr: $n = 51$	VAS	Total pain relief rate ($P < 0.05$): Tx: 93.15%, Ctr. 74.51%; Tx: AR-75.34%, PR-17.81%; Ctr: AR-45.10%, PR-29.41%	Tx: Shi-tong-tang + Morphine or Indometacin for 7 days; Ctr: Morphine or Indometacin for 7 days	Not reported

Table 8.2 (continued)

References	Study type	Type of cancer	Number of patients	Evaluation methods and pain assessment	Benefit reported	Administration methods	Adverse effects (number of patients)
Chen et al. (2005)	RCT	Lung, liver, breast gastric, esophageal cancer, pancreatic, colorectal cancer	$N = 50$ Tx: $n = 25$ Ctr: $n = 25$	VRS, VAS Tx: I:7, II:8, III:10 Ctr: I:7, II:9, III:9	Pain relief ($P <$ 0.05): Tx: CR-12, PR-8, MR-4 Ctr: CR-6, PR-7, MR-11 Total rate of pain relief ($P < 0.05$): Tx: 80%, Ctr: 52%	Tx: I: Zhongyao-zhitong capsule 4 capsules, 3 times daily; II: Zhongyao-zhitong capsule 4 capsules, 3 times daily + Tramal 100 mg 2 times daily; III: Zhongyao-zhitong capsule 4 capsules, 3 times daily + Morphine 30 mg 2 times daily; Ctr: I:	Tx: constipation (3), dizziness (2), nausea (5), somnolence (2): Ctr: Stomach upset (2), constipation (11), dizziness (2), nausea (7), somnolence (5)

Table 8.2 (continued)

References	Study type	Type of cancer	Number of patients	Evaluation methods and pain assessment	Benefit reported	Administration methods	Adverse effects (number of patients)
						Indometacin 25 mg 3 times daily; II: Tramal 100 mg 2 times daily; III: Morphine 30 mg 2 times daily; Treatment period: 14 days	
Lin et al. (2005)	RCT	Primary hepatocellular carcinoma	$N = 48$ Tx: $n = 26$ Ctr: $n = 22$	Not reported	Pain relief rate ($P < 0.01$): Tx: 80.76%, Ctr: 36.36%	Tx: Shen-qi mixture 20 ml p.o. 3 times a day for 1 month + microwave coagulation 60 W, 800 s once a week for 2 weeks; Ctr: Microwave coagulation 60 W, 800 s once a week for 2 weeks	Tx: Severe right upper abdominal pain (2); Ctr: Severe right upper abdominal pain (1), nausea, vomiting and constipation (3)

Table 8.2 (continued)

References	Study type	Type of cancer	Number of patients	Evaluation methods and pain assessment	Benefit reported	Administration methods	Adverse effects (number of patients)
Shi et al. (2005)	RCT	Liver, lung, gastric	$N = 180$ Tx: $n = 90$ Ctr: $n = 90$	Intensity (WHO 1987): Tx: 26.5 ± 12.2 Ctr: 24.3 ± 11.5	Pain relief: Tx: AR-42, PR:30; Ctr: AR-45, PR-33 Rate of pain relief ($P > 0.05$): Tx: 80.0%, Ctr: 87.7% Initiation of analgesia (min) ($P > 0.05$): Tx: 48.8 ± 11.5, Ctr: 45.9 ± 10.6 Analgesic duration (h) ($P < 0.05$): Tx: 7.8 ± 2.2, Ctr: 6.6 ± 1.7	Tx: Ai-tong-ning pill, 1.5 g, twice a day for 14 days; Ctr: Tramal 50 mg, twice a day for 14 days	Not reported

Table 8.2 (continued)

References	Study type	Type of cancer	Number of patients	Evaluation methods and pain assessment	Benefit reported	Administration methods	Adverse effects (number of patients)
Wu et al. (2005)	RCT	Liver, lung, colon, gastric, pancreatic	$N = 60$ Tx: $n = 30$ Ctr: $n = 30$	VRS, NRS Tx: I:7, II:17, III:6 Ctr: I:6, II:16, III:8	Tx: no pain 4, mild pain 15, moderate pain 6, severe pain 5; Ctr: no pain 3, mild pain 14, moderate pain 6, severe pain 7 ($P < 0.05$) Initiation of analgesic action in hours ($P > 0.05$): Tx: 0.58 ± 0.33, Ctr: 0.53 ± 0.28 Analgesic duration in hours ($P > 0.05$): Tx: 3.66 ± 1.82, Ctr: 3.83 ± 2.13	Tx: Ai-tong-ping capsule 1.6 g, 3 times a day for 7 days; Ctr: Diclofena 40 mg, p.o. 3 times a day for 7 days	Ctr: Nausea, vomiting and constipation (3)

Table 8.2 (continued)

References	Study type	Type of cancer	Number of patients	Evaluation methods and pain assessment	Benefit reported	Administration methods	Adverse effects (number of patients)
Cao and Xu (2006)	RCT	Bone	$N = 82$ Tx: $n = 41$ Ctr: $n = 41$	VRS Tx: I:15, II:19, III:7 Ctr: I:16, II:18, III:7	Pain relief ($P <$ 0.05): Tx: CR-19, PR-13, MR-8 Ctr: CR-7, PR-14, MR-14 Prolonged analgesic duration (t/h) ($P < 0.01$): Tx: 7.83 ± 2.46, Ctr: 5.71 ± 2.24	Tx: I: Zhuang-gu-zhi-tong-san + Aspirin 0.3 g, 4 times daily; II: Zhuang-gu-zhi-tong-san + Tramal tablet 50 mg, 4 times daily; III: Zhuang-gu-zhi-tong-san + Pethidine 50 mg, 4 times daily; Ctr: I: Aspirin 0.3 g, 4 times daily; II: Tramal tablet, 50 mg, four times daily; III: pethidine 50 mg, 4 times daily	Tx: Nausea (8), vomiting (7), dizziness (6), constipation (7); Ctr: Nausea (13), vomiting (8), dizziness (7), constipation (18)

Table 8.2 (continued)

References	Study type	Type of cancer	Number of patients	Evaluation methods and pain assessment	Benefit reported	Administration methods	Adverse effects (number of patients)
Zhang et al. (2006)	RCT	Lung, gastric, liver, esophagus, large intestine cancer	$N = 84$ Tx: $n = 41$ Ctr: $n = 43$	VRS, VAS	Total pain relief ($P < 0.05$): Tx: 92.0%, Ctr: 83.0% Tx: CR-7, PR-17, MR-14, NR-3 Ctr: CR-3, PR-11, MR-23, NR-6 Analgesic primary time (h) ($P < 0.05$): Tx: 2.92 ± 1.46, Ctr: 3.58 ± 2.35	Tx: Nourishing yin and unblocking meridians Recipe 100 ml p.o. 2 times a day + Morphine (same as Ctr) for 14 days; Ctr: Morphine hydrochloride sustained-release tablets 30 mg q12 h for 14 days	Tx: Nausea and vomiting (1), constipation (1): Ctr: Burning sense on back (1), nausea and vomiting (3)
C. Intravenous infusions for cancer pain							
Luo and Kong (2001)	RCT	Esophageal carcinoma at advanced stage	$N = 34$ Tx: $n = 18$ Ctr: $n = 16$	Evaluation methods didn't report Tx: I:6, II:8, III:4 Ctr: I:2, II:11, III:3	Total pain relief rate: Tx: 88.89%, Ctr: 43.75%	Tx: Kang-lai-te injection 200 ml i.v. once daily, 20 days/month for 2 months Ctr: Chemotherapy: 5-FU + Cisplatin + Pingyangmycin for 2 course	Not reported

Table 8.2 (continued)

References	Study type	Type of cancer	Number of patients	Evaluation methods and pain assessment	Benefit reported	Administration methods	Adverse effects (number of patients)
Shi et al. (2002)	RCT	Gastric, pancreatic, liver, colon cancer	$N = 32$ Tx: $n = 17$ Ctr: $n = 15$	VRS TX: I:5, II:7, III:5 Ctr: I:3, II: 6, III:6	Total pain relief rate: Tx: 64.70%, Ctr: 33.33% Initiation time of analgesic action (t/min): Tx: 20.62 ± 7.15, Ctr: 31.42 ± 8.06 ($P > 0.05$) Analgesic duration (t/h) ($P < 0.05$): Tx: 25.13 ± 3.99, Ctr: 9.47 ± 1.97	Tx: Hua-chan-su injection at acupuncture point ST36 (Zusanli) 1 ml i.m. each side every other day for 10 days Ctr: 0.9% saline at acupuncture point ST36 (Zusanli) 1 ml i.m. each side every other day for 10 days	Tx: Arrhythmia (1), skin rash (1)

Table 8.2 (continued)

References	Study type	Type of cancer	Number of patients	Evaluation methods and pain assessment	Benefit reported	Administration methods	Adverse effects (number of patients)
Wang et al. (2002)	RCT	Lung, liver, breast, colon-rectal cancer at III–IV stage	$N = 56$ Tx: $n = 29$ Ctr: $n = 27$	Not reported	Total pain relief rate ($P < 0.01$): Tx: 75.9%, Ctr: 29.6%	Tx: Kang-lai-te injection 200 ml i.v. once daily, 20 days/cycle for 3 cycles plus chemotherapy or radiotherapy Ctr: Chemotherapy or radiotherapy (different regimen for different primary cancer)	Skin reaction at the injection site (4)
An and Wang (2003)	RCT	Lung, breast, rectal, gastric, liver cancer at advanced stage	$N = 81$ Tx: $n = 39$ Ctr: $n = 42$	Not reported	Total pain relief rate ($P < 0.01$): Tx: 35.9%, Ctr: 4.8% Tx: CR-2, PR-10; Ctr: CR-0, PR-1	Tx: Supportive care plus Compound Ku-shen injection 20 ml i.v. once daily for 30 days Ctr: Supportive care (drug name didn't report)	Not reported

Table 8.2 (continued)

References	Study type	Type of cancer	Number of patients	Evaluation methods and pain assessment	Benefit reported	Administration methods	Adverse effects (number of patients)
Luo et al. (2003)	RCT	Liver, lung, breast gastric cancer, pancreatic cancer, bladder, ovarian cancer	$N = 102$ *A*: $n = 32$ *B*: $n = 70$	NRS A: I:20, II:12 B: II:38, III:32	A: Total pain relief rate ($P > 0.05$): Tx: 56.3%, Ctr: 71.9% Tx: CR-10, PR-8; Ctr: CR-16, PR-7 B: Total pain relief rate ($P > 0.05$): Tx: 57.1%, Ctr: 42.9%	A: WHO 3 step analgesic treated 2 or 3 days, discontinued and exchanged to Yan-shu 20–40 ml i.v. once daily for 5–10 days B: WHO 3 step analgesic treated 2 or 3 days plus Yan-shu 20–40 ml i.v. once daily for 5–10 days	A: Tx: 12.5%, Ctr: 31.2%; B: Tx: Constipation11.4%, nausea 4.3%, vomiting 2.9%, urinary retention 1.4%, abdominal distension 2.9%, anorexia 2.9%, headache 4.3%, itch 2.9%, diaphoresis 2.9%, flustered 1.4%

Table 8.2 (continued)

References	Study type	Type of cancer	Number of patients	Evaluation methods and pain assessment	Benefit reported	Administration methods	Adverse effects (number of patients)
						Tx: After Yan-shu treatment; Ctr: Before Yan-shu treatment I & II: Yan-shu 20–30 ml i.v. once daily for 5–7 days III: Yan-shu 40 ml i.v. once daily for 7–10 days WHO 3 step analgesic's name didn't report	B: Ctr: Constipation17.4%, nausea 7.1%, vomiting 7.1%, urinary retention 4.3%, abdominal distension 4.3%, anorexia 4.3%, headache 4.3%, itch 1.4%, diaphoresis 2.9%, flustered 2.9%
Zeng et al. (2003)	RCT	Gastrointestinal cancer	$N = 35$ Tx: $n = 20$ Ctr: $n = 15$	Not reported	Pain relief: Tx: CR-7, PR-10, MR-3; Ctr: not reported Tumour control: Tx: CR-2, AR-7; Ctr: CR-1, AR-5	Tx: Yan-shu 20 ml i.v. once daily for 10 days plus chemotherapy (5-FU + CF) Ctr: Chemotherapy (5-FU + CF)	Not reported

Table 8.2 (continued)

References	Study type	Type of cancer	Number of patients	Evaluation methods and pain assessment	Benefit reported	Administration methods	Adverse effects (number of patients)
Jin et al. (2004)	RCT	Lung cancer	$N = 87$ A: Tx: $n = 21$ Ctr: $n = 19$ B: Tx: $n = 26$ Ctr: $n = 21$	NRS	A: Total pain relief rate ($P < 0.01$): Tx: 80.95%, Ctr: 52.63% Tx: CR-8, PR-9, MR-3; Ctr: CR-4, PR-6, MR-5 B: Total pain relief rate ($P < 0.05$): Tx: 65.38%, Ctr: 52.38% Tx: CR-6, PR-11, MR-5; Ctr: CR-4, PR-7, MR-8	A: Tx: Radiotherapy 60Co 40–60 Gy 30 days plus Compound Ku-shen injection 20 ml i.v. once a day for 10 days; Ctr: Radiotherapy 60Co 40–60 Gy 30 days	Tx: Chest distress (1)

Table 8.2 (continued)

References	Study type	Type of cancer	Number of patients	Evaluation methods and pain assessment	Benefit reported	Administration methods	Adverse effects (number of patients)
						B: Tx: CBP 300 mg/m^2 i.v. d1, VP16 0.1 i.v. d1–d5, 2 course plus Compound Ku-shen injection 20 ml i.v. once a day for 10 days; Ctr: CBP 300 mg/m^2 i.v. d1, VP16 0.1 i.v. d1–d5, 2 course	

Table 8.2 (continued)

References	Study type	Type of cancer	Number of patients	Evaluation methods and pain assessment	Benefit reported	Administration methods	Adverse effects (number of patients)
Ma (2004)	RCT	Multiple myeloma	$N = 26$ Tx: $n = 13$ Ctr: $n = 13$	VRS	Total pain relief rate ($P < 0.01$): Tx: 92.3%, Ctr: 38.5% Tx: CR-8, PR-4; Ctr: CR-1, PR-4 Initiation time of analgesic action (t/day): Tx: 1–3 day:7, 4–10 day:4 Ctr: 1–3 day:1, 4–10 day: 3 ($P < 0.01$)	Tx: Chemotherapy + Pamidronati sodium 90 mg i.v. every other 2–4 weeks + Shenfu injection 40 ml i.v. once daily Ctr: Chemotherapy + Rotundine 60 mg i.m. twice daily	Tx: Nausea and anorexia (1); Ctr: Fever (2)

Table 8.2 (continued)

References	Study type	Type of cancer	Number of patients	Evaluation methods and pain assessment	Benefit reported	Administration methods	Adverse effects (number of patients)
						Chemotherapy: Carmustine 0.5–1 $mg \cdot kg^{-1}$ i.v. at day 1, Cyclophosphamide 10 $mg \cdot kg^{-1}$ i.v. at day 1, L-Sarcolysinum 0.1 $mg \cdot kg^{-1}$ i.v. at day 7, Prednisone 1 $mg \cdot kg^{-1}$ p.o. from day 1 to day 14, Vincristine 0.031 $mg \cdot kg^{-1}$ i.v. at day 21	

Table 8.2 (continued)

References	Study type	Type of cancer	Number of patients	Evaluation methods and pain assessment	Benefit reported	Administration methods	Adverse effects (number of patients)
Wang et al. (2004)	RCT	Lung, liver, gastric, colon, breast cancer	$N = 208$ Tx: $n = 110$ Ctr: $n = 98$	VRS	Total pain relief rate ($P < 0.05$): Tx: 85.5%, Ctr: 82.7% Tx: CR-34, PR-36, MR-24 Ctr: PR-23, MR-32, MR-26 Initiation time of analgesic action (t/h): Tx: 2.9 ± 1.3, Ctr: 2.7 ± 1.0 ($P <$ 0.05) Analgesic duration (t/h) ($P < 0.05$): Tx: 4.1 ± 1.9, Ctr: 4.5 ± 1.9	Tx: Compound Ku-shen injection 20 ml i.v. once daily for 30 days; Ctr: First WHO 3 step analgesic (name didn't report), then Compound Ku-shen injection 20 ml i.v. once daily for 30 days	Not reported

Table 8.2 (continued)

References	Study type	Type of cancer	Number of patients	Evaluation methods and pain assessment	Benefit reported	Administration methods	Adverse effects (number of patients)
Liu and Kuang (2005)	RCT	Lung, liver, gastric, colon, pancreatic, bladder, ovarian cancer	$N = 44$ Tx: $n = 23$ Ctr: $n = 21$	VRS Tx: I:6, II:11, III:6 Ctr: I:6, II:10, III:5	Total pain relief rate ($P > 0.05$): Tx: 73.91%, Ctr: 80.95% Tx: CR-8, PR-9; Ctr: CR-9, PR-8	Tx: Hua-chan-su injection 30 ml i.v. once daily for 28 days Ctr: Morphine 10 mg or 30 mg p.o. twice daily for 28 days	Tx: Fever (1 cases), skin reactions at the injection site (2); Ctr: Nausea and vomiting (3), constipation (5)

Table 8.2 (continued)

References	Study type	Type of cancer	Number of patients	Evaluation methods and pain assessment	Benefit reported	Administration methods	Adverse effects (number of patients)
Guan et al. (2006)	RCT	Liver cancer at III stage	$N = 94$ A: Tx: $n = 28$ Ctr: $n = 28$ B: Tx: $n = 12$ Ctr: $n = 10$ C: Tx: $n = 8$ Ctr: $n = 8$	Not reported	A: Total pain relief rate: Tx: 96.4%, Ctr: 85.7% Tx: CR-23, AR-4, MR-1 Ctr: CR-21, AR-3, MR-4 B: Total pain relief rate: Tx: 100%, Ctr: 90% Tx: CR-9, AR-3, MR-0 Ctr: CR-5, AR-4, MR-1 C: Total pain relief rate: Tx: 87.5%, Ctr: 62.5% Tx: CR-5, AR-2, MR-1 Ctr: CR-3, AR-2, MR-2 Total pain relief rate (A + B + C): Tx: 95.8%, Ctr: 82.6% ($P < 0.05$)	A: Tx: Transcatheter arterial chemoembolization plus Yan-shu 20 ml i.v. once daily, 15 day/cycle, 3–4 cycle; Ctr: TACE: (1) 5-FU + Tegafur + Adriamycin or (2) Pirarubicin + Cisplatin/Carboplatin	Not reported

Table 8.2 (continued)

References	Study type	Type of cancer	Number of patients	Evaluation methods and pain assessment	Benefit reported	Administration methods	Adverse effects (number of patients)
						B: Tx: Chemotherapy plus Yan-shu 20 ml i.v. once daily, 15 day/cycle, 3–4 cycle; Ctr: Chemotherapy: (1) Gemzar + Tegafur/5-FU + Pirarubicin or (2) Hydroxycamptothecin + Tegafur + Pirarubicin or (3) Gemzar + Oxaliplatin C: Tx: ATX + BTX; Ctr: A Ctr + B Ctr	

Table 8.2 (continued)

References	Study type	Type of cancer	Number of patients	Evaluation methods and pain assessment	Benefit reported	Administration methods	Adverse effects (number of patients)
Zhuang and Gu (2006)	RCT	Liver, gastric, colon-rectal, breast cancer at advanced stage	$N = 38$ Tx: $n = 18$ Ctr: $n = 20$	Not reported	Total pain relief rate ($P < 0.01$): Tx: 38.8%, Ctr: 5% Tx: CR-2, PR-5; Ctr: CR-0, PR-1	Tx: Supportive care plus Compound Ku-shen injection 30 ml i.v. once daily for 30 days Ctr: Supportive care (drug name didn't report)	Not reported

RCT: randomized controlled trial I: The patient feels mild, tolerable pain, sleep is good, movement is unrestricted, facial expression is good; II: The patient feels moderate, tolerable pain, sleep is poor due to pain; movement is limited, facial expression shows pain; III: The patient feels severe, intolerable pain, cannot sleep due to pain, movement is limited, facial expression shows pain and he/she groans constantly.

VAS: visual analog scale: The visual analog scale is a straight line (100 mm) with the left end of the line representing no pain and the right end of the line representing the worst pain. Patients are asked to mark on the line where they think their pain is.

NRS: numerical rating scale: On the numerical rating scale, the patient is asked to identify how much pain they are having by choosing a number from 0 (no pain) to 10 (the worst pain imaginable).

* Tx: treatment group; Ctr: control group; Op: open group.

□ CR: complete relief; AR: apparent relief; PR: partial relief; MR: moderate relief; NR: no relief.

Table 8.3 Formula and herbal information used in various randomized clinical trials (Xu et al. 2007)

Formula name	Herbal name
Ai-li-tong transdermal plaster	*Bufo bufo gargarizans, Strychnos nux-vomica, Moschus berezovskii, Cynanchum paniculatum, Dryobalanops aromatica*
Ai-tong waistcloth	*Hedyotis diffusa, Sparganium stoloniferum, Curcuma zedoaria, Scutellaria barbata, Scolopendra subspinipes mutilans, Eupolyphaga sinensis, Boswellia carterii, Commiphora molmol, Salvia miltiorrhiza, Rheum palumatum, Carthamus tinctorius, Moschus berezovskii*
Ai-tong-ning pill	*Corydalis turtschaninovii, etc*
Ai-tong-ning transdermal plaster	*Boswellia carterii, Commiphora molmol, Panax notoginseng, Typha angustifolia, Hedyotis diffusa*
Ai-tong-ping capsule	*Polygonum bistorta, Armadillidium vulgare, Arisaema heterophyllum, Typhonium giganteum, Boswellia carterii, Corydalis turtschaninovii, Piper longum*
Chinese medicine tincture	*Daemonorops draco, Boswellia carterii, Commiphora molmol, Dryobalanops aromatica*
Compound Chanshu powder	*Bufo bufo gargarizans, Moschus berezovskii, Dryobalanops aromatica, Cinnamomum cassia, Asarum heterotropoides, Aconitum kusnezoffii, Daemonorops draco, Prunus persica, Sparganium stoloniferum, Curcuma zedoaria, Baphicacanthus cusia, Locopus lucidus, Phellodendron amurense, Rubia cordifolia*
Compound Ku-shen injection	*Sophora flavescens, Cremastra variabilis, Trogopterus xanthipes, Polygonum multiflorum*
Compound strychnos capsule	*Strychnos nux-vomica, Glycyrrhiza uralensis*
Gui-shen analgesic mixture	*Cinnamomum cassia, Asarum heterotropoides, Codonopsis pilosula, Eucommia ulmoides*
Hua-chan-su injection	*Bufo bufo gargarizans*

Table 8.3 (continued)

Formula name	Herbal name
Hua-jian-ba-du-mo	*Eupolyphaga sinensis, Momordica cochinchinensis, Rheum palumatum, Curcuma longa, Dryobalanops aromatica*
Jia-wei-bao-an-ke-li	*Rheum palumatum, Aconitum carmichaeli, Amyda sinensis, Arisaema heterophyllum, Paeonia lactiflora, Glycyrrhiza uralensis*
Jia-wei-nian-tong capsule	*Corydalis turtschaninovii, Cyperus rotundus, Panax notoginseng, Aquilaria agallocha, Curcuma zedoaria, Citrus reticulata, Nardostachys chinensis, Cinnabaris, Rheum palumatum, Dryobalanops aromatica*
Kang-fu-zhi-tong adhesive plaster	*Rheum palumatum, Bufo bufo gargarizans, Euphorbia pekinensis, Cremastra variabilis, Aconitum carmichaeli, Aconitum carmichaeli, Arisaema heterophyllum, Eupolyphaga sinensis, Gleditsia sinensis, Dryobalanops aromatica, Boswellia carterii, Commiphora molmol, Sparganium stoloniferum, Curcuma zedoaria*
Kang-lai-te injection	*Coix lachryma-jobi*
Kang-sai-de-zhi-tong decoction	*Cinnamomum cassia, Codonopsis pilosula, Atractylodes macrocephala, Poria cocos, Eucommia ulmoides, Epimedium grandiflorum, Asarum heterotropoides, Paeonia lactiflora, Cyperus rotundus, Citrus reticulata, Crataegus cuneata, Ziziphus jujuba*
Lamiophlomis Rotata Kudo capsule	*Lamiophlomis rotata*
Nourishing yin and unblocking meridians Recipe	*Asparagus cochinchinensis, Ophiopogon japonicus, Scrophularia ningpoonsis, Rehmannia glutinosa, Bupleurum chinense, Anemarrhena asphodeloides, Corydalis turtschaninovii, Paeonia lactiflora, Angelica sinensis, Panax notoginseng, Citrus reticulata, Prunus persica, Glycyrrhiza uralensis*

Table 8.3 (continued)

Formula name	Herbal name
She-bin-zhi-tong transdermal plaster	*Moschus berezovskii, Corydalis turtschaninovii, Angelica sinensis, Salvia miltiorrhiza, Lindera strychnifolia, Dryobalanops aromatica, Eupolyphaga sinensis, Daemonorops draco, Bufo bufo gargarizans, Rheum palumatum, Cinnabaris, Citrus reticulata, Polygonum bistorta, Euphorbia kansui*
Shen-fu injection	*Panax ginseng, Aconitum carmichaeli*
Shen-qi mixture	*Pseudostellaria heterophylla, Astragalus membranaceus, Poria cocos, Paeonia lactiflora, Rehmannia glutinosa, Atractylodes macrocephala, Dendrobium nobile, Angelica sinensis, Hedyotis diffusa, Lobelia chinensis, Zingiber officinale, Glycyrrhiza uralensis*
Shi-tong decoction	*Bupleurum chinense, Citrus aurantium, Magnolia officinalis, Rheum palumatum, Salvia miltiorrhiza, Paeonia veitchii, Typha angustifolia, Curcuma zedoaria, Panax notoginseng, Corydalis turtschaninovii, Coptis chinensis, Hedyotis diffusa, Scutellaria barbata*
Shuang-bai powder	*Phellodendron amurense, Platycladus orientalis, Rheum palumatum, Mentha haplocalyx, Locopus lucidus*
Tian-chan capsule	*Rhizoma corydalis decumbentis, Aconitum carmichaeli, Bufo bufo gargarizans, Giraldi daphne, Angelica dahurica, Paeonia lactiflora, Chelidonii herba, Gentiana macrophylla, Ligusticum chuanxiong, Glycyrrhiza uralensis*
Tong-kuai-xiao cataplasma	*Corydalis turtschaninovii, Lindera strychnifolia, Curcuma longa, Iron pyrites, Taraxacum mongolicum, Polygonum bistorta, Sinapisca alba, Vaccaria segelalis, Boswellia carterii, Dryobalanops aromatica*

Table 8.3 (continued)

Formula name	Herbal name
Tong-shu plaster	*Kronopolites millepeda, Aconitum carmichaeli, Aconitum kusnezoffii, Typhonium giganteum, Strychnos nux-vomica, Sophora flavescens, Gleditsia sinensis*
Yuan-she-zhi-tong physic liquor	*Corydalis turtschaninovii, Moschus berezovskii, Bufo bufo gargarizans, Bos taurus domesticus, Dryobalanops aromatica*
Zhong-yao-tu-bu-ji transdermal plaster	*Aconitum carmichaeli, Bufo bufo gargarizans, Spatholobus suberectus, Curcuma zedoaria, Typhonium giganteum, Eugenia caryophyllata*
Zhong-yao-zhi-tong capsule	*Asarum heterotropoides, Paeonia lactiflora, Ligusticum chuanxiong, Cynanchum paniculatum*
Zhong-yao-zhi-tong plaster	*Papaver somniferum, Corydalis turtschaninovii, Paeonia veitchii, Paeonia lactiflora, Carthamus tinctorius, Curcuma zedoaria, Coix lachryma-jobi*
Zhuang-gu-zhi-tong powder	*Angelica sinensis, Rehmannia glutinosa, Taxillus chinensis, Manis pentadactyla, Psoralea corylifolia, Drynaria fortunei, Paeoniae alba, Paeonia lactiflora, Corydalis turtschaninovii, Panax notoginseng, Curcuma zedoaria, Arisaema heterophyllum, Scolopendra subspinipes mutilans, Pheretima aspergillum, Buthus martensii, Citrus reticulata*

A number of RCTs have also been conducted to examine the analgesic effect of intravenous Chinese herbal medicines, particularly Hua-chan-su. Studies have that the pain relief from Hua-chan-su was equivalent in the two intervention groups, but with Chinese herbal group patients had a better quality of life based on the Karnofsky criteria (Liu and Kuang 2005). However, again the study results should be interpreted with caution given its small sample size (60 patients in total), lack of randomization and blinding design.

8.2.2.4 Adverse Effects

The common side effects reported in the clinical trials include skin rash, pruritus, blisters, nausea and vomiting associated with external applications of herbal medications; nausea, vomiting, dizziness and drowsiness with oral herbal medicines; and low-grade fever, fatigue, dry mouth, skin rash with intravenous herbal medicine infusion. Severe side effects include neuromuscular symptoms such as tremors in oral muscles and tongue numbness with oral medications, and chest distress, dyspnea and arrhythmia with intravenous infusion have also been reported. Most side effects were generally transient and self-limited, and did not require medical intervention. Studies have suggested that the side effects caused by herbal medicines were less than those caused by conventional medicines (Xu et al. 2007).

8.2.2.5 Conclusion

While few Chinese herbal regimens appear promising as therapies for cancer related pain, based on the current scientific evidence, it cannot be recommended for routine clinical practice yet for multiple reasons. Most studies had a small sample size, lacked a statistical section and effective randomization or blinding design. The interaction of Chinese herbal regimens with chemotherapy drugs or conventional analgesic drugs has not been established. Moreover, most of the trials were not written in English and were not listed in Medline database. Finally, each trial used a different Chinese herbal formula, which makes it difficult to confirm the effect of any formula. These factors make it difficult to draw any firm conclusions about the efficacy and safety of Chinese herbal medicines. There is a need for well designed trials to establish the role of Chinese herbal medicine in alleviating pain in cancer patients.

8.2.3 Qigong

8.2.3.1 Overview

Qigong refers to the exercise of qi, the vital energy circulating along the energy channels in the body with the goal of helping the body to reach harmony and building up qi. It is a type of mind-body intervention that has minimum side effects, unclear mechanism and potential significant benefit. It originated in China and has been widely used among Chinese to prevent disease and strengthen health. It has also been reported to decrease pain by raising pain threshold. Qigong therapy can be divided into two types: internal qigong and external qigong. Internal qigong refers to qigong exercise that is performed by the patients themselves to achieve therapeutic effect, whereas external qigong refers to qigong therapy applied to the patients by qigong master – someone who has been practicing internal qigong for years and is able to use their qi to direct the patient's qi flow and achieve therapeutic effect.

8.2.3.2 Scientific Basis for Analgesic Effect

The mechanism of qigong induced self-healing is unclear and warrants further research. Chinese literature did suggest that qigong might have induced improving immune function, raising pain threshold, and increasing microcirculation.

8.2.3.3 Review of Clinical Studies

There have been a number of case reports, and case series in Chinese reporting the effect of qigong therapy in oncology patients. Chen and Yeung (2002) reviewed 21 studies of qigong in cancer patients. Most were observational studies with or without controls and very few trials explore the effect of qigong in reducing cancer pain. This review article did identify two clinical trials on qigong and pain control. One single armed study of 55 patients showed that pain threshold in the joints was significantly increased during internal qigong practice (Wang and Li 1989). Another study showed that external qigong increased skin pain threshold (Zhang et al. 1990).

Additional literature search at MEDLINE database produced two case reports (Zhang et al. 1990; Lee et al. 2005) and one non-randomized controlled trial on qigong and cancer pain (Lee et al. 2006). Lee et al. (2006) from Taiwan reported a non-RCT on the effect of Chan-Chuang qigong on reducing symptoms related to chemotherapy in 67 breast cancer patients undergoing first cycle of chemotherapy. In this study, 32 patients were assigned to Chan-Chuang qigong group and 35 patients to the control group. In the qigong group, the patients were asked to practice Chan-Chuang qigong for 15–60 min every day during the 21 days of first cycle of chemotherapy. The study showed that the mean symptoms stress scores on McCorkle and Yang's symptom distress scale peaked at 1.61 on day 8, and plateaued to 1.37 and 1.41 on days 15 and 22 in the control group. In the qigong group, it peaked at 1.43 on day 8 and plateaued to 1.24 and 1.22 on days 15 and 22. Statistically significant difference in pain score were noticed on days 15 and 22 between the qigong and control groups ($P < 0.05$). Similar difference between the two groups was noticed in other symptoms such as numbness, heartburn and dizziness. The study concluded that Chan-Chuang qigong has the potential to decrease chemotherapy induced symptoms stress such as pain, numbness, heartburn and dizziness. This study is limited by its small sample size, lack of randomization or blinding design.

8.2.3.4 Adverse Effects

None have been reported.

8.2.3.5 Conclusion

The idea of qigong reducing cancer pain is quite stimulating as this is an intervention with minimal risk and potential significant benefit. The research in this area is quite limited as there have only been a couple of case reports and clinical trials available. In addition, there has been very little unbiased research explaining how qigong works. High quality, well designed RCTs that also explore the mechanism of qigong are needed.

8.2.4 Dietary Intervention

Dietary intervention is a very important part of TCM. Unfortunately, after careful literature search, we were unable to identify any clinical studies showing any relationship between dietary intervention and cancer pain.

8.2.5 Massage

8.2.5.1 Overview

Massage is one of the oldest and most popular complementary interventions among oncology patients. It involves putting pressure and traction in the soft tissue in the body with therapeutic intent. It is not only an important part of TCM, but also an important part of other types of complementary medical cultures, such as Indian medicine and reflexology.

8.2.5.2 Scientific Basis for Analgesic Effect

Massage produces various physiological effects on the body including increasing blood circulation, increasing cardiac output, reducing edema, relieving muscle spasm and preventing scar adhesions. It is postulated that it has analgesic effects through activation of inhibitory control mechanisms and its relaxing effects.

8.2.5.3 Review of Clinical Studies

There have been many clinical trials assessing the effect of massage on cancer pain. Most studies were limited by its small sample size and inadequate study design that was lack of randomization, control or blinding method (Ernst 2009).

A recently published, relatively well designed multi-centered RCT involved 380 adults with different types of advanced cancer (Kutner et al. 2008). They were randomized into two groups, with one receiving 6 massage sessions (30 min each) in 2 weeks and another group receiving sham massage with light touch at the same schedule. Memorial pain assessment card and brief pain inventory were used to evaluate their pain at baseline, right after each treatment and weekly afterwards for 3 weeks. Both groups experienced immediate improvement in pain reduction, with massage group had statistically significant pain reduction compared to the sham massage control group –1.87 (95% CI –2.07 to –1.67) versus –0.97 (–1.18 to 0.76) with inter-group difference $P < 0.001$. This study is however limited by potential reporting bias as the immediate outcome measured were obtained by the unblinded study therapists.

8.2.5.4 Adverse Effects

A potential concern in using massage therapy is that it might promote metastatic spread of tumour cells through increased lymph flow. There is however no evidence to support such thinking. The adverse effects of massage are few. A recent review on the safety of massage found that most of adverse effects were associated with exotic types of manual massage or massage delivered by laymen, while massage therapists rarely caused adverse effects (Sun et al. 2006). The reported adverse events included cerebrovascular accidents, displacement of a ureteral stent, embolization of a kidney, hematoma, leg ulcers, nerve damage, posterior interosseous syndrome, pseudoaneurysm, pulmonary embolism, ruptured uterus, strangulation of neck, thyrotoxicosis and various pain syndromes. Serious adverse effects were rare and included fracture of osteoporotic bones and rupture liver. The contraindications of massage therapy include phlebitis, deep vein thrombosis, burns, skin infections, eczema, open wounds, bone fractures and advanced osteoporosis.

8.2.5.5 Conclusion

While there is a lack of a large well designed placebo/sham controlled study evaluating massage therapy, small studies do suggest that massage is a promising therapy for control of cancer related pain, particularly short term benefit. Moreover, massage is generally well tolerated and can elevate the mood of the recipient. Since pain is a subjective phenomenon, it is said patient preference is important for optimal pain management. Thus, even if placebo response these therapies could be offered if patient desire so and risk/benefit ratio is favorable. Nevertheless from a pure scientific perspective, larger well designed studies assessing the effect of massage on cancer pain are needed. Also, research should be standardized with clear definitions of massage procedures, area of body massaged, massage time and a standard outcome.

8.3 Summary

Cancer related pain is a common, complex and can be a difficult problem to manage. The current treatments are limited to oral analgesics and occasional surgical intervention, which have limited response and with significant side effects. Traditional Chinese medicine has the potential to provide effective complementary therapy to decrease cancer pain. However, the current research in different TCM modalities in treating cancer pain are limited by methodological weaknesses such as small sample size, lack of standard outcome measurement, and lack of effective randomization and blinding method.

While testing TCM therapies do pose unique methodological challenges (therapies are difficult to standardize, designing placebo is often difficult, therapies cannot be patented, lack of funding from industry, etc), randomized placebo-controlled trials remain the gold standard to test efficacy of a therapy and many multi-institutional trials related to TCM, such as acupuncture have been completed successfully. Thus future research should focus on methodologically strong RCTs. The studies should be well designed with adequate sample size, have sufficient duration, have good sham control groups, involve multiple institutions and adequately monitor, and report adverse effects. Research should be standardized with clear definitions of procedures, area of intervention on body (if any), duration of intervention, standardized instrument for pain assessment and a standard outcome. Finally, there is also a need to understand the scientific mechanism by which these therapies are beneficial. This would optimize the likelihood of success, and would help remove the label of soft science that is often applied to these potentially useful therapies.

References

Alimi D, Rubino C, Leandri EP et al. Analgesic effects of auricular acupuncture for cancer pain. J Pain Symptom Manage. 2000;19:81–2.

Alimi D, Rubino C, Pichard-Leandri E et al. Analgesic effect of auricular acupuncture for cancer pain: a randomized, blinded, controlled trial. J Clin Oncol. 2003;21:4120–6.

An YZ, Wang XH. Treatment of 56 cases of advanced cancer with Compound Kushen Injection. Shanghai J Tradit Chin Med. 2003;37:15–6.

Banning A, Sjogren P, Henriksen H. Pain causes in 200 patients referred to a multidisciplinary cancer pain clinic. Pain. 1991;45:45–8.

Bardia A, Barton DL, Prokop LJ et al. Efficacy of complementary and alternative medicine therapies in relieving cancer pain: a systematic review. J Clin Oncol. 2006;24:5457–64.

Brescia FJ, Portenoy RK, Ryan M et al. Pain, opioid use, and survival in hospitalized patients with advanced cancer. J Clin Oncol. 1992;10:149–55.

Cao JX, Xu GY. Clinical observation on treatment of 41 cases of pain induced to bone metastasis cancer with Zhuang-gu-zhi-tong-san and Western medicine. Chin J Tradit Med Sci Technol. 2006;48:49.

Chen CH, Sun GZ, Tang WX et al. Clinical observation on treatment of cancer pain with Guishen analgesic mixture. Chin J New Drugs. 2000;9:196–200.

Chen GY, Liu YQ, Gao P et al. Clinical study of Zhongyao Zhitong Capsule on 25 cases with cancer pain. Jiangsu J Tradit Chin Med. 2005;16:17.

Chen K, Yeung R. Exploratory studies of qigong therapy for cancer in China. Integr Cancer Ther. 2002;1:345–70.

Chen MX, Huang LZ, He YH et al. A clinical study on the analgesic effect of compound Chanshu powder on cancerous pain used in a way of external application – a report of 60 cases. J Tradit Chin Med Univ Hunan. 2004;24:37–9.

Chen SQ, Wang ZX, Zhao SR et al. Clinical and experimental study on effects of Kangfu Zhitong Adhesive Plaster in treating cancer pain. Shandong J Tradit Chin Med. 2001;20:332–3.

Cleeland CS, Gonin R, Hatfield AK et al. Pain and its treatment in outpatients with metastatic cancer. N Engl J Med. 1994;330:592–6.

Coyle N, Adelhardt J, Foley KM et al. Character of terminal illness in the advanced cancer patient: pain and other symptoms during the last four weeks of life. J Pain Symptom Manage. 1990;5:83–93.
Dang W, Yang J. Clinical study on acupuncture treatment of stomach carcinoma pain. J Tradit Chin Med. 1998;18:31–8.
Deng G, Rusch V, Vickers A et al. Randomized controlled trial of a special acupuncture technique for pain after thoracotomy. J Thorac Cardiovasc Surg. 2008;136:1464–9.
Ernst E. Massage therapy for cancer palliation and supportive care: a systematic review of randomised clinical trials. Support Care Cancer. 2009;17:333–7.
Foley KM. Pain syndromes in patients with cancer. In: Advances in pain research and therapy. New York: Raven Press; 1979.
Foley KM. The treatment of cancer pain. N Engl J Med. 1985;313:84–95.
Gao TJ, Shi HL, Lu Z. Clinical treatment of cancer's Anodyne Kangsaide Zhitong Tang. Tuberculosis Chest Tumor. 1998;2:18–21.
Guan CN, Cai LZ, Yue LQ et al. Clinical study on treatment of advanced primary liver cancer by Yanshu injection combining with chemotherapy. China J Chin Mater Med. 2006;31:510–2.
He JG. Treatment of 33 cases of bone metastasis cancer with Zhitong plaster and radiotherapy. Shangdong J Tradit Chin Med. 2005;24:20–1.
He JP, Friedrich M, Ertan AK et al. Pain-relief and movement improvement by acupuncture after ablation and axillary lymphadenectomy in patients with mammary cancer. Clin Exp Obstet Gynecol. 1999;26:81–4.
Ji YF, Huang JH, Liang HJ et al. Clinical observation on 26 cases of treatment over pain caused by liver cancer spread with Shebin Zhitong Gao. J Jiangxi Univ Tradit Chin Med. 2005;17: 31–2.
Jia YJ, Liu Y, Sun YY et al. Clinical observation on 80 cases of moderate cancerous pain treated by Hua Jian Ba Du Mo. J Tianjin Univ Tradit Chin Med. 2002;21:11–2.
Jin SY, Ge RG, Quan XL et al. Clinical observation of compound Kushen Injection in treating elderly patients of lung cancer pain. Chin J Misdiagn. 2004;10:1675–6.
Kou SL, Bo LY, Li ZP et al. Clinical observation on 38 cases of cancer pain with Yuanshezhitong physic liquor. J Emerg Tradit Chin Med. 2003;12:421–32.
Kutner JS, Smith MC, Corbin L et al. Massage therapy versus simple touch to improve pain and mood in patients with advanced cancer: a randomized trial. Ann Intern Med. 2008;149:369–79.
Lao L, Hamilton GR, Fu J et al. Is acupuncture safe? A systematic review of case reports. Altern Ther Health Med. 2003;9:72–83.
Lao L. Traditional Chinese medicine. In: Essentials of complementary and alternative medicine. Philadelphia: Lippincott Williams & Wilkins; 1999.
Lee MS, Yang SH, Lee KK et al. Effects of qi therapy (external qigong) on symptoms of advanced cancer: a single case study. Eur J Cancer Care (Engl). 2005;14:457–62.
Lee TI, Chen HH, Yeh ML. Effects of chan-chuang qigong on improving symptom and psychological distress in chemotherapy patients. Am J Chin Med. 2006;34:37–46.
Li HL, Hao MA, Wang BT et al. The analgesic effect of traditional Tibetan herb Lamiophlomis rotata on cancer pain. Hebei Med J. 2002;26:146–7.
Li QS, Cao SH, Xie GM et al. Combined traditional Chinese medicine and Western medicine. Relieving effects of Chinese herbs, ear-acupuncture and epidural morphine on postoperative pain in liver cancer. Chin Med J (Engl). 1994;107:289–94.
Li YH. Pain of liver cancer treated by application with Shuangbai Power. J External Ther Tradit Chin Med. 2004;13:26–7.
Lin D, Li F, Chen LS et al. Treatment of cancer pain by Jiawei Niantong Capsule: A clinical observation of 30 cases. N J Tradit Chin Med. 2001;33:18–9.
Lin JJ, Jin CN, Zheng ML et al. Clinical study on treatment of primary hepatocellular carcinoma by Shenqi mixture combined with microwave coagulation. Chin J Integr Med. 2005;11:104–10.
Liu YX, Kuang TH. Clinical observation on improving quality of life of advanced cancer patients with Huachansu injection. Chin J Tradit Med Sci Technol. 2005;45:46.

Liu ZL, Xu M, Zhen L. Treatment of bone metastasis cancer with external using Chinese medicine and radiotherapy. J Emerg Tradit Chin Med. 2006;15:142.
Luo J, Lin HS, Liu SJ et al. Clinical study on treatment of cancer pain at IV stage with Yanshu injection. J Tradit Chin Med Univ Hunan. 2003;23:40–2,50.
Luo ZH, Kong LY. The clinical study of life qualify improvement of advanced esophageal carcinoma patient by using Kanglalte. Chin J Cancer Prev Treat. 2001;8:418–9.
McMahon S. Mechanisms of cutaneous, deep, and visceral pain. In: Textbook of pain. New York: Livingstone; 1994.
Ma TX, Li XL, Song ZH et al. Clinical study about the ache caused by stomach tumor treated with Jiaweibaoankeli. Chin J Cancer Prev Treat. 2003;10:297–9.
McMillan SC, Tittle M, Hagan S et al. Management of pain and pain-related symptoms in hospitalized veterans with cancer. Cancer Nurs. 2000;23:327–36.
Mehling WE, Jacobs B, Acree M et al. Symptom management with massage and acupuncture in postoperative cancer patients: a randomized controlled trial. J Pain Symptom Manage. 2007;33:258–66.
Portenoy RK, Foley KM, Inturrisi CE. The nature of opioid responsiveness and its implications for neuropathic pain: new hypotheses derived from studies of opioid infusions. Pain. 1990;43: 273–86.
Richardson MA, Sanders T, Palmer JL et al. Complementary/alternative medicine use in a comprehensive cancer center and the implications for oncology. J Clin Oncol. 2000;18:2505–14.
Shi HC, Liu XY, Shi KG et al. Clinical observation on the treatment of 90 cases of pain caused by malignant tumor with Aitongning. Guide J Tradit Chin Med. 2005;11:21–2.
Shi J, Xu L, Wei PK. Clinical observation on treatment of 17 cases of cancer pain with injection ad acumen of Huachansu injection. Chin J Integr Tradit West Med. 2002;22:121.
Sun JF, Lu LJ, Zuang JH, et al. Clinical observation of Tongshugao on cancer pain. Chin J Info Tradit Chin Med. 2006;13:56.
Sun YB, Zhou YN, Zhang CG, et al. 45 cases of cancer patients treated with external application of Aitongning. Chin Arch Tradit Chin Med. 2005;23:728–729.
Tian HQ, Huang HQ, Huang ZQ et al. 60 cases of cancer pain treated with Ailitong. Shaanxi J Tradit Chin Med. 2004;25:232–5.
Wan DG, Li PW. Clinical study on treatment of cancerous pain with Tongkuaixiao Cataplasma. Chin J Info Tradit Chin Med. 2005;12:68–9.
Wang JS, Li DZ. Experimental study of compound analgesia by qigong information treating instrument and acupuncture. Second International Conference on Qigong. Xi'an, China; 1989.
Wang YH, Han H, Fu J et al. Clinical therapeutic evaluation of combined use of Kanglaite (KLT) and chemo-or radio-therapy in late cancer. Chin J Cancer Prev Treat. 2002;9:340–1.
Wei L, Yang CG, Miao WH. Observation of the efficacy and safety of Tian chan capsule in the treatment of cancer pains. Chin J N Drugs. 2003;12:663–5.
Wells N. Pain intensity and pain interference in hospitalized patients with cancer. Oncol Nurs Forum. 2000;27:985–91.
Wong RH, Lee TW, Sihoe AD et al. Analgesic effect of electroacupuncture in postthoracotomy pain: a prospective randomized trial. Ann Thorac Surg. 2006;81:2031–6.
Wu MH, Zhou XP, Chen HB et al. Clinical study on Aitongping capsule in treating cancerous pain. Chin J Integr Tradit West Med. 2005;25:218–21.
Xu L, Lao LX, Ge A et al. Chinese herbal medicine for cancer pain. Integr Cancer Ther. 2007;6:208–34.
Yang XF, Yu C. The effect of Zhongyao Tubu Ji on 68 cases with cancer pain. Chinas Naturopathy. 2003;11:24–5.
Yuan M, Huang GL, Bian WG et al. Clinical observation of Aitong waistcloth on liver cancer pain. J Sichuan Tradit Chin Med. 2005;23:49–50.
Zech DF, Grond S, Lynch J et al. Validation of World Health Organization Guidelines for cancer pain relief: a 10-year prospective study. Pain. 1995;63:65–76.

Zeng JY, Lan BY, Li ZH et al. Clinical observation of the treatment of gastrointestinal malignant tumor by chemotherapy combined with composite Kusheng Injection. Guangxi Med J. 2003;25:1657–8.

Zhang M. Observation of therapeutic effect of "Compound Strychnos Capsules" in treating cancerous pain. Acta Univ Tradit Med Sins Pharmacol Shanghai. 2001;15 :31–2.

Zhang JM, Chen YF, He JH et al. Analgesic effect of emitted qi and the preliminary study of its mechanism. Third National Academic Conference on Qigong Sciences. Guangzhou, China; 1990.

Zhang T, Ma SL, Xie GR et al. Clinical research on nourishing yin and unblocking meridians Recipe combined with opioid analgesics in cancer pain management. Chin J Integr Med. 2006;180:184.

Zhou Y. Clinical and experimental study on treatment of cancer pain with Aitonglin spray. Tradit Chin Med Res. 1995;17:19.

Zhuang GF, Gu BQ. Clinical observation on treatment of advanced malignant tumor with Compound Kushen Injection. Shanghai Med Pharm J. 2006;27:323–4.

Chapter 9
Novel Developments on Artemisinin and Its Derivatives for Cancer Therapy

Serkan Sertel, Peter K. Plinkert, and Thomas Efferth

Abstract The lack of effective long-term anticancer therapy highlights the necessity to identify new potent anticancer compounds. Many biocompounds of naturally occurring medicinal plants have pharmacological activities and, thus, represent a source of molecules that may have anti-proliferative effects on a variety of cancers. During the past 10 years, we have systematically analyzed medicinal plants used in traditional Chinese medicine and focused our interest on *Artemisia annua* (sweet wormwood herb). The active principle of sweet wormwood herb is Artemisinin, a sesquiterpene, which exerts not only anti-malarial activity but also profound cytotoxicity against tumour cells. The anti-tumour mechanism shares similarities to the anti-malarial mechanism: the Artemisinin molecule contains an endoperoxide bridge that reacts with an iron atom to form free radicals causing macromolecular damage and cell death. The anticancer activity of artesunate, a semi-synthetic derivative of Artemisinin, has also been shown in human xenograft tumours in mice and dogs. First encouraging experience in the clinical treatment of patients suffering from laryngeal carcinoma, uveal melanoma, pituitary macroadenoma and non-small cell lung cancer calls for comprehensive clinical trials with artesunate for cancer treatment in the near future. In this chapter, we summarize novel developments on Artemisinin and its derivatives concerning mode of action, metabolism, toxicity, in vivo effects, clinical application and biotechnological production methods.

9.1 Introduction

Artemisia annua (sweet wormwood herb) is an annual medicinal plant native of Asia and has been used for many centuries for the treatment of fever and malaria. Here, we give an introduction of the medicinal herb and its main bioactive compound, Artemisinin, as far as origin, botany, history and chemical structure are concerned.

T. Efferth (✉)
University of Mainz, Germany
e-mail: efferth@uni-mainz.de

W.C.S. Cho (ed.), *Supportive Cancer Care with Chinese Medicine*,
DOI 10.1007/978-90-481-3555-4_9,

9.1.1 Traditional Chinese Medicine

Artemisia annua is also known as sweet wormwood, sweet annie, sweet sagewort or annual wormwood (Chinese pinyin: Qīnghāo). It belongs to the medicinal herbs used in traditional Chinese medicine (TCM).

Medicinal herbs from TCM hold a unique position since an enormous variety of drugs from plant origin are founded on more than 5,000 years of tradition (Tang et al. 2003a, b). Hence, it is assumed that many ineffective prescriptions have disappeared, thereby significantly improving the prospect for identifying novel active constituents from TCM (Boik 2001; Newman et al. 2003). Our interest in natural products from TCM was triggered in the 1990s by sesquiterpene lactones of the Artemisinin type from sweet wormwood herb (Efferth et al. 1996). The sweet wormwood herb genus is known to contain many bioactive compounds (Tan et al. 1998).

9.1.2 Botany of Sweet Wormwood Herb

This plant belongs to the family of Asteraceae. It has a single stem of 50–200 cm in height with fern-like leaves, bright yellow blossoms and a camphor-like scent. The leaves of sweet wormwood herb contain 89% of the total Artemisinin in the plant with the uppermost foliar portion of the plant containing almost double that of the lower leaves (Charles et al. 1990).

The reproduction occurs through cross-pollination by insect or wind distribution. The plant represents a typical neophyte in lowlands and hill countries in Asia and Europe, continental to sub-continental climate. However, sweet wormwood herb was only recognized in China as a medicinal plant.

9.1.3 History of Artemisinin

Sweet wormwood herb has been used as a traditional medicine for at least 2,000 years in China. The earliest written record in silk so far discovered is the Recipes for 52 Kinds of Diseases, which was found in the Mawangdui Tomb of the West Han Dynasty (168 BC) in Changsha, Hunan Province (van Agtmael et al. 1999). The first record of sweet wormwood herb for the treatment of fever and chills was described in the Handbook of Prescriptions for Emergencies (Zhouhou Beiji Fang) written by Ge Hong (261–341). The next historical tradition is from the year 1086, written by Shen Gua. Since then a series of Chinese medicine books including the most famous book Compendium of Materia Medica (Bencao Gangmu) published by Li Shizen in 1596 cited Ge Hong's prescription.

In the course of the Vietnam War, the Chinese government started an anti-malarial research program to systematically search for anti-malarial TCM plants to support the Vietnamese army. As a result, Artemisinin (Qinghaosu) was identified in 1972 as the active anti-malarial constituent of sweet wormwood herb (Klayman 1985; Li and Wu 1998). Today, Artemisinin is widely used worldwide to combat otherwise drug-resistant *Plasmodium* strains, cerebral malaria and malaria in children (Yeung et al. 2004). While sweet wormwood herb and Artemisinin were regarded by the World Health Organization (WHO) with much reluctance for a long time, the full potential was recently recognized. In the meantime, the WHO officially recommends Artemisinin and its derivatives for the treatment of malaria, particularly as a part of combination therapies with other anti-malarial drugs, called Artemisinin-based combination therapies (ACTs).

9.1.4 Chemical Structure of Artemisinin and Its Derivatives

Artemisinin is the parent compound of an emerging class of anti-malarial drugs of importance in the treatment of malaria in areas with multidrug-resistant *Plasmodium falciparum.* Artemisinin is a sesquiterpene lactone with an internal peroxide bridge (Fig. 9.1), necessary for its anti-parasitic effect (Klayman 1985). Systematically, it is named [3R-(3α,5αβ,6β,9α,12β,1αR*)]-octahydro-3,6,9-trimethyl-3,12-epoxy-12H-pyrano[4,3-j]-1,2 benzodioxepin-10(3H)-one. Therapeutically used semi-synthetic derivatives of Artemisinin in malaria treatment are artesunate (ART), artemether (ARM) and arteether (ARE) (Fig. 9.1).

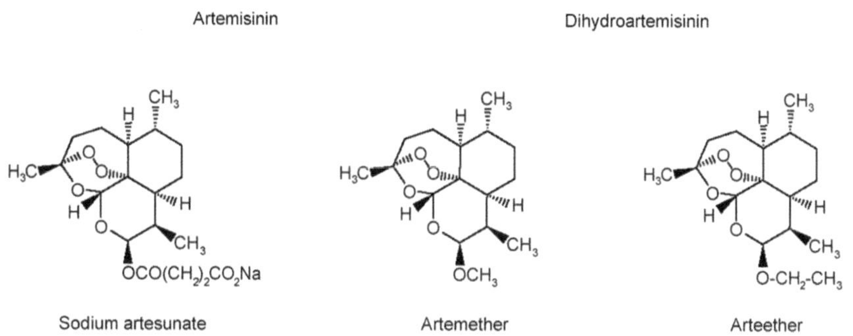

Fig. 9.1 Chemical structure of Artemisinin and its semi-synthetic derivatives

9.2 Molecular Mode of Action in Cancer Cells

Here, we elucidate various molecular mechanisms of Artemisinin and its analogues in cancer cells with the focus on inhibition of angiogenesis and metastasis. Moreover, Artemisinins' impact on protein kinases and transferrin-/estrogen receptors (ERs) in anticancer activity are reviewed.

9.2.1 Chemical Structure of Artemisinin and Its Derivatives

Anti-tumour activity is frequently determined by multiple factors (Efferth et al. 1992; Efferth and Volm 1993; Volm et al. 1993; 2002a, b). Although anticancer drugs are extremely divergent in their chemical and physical structures and biological actions, a synopsis of the relevant mechanisms influencing drug effects allows their categorization into (I) those acting upstream of the actual drug target, (II) those acting at critical target sites or (III) those acting downstream of them (Efferth and Grassmann 2000; Efferth and Volm 2005).

Mechanisms acting upstream include transporter proteins for uptake or excretion (i.e. ATP-binding cassette transporters (ABC transporter), reduced folate carriers and nucleoside transporters) and drug-metabolizing enzymes that activate, inactivate or detoxify drugs (i.e. phase I/II enzymes). Metabolizing enzymes and transporter molecules often do not exhibit specificity for certain anticancer drugs, but are operative towards a wide range of different xenobiotic drugs including anticancer agents. Drug-metabolizing enzymes may influence pharmacokinetics and dynamics. Drug target sites for alkylating agents and platinum drugs are DNA (and DNA repair mechanisms), RNA (RNA synthesis inhibitors, e.g. actinomycin D) and specific proteins such as DNA topoisomerases I/II (camptothecins, anthracyclines, and epipodophyllotoxins), tubulins (*Vinca* alkaloids and taxanes) or enzymes of DNA biosynthesis (antimetabolites).

Mechanisms downstream of the actual drug targets and at distinct intracellular locations are operative after injury by drugs has been taken place. The most important downstream mechanisms are the diverse apoptosis pathways. Their deregulation may lead to drug resistance and survival of cancer cells despite target molecules have been successfully targeted by anticancer drugs (Efferth et al. 1997; Pommier et al. 2004). Apoptosis is not only regulated by the proteins directly involved in the apoptotic cascade but also by external factors, i.e. by chemokines that act as "survival factors" involved in prevention of apoptosis and, hence, contributing to survival and drug resistance of tumour cells after chemo-therapeutic insult (Lotem and Sachs 1996; Efferth et al. 2002a).

It is, therefore, reasonable to propose that the same is true for cytotoxic compounds from TCM such as Artemisinin and its derivatives. The remarkable anticancer activity of ART, ARE and ARM (Woerdenbag et al. 1993; Efferth et al. 2001; 2002c) is associated with the basal mRNA expression of genes, which most probable affect the proliferation of cells (cell cycle regulating genes, growth factors with their receptors, oncogenes and tumour suppressor genes) (Efferth et al. 2002b). By microarray and hierarchical cluster analyses, a set of apoptosis-regulating genes was identified whose mRNA expression significantly correlated with the IC_{50} valucs for ART in the National Cancer Institute (NCI) cell lines. Furthermore, ART acts via *p53*-dependent and -independent pathways in isogenic *p53+/+ p21*WAF1/CIP1+/+, *p53 −/− p21*WAF1/CIP1+/+, and *p53+/+ p21*WAF1/CIP1/colon carcinoma cells (Efferth et al. 2003b).

Dihydroartemisinin (DHA) is the first metabolite of ART, ARM or ARE and reveals considerable cytotoxicity towards cancer cells. DHA has exhibited the strongest anticancer activity among the derivatives of Artemisinin. A number of studies have investigated the use of DHA to inhibit growth and/or to induce apoptosis of cells of breast cancer (Singh and Lai 2001), cervical cancer, uterus chorion cancer, embryo transversal cancer, ovarian cancer (Chen et al. 2003; Jiao et al. 2007; Chen et al. 2009), glioma (Huang et al. 2007), lung cancer (Mu et al. 2007; 2008), leukemia (Singh and Lai 2005; Lee et al. 2006), fibrosarcoma (Singh and Lai 2004), osteosarcoma (Fujita et al. 2008) and oral cancer (Nam et al. 2007). These compounds have also been used in vitro for enhancing radiosensitivity of glioma cells (Kim et al. 2006), cytotoxicity of pirarubicin and doxorubicin in leukemia and lung cancer cells (Reungpatthanaphong and Mankhetkorn 2002), cytotoxicity of sodium butyrate in leukaemia cells (Singh and Lai 2005) and cytotoxicity of temozolomide for glioma cells (Huang et al. 2008). More recently, DHA has displayed significant cytotoxic effects towards human hepatoma cells with minimal effects on normal cells (Hou et al. 2008). Mechanisms that might explain the cytotoxic activity of DHA include its ability to induce apoptosis of lymphatic endothelial cells by regulating apoptosis-related proteins and down-regulating vascular endothelial growth factor (VEGF)-3, thus inhibiting lymphangiogenesis (Wang et al. 2007a). In lung cancer cells, an activation of P38 mitogen-activated protein kinase and increase of intracellular Ca^{2+} (Mu et al. 2008) or down-regulating survivin expression was observed (Mu et al. 2007). Ovarian cancer cells have been reported to be regulated by the apoptosis-related proteins of the Bcl-2 family (Jiao et al. 2007). DNA fragmentation in U2OS osteosarcoma cells by interfering with fortilin (Fujita et al. 2008) was found. Growth inhibition of C6 glioma cells was associated with an increase of reactive oxygen species and inhibition activation of hypoxia-inducible factor-1 alpha (HIF1α) (Huang et al. 2007). Other investigations point to the inhibition of angiogenesis by reducing extracellular signal-regulated kinase 1/2 activation (Wu et al. 2006), down-regulation of VEGF expression (Lee et al. 2006) and inhibition of proliferation, migration and tube formation of vascular endothelial cells (Chen et al. 2003). More importantly, DHA revealed selective toxicity on breast cancer cells, but not on normal human breast cells (Singh and Lai 2001) and exerted potent cytotoxicity on ovarian carcinoma cells with minimal effects on non-tumourigenic human ovarian surface epithelial cells (Chen et al. 2009). This suggests that DHA might be well tolerated in a clinical setting and represents a potent promising therapeutic agent to treat cancers.

9.2.2 Angiogenesis Inhibition

In the angiogenic process, the formation of new blood vessels from pre-existing ones is essential for the supply of tumours with oxygen and nutrients and for the spread of metastatic cells throughout the body (Folkman 1992). Angiogenesis is promoted by numerous factors including cytokines, VEGF, fibroblast growth factor-basic, platelet-derived growth factor, etc. and negatively regulated by angiostatin, endostatin, thrombospondin, tissue inhibitor of metalloproteinase and others. These factors, which are produced in tumour cells as well as in surrounding stromal cells, act in a balance to promote either pro-angiogenic or anti-angiogenic processes (Relf et al. 1997). Inhibitors of angiogenesis that block angiogenic signals have been developed, and anti-angiogenic therapy strategies have raised considerable interest as valuable adjuncts to cytostatic and cytotoxic chemotherapy (Kerbel and Folkman 2002; Broxterman et al. 2003; Shimizu and Oku 2004).

Artemisinin and DHA significantly inhibited angiogenesis in a dose-dependent manner as demonstrated by measurement of proliferation, migration and tube formation of human umbilical vein endothelial cells (HUVEC) (Chen et al. 2003). DHA markedly reduced VEGF binding to its receptors on the surface of HUVEC and reduced the expression levels of two major VEGF receptors, Flt-1 and kinase-insert-containing receptor (KDR)/flk-1, on HUVEC. Chicken chorioallantoic membrane neovascularization was significantly inhibited by DHA (Chen et al. 2004a). The inhibitory effect of Artemisinin on HUVEC proliferation was stronger than that on HeLa, JAR, HO-8910 cancer cells, NIH-3T3 fibroblast cells and human endometrial cells (Chen et al. 2004b).

VEGF produced by tumour cells is a potent angiogenic factor that has been strongly implicated in tumour neo-vascularization. It binds to endothelial cell surface receptors and activates various functions of the cell including stimulation of endothelial cell ingrowths into the tumour and angiogenesis. One of the major VEGF receptors expressed preferentially on vascular endothelial cells is KDR/Flk-1. Anti-angiogenic effects were also shown for ART. It significantly inhibited chorioallantoic membrane angiogenesis and proliferation. Moreover, ART inhibited the differentiation of human microvascular dermal endothelial cells in a dose-dependent manner and reduced Flt-1 and KDR/flk-1 expression (Huan-huan et al. 2004). ART strongly reduced angiogenesis in vivo in terms of vascularization of Matrigel plugs injected subcutaneously into syngenic mice (Dell'Eva et al. 2004). ART also retarded growth of human ovarian cancer HO-8910 xenografts in nude mice. Microvessel density was reduced following drug treatment with no apparent toxicity to the animals. ART also markedly lowered VEGF expression in tumour cells and KDR/flk-1 expression in endothelial cells as well as tumour cells (Chen et al. 2004b). ART could inhibit the VEGF expression, correlated well with the level of VEGF secreted in conditioned media (Zhou et al. 2007). The microarray-based mRNA expression of 30 out of 89 angiogenesis-related genes correlated significantly with the cellular response to several Artemisinins. Among this panel were many fundamental angiogenic regulators such as vascular endothelial growth factor C (VEGF-C), fibroblast growth factor-2, matrix metalloproteinase 9, thrombospondin-1, HIF1α, angiogenin and others. By means of hierarchical cluster analysis, expression profiles were identified that determined significantly the cellular response to ART, ARE, ARM and dihydroartemisinylester stereoisomer 1. A borderline significance ($0.05 < P < 0.1$) was observed to dihydroartemisinylester stereoisomer 2 and Artemisinin (Anfosso et al. 2006). The fact that sensitivity and resistance of tumour cells could be predicted by the mRNA expression of angiogenesis-related genes indicates that Artemisinins reveal their anti-tumour effects at least in part by inhibition of tumour angiogenesis. Thioacetal Artemisinin derivatives also inhibited HUVEC tube formation and exhibited anti-angiogenic effects (Oh et al. 2004). Endothelial cell proliferation and vessel like formation were inhibited in a dose-dependent fashion by both DHA and artemisone. The effect of artemisone was significantly less pronounced than that of DHA (D'Alessandro et al. 2007).

Tumour hypoxia activates the transcription factor HIF1α. This adaptation increases tumour angiogenesis to support the survival of poorly nourished cancer cells. Hypoxic tumours are resistant to radiation and many anticancer agents (Yu et al. 2002; Wouters et al. 2004). HIF1α is not only activated during angiostatic therapy, but also up-regulates the transferrin receptor expression (McCarty 2003). Since Artemisinin is selectively toxic to iron-loaded cells, radio- and drug-resistant tumours might be selectively susceptible to the attack of iron-loading/Artemisinin strategies.

Artemisinin dose-dependently inhibits angiogenesis in mouse embryonic stem cell-derived embryoid bodies through inhibiting HIF1α and VEGF, and raising the level of intracellular reactive oxygen species. Furthermore, Artemisinin increases cell permeability by interfering organization of the extracellular matrix component laminin and varying expression patterns of MMP1, 2 and 9 (Wartenberg et al. 2003). Inhibition of angiogenesis and increasing cell permeability for chemotherapeutics are both valuable features of Artemisinin that qualify for usage in clinical oncology.

In light of these results, it is reasonable to state that inhibition of tumour angiogenesis represents an important determinant of the anti-tumour effects of Artemisinin and its derivatives.

9.2.3 Metastasis

Metastasis is the spread of malignant tumour cells from a primary tumour via lymphatic and blood vessels to regional lymph nodes and other organs of the body. Most malignant tumours can metastasize, although in varying degrees (e.g. glioma and basal cell carcinoma rarely metastasize). Lymph node involvement is clinically identified as a key factor in staging of cancers and considered as an important prognostic factor in human cancers (Tuttle 2004). Tumour-induced lymphangiogenesis can promote metastatic spread of cancer cells and influence prognosis and overall survival of cancer patients (McColl et al. 2005). There have been various lymphangiogenic molecules identified, such as VEGF-C and VEGF-D that are the most important lymphangiogenic growth factors. Both are able to stimulate growth, migration and tube-like formation of lymphatic endothelial cells and induce lymphangiogenesis by activating VEGF receptor 3 tyrosine kinase signals (Joukov et al. 1996; Achen et al. 1998).

DHA inhibits lymphangiogenesis under induction of cell apoptosis, inhibition of the migration and formation of tube-like structures in lymphatic endothelial cells by down-regulating VEGFR-3/Flt-4 (Wang et al. 2007a). Artemisinin inhibits lymph node and lung metastasis via down-regulating VEGF-C and reducing tumour lymphangiogenesis (Wang et al. 2008).

In colorectal tumour xenografts, ART not only decreases tumour growth, but also delays spontaneous liver metastasis. These anti-tumour and anti-metastasis effects are induced by the membranous translocation of β-catenin and the inhibition of the unrestricted activation of Wnt/β-catenin pathway (Li et al. 2007). Other evidence for the relevance of the Wnt/β-catenin pathway comes from microarray-based mRNA expression profiling (Konkimalla et al. 2008). This observation is very interesting, since this pathway plays an important role in colon cancer (Segditsas and Tomlinson 2006), and colon cancer cell lines are most sensitive towards ART among all solid tumour types tested (Efferth et al. 2001).

9.2.4 Transferrin Receptor

Cancer cells require and uptake a large amount of iron to proliferate. Iron is an essential micronutrient for cell growth that plays an important role in energy metabolism and DNA synthesis, and iron levels are much higher in cancer cells compared with normal cells (Reizenstein 1991). Artemisinin contains an endoperoxide group that can be activated by intracellular iron to generate cytotoxic radical species and radical molecules. Thus, cancer cells are more susceptible to the cytotoxic effect of Artemisinin than normal cells. Oxidative stress, induced by Artemisinin-type drugs provokes oxidative stress response gene expression in cancer cells (Efferth et al. 2003a; Efferth and Oesch 2004; Efferth and Volm 2005). Oxidative stress-mediated DNA damage may explain the cytotoxicity of this type of compounds towards cancer cells (Li et al. 2008).

The cytotoxic effect of Artemisinin is specific to cancer cells because most cancer cells express a high concentration of transferrin receptors (TfRs) on cell surface and have higher iron ion influx than normal cells via transferrin mechanism. It has been shown that the susceptibility of tumour cells to Artemisinins can further be enhanced by the addition of transferrin or ferrous iron (Moore et al. 1995; Efferth et al. 2004). TfR is involved in iron uptake by internalization of transferrin and is over-expressed in rapidly growing tumours.

Another mechanism of intracellular iron ion uptake is the transportation with ABC transporters ABCB6 and ABCB7. ABCB6 is involved in the biosynthesis of heme via interaction with ferrochelatase, which is regulated by iron (Taketani et al.

2003). Microarray-based mRNA expression of ABCB6, but not of ABCB7 correlates with IC_{50} values for ART in the NCI cell line panel. ART treatment induces ABCB6 but down-regulates ABCB7 expression in MCF7 and CCRF-CEM cells. Consequently, ABCB6 may have a role in determining sensitivity to ART (Kelter et al. 2007).

TfR play another important role in tumour biology, as cancer cells express a large concentration of cell surface TfR that facilitate uptake of the plasma iron-carrying protein transferrin via endocytosis. By covalently tagging Artemisinin to transferrin, Artemisinin is selectively picked up and concentrated by cancer cells. Furthermore, both Artemisinin and iron are transported into the cell in one package. Once an Artemisinin-tagged transferrin molecule is endocytosed, iron is released and reacts with Artemisinin moieties tagged to transferrin. Formation of free radicals kills the cancer cell. Artemisinin-tagged transferrin is highly selective and potent in killing cancer cells. Thus, Artemisinin and Artemisinin-tagged iron-carrying compounds could be developed into powerful anticancer drugs (Lai et al. 2005).

Artemisinin tagged to transferrin via carbohydrate chain has also been shown to have high potency and specificity against cancer cells. The conjugation enables targeted delivery of Artemisinin into cancer cells (Nakase et al. 2008). Artemisinin-tagged transferrins showed cytotoxic activity against the prostate carcinoma cell line DU 145 by the mitochondrial pathway of apoptosis (Nakase et al. 2009).

Artemisinin can be enabled to co-internalize with receptor-bound transferrin by covalent conjugation to HAIYPRH, a TfR-targeting peptide that binds to a cavity on the surface of TfR. The iron released from transferrin activates Artemisinin to generate cytotoxic radical species. The Artemisinin-peptide conjugates show potent anti-cancer activity against MOLT-4 leukemia cells with a significantly improved cancer/normal cells selectivity (Oh et al. 2009).

DHA enhances cytotoxicity towards myeloid leukemia K562 cells growth by iron. In contrast, DHA down-regulates TfR and VEGF expression (Lee et al. 2006; Zhou et al. 2008). Furthermore, DHA induces HL-60 leukemia cell apoptosis by down-regulation of TfR (Zhou et al. 2008), indicating a potential novel anti-leukemic strategy.

9.2.5 Estrogen Receptor

Breast cancer cells frequently over-express estrogen receptor α (ERα) in relation to ERβ compared to normal breast tissues. This observation has lead to investigate the potential effects of Artemisinin on ER expression in human breast cancer cells. Artemisinin selectively down-regulates ERα expression without altering ERβ levels and disrupts ERα-responsive growth and gene expression. Artemisinin switches highly proliferative human breast cancer cells from expressing a high ERα:ERβ ratio to a growth-arrested state in which expression of ERβ is significantly greater to that of ERα which parallels the physiological state linked to anti-proliferative events in both normal mammary epithelium and in breast cancer (Sundar et al. 2008).

Artemisinin could potentially be used in combinational therapies with well-established anti-estrogens. In this regard, tamoxifen, a selective ER modulator (Gallo and Kaufman 1997), is currently used for the treatment of both early and advanced ER^+ (estrogen receptor positive) breast cancer. Thus, Artemisinin has the potential to be a strong candidate for adjuvant therapy with tamoxifen. Patients could also benefit from lowering the systemic exposure of the patient to anti-estrogens and minimizing undesirable side effects due to Artemisinin-anti-estrogen cooperativity.

9.2.6 Signal Transduction

Protein kinases not only play a crucial role for many fundamental cellular processes such as proliferation, apoptosis, differentiation, etc. (Grant et al. 2002; Shaul and Seger 2007), but are also involved in signal transduction related to resistance towards established anticancer drugs (Navolanic et al. 2003; McCubrey et al. 2007). As EGFR confers resistance to ART (Efferth et al. 2003b), protein kinases were hypothesized to play a role for ART's cytotoxicity towards cancer cells (Konkimalla et al. 2009). AKT1 as a key molecule in the EGFR signaling is involved in ART resistance. There is also a significant relationship between *MYC* expression and ART response. *MYC*, represents an important transcription factor and oncogene, which is a downstream element in the EGFR signaling route and which regulates the cell cycle machinery also affecting cytotoxic cancer therapy. In contrast, there is no correlation between codes a protein exhibiting the SH2 domain, abelson murine leukemia viral oncogene homolog 1 and ART resistance. The AKT1- and mitogen-activated protein kinase-pathways seem to be the most relevant ones associated with resistance of cancer cells to ART.

9.2.7 Cell Cycle Effects

Cell cycle by flow cytometry results show that 5-FU treated human gingival epithelial cells demonstrate a significant S-phase rate increase to 45% versus only 21% of DHA-treated cells. This in conclusion supports the less intense cytotoxicity of DHA, through induction of apoptosis, while 5-FU is cytotoxic primarily through cell toxicity (Yamachika et al. 2004).

Critical components of the cell cycle machinery are the cyclin-dependent kinases (CDKs), their activating binding partners called cyclins and a variety of cyclin-dependent kinase inhibitors. CDKs bind to specific cyclin subunits to achieve the kinase activity necessary for the phosphorylation of substrates needed for the progression of the cell cycle. Artemisinin signaling pathways inhibit prostate cancer cell growth in part by targeting the transcription of CDK4 and CDK2, thereby induces a G1 block in cell cycle progression. The key event of Artemisinin's anti-proliferative effect in prostate cancer cells is the transcriptional down-regulation of CDK4 expression by disruption of Sp1 interactions with the CDK4 promoter (Willoughby et al. 2009).

9.2.8 Apoptosis

ART and DHA show significant cytotoxicity towards human hepatoma cells, regardless of p53 status, with minimal effects on normal cells. The underlying mechanisms are inhibition of cell proliferation, induction of G1-phase arrest, decreased cyclin D1, cyclin E, CDK 2, 4 and E2F1 levels. In addition, both the levels of Cip1/p21 and Kip1/p27 increase. ART and DHA induce apoptosis, activate caspase-3, increase the Bax/Bcl-2 ratio and poly (ADP-ribose) polymerase and down-regulate MDM2. Furthermore, DHA potentiates the efficacy of the chemotherapeutic agent gemcitabine (Hou et al. 2008).

Artemisinin and its derivatives also act immunosuppressive. ARM shows immunosuppressive effects directed towards T-cells both in vitro and in vivo by inhibiting the activation of the Ras-Raf1-ERK1/2 protein kinase cascade in T-cells (Wang et al. 2007c). SM905, a new water-soluble Artemisinin derivative suppresses T-cell activation both in vitro and in vivo associated with the inhibition of MAP kinases and Ras activation. It remains to be further analyzed, whether Artemisinin-type compounds represent a novel option for treating T-cell-mediated immune disorders (Wang et al. 2007b).

9.3 Hepatic Metabolism of Artemisinin

The liver is responsible for concentrating and metabolizing the majority of drugs and toxins that are introduced into the body. These compounds are processed by a variety of soluble and membrane-bound enzymes, predominantly by the cytochrome P450 superfamily in the hepatocyte endoplasmic reticulum. Here, we point to the role of hepatic enzymes in the metabolism of Artemisinin and its derivatives. Hepatic metabolism is presumably the reason for their biological effect in patients.

After absorption, Artemisinin derivatives such as ART are metabolized in the liver by phase II enzymes (cytochrome P450 monoxygenases) to DHA, which retains its bioactivity. Artemisinin itself was not converted to DHA (Haynes 2001; Woodrow et al. 2005). The metabolism of Artemisinin in human liver microsomes is primarily mediated by cytochrome P450 monooxygenase enzyme (CYP) 2B6, with a secondary contribution by CYP3A4 in individuals with low CYP2B6 expression. The contribution of CYP2A6 to Artemisinin metabolism is likely of minor importance (Svensson and Ashton 1999). There is a large body of evidence suggesting that Artemisinin influences the CYP activity, which can result in drug-drug interactions (Sukhija et al. 2006). An induction of activity by Artemisinin was reported for CYP2A5, CYP2A6, CYP2B1, CYP2B6, CYP2B10, CYP2C19 and CYP3A4 (Mihara et al. 1999; Giao and de Vries 2001; Li et al. 2003; Svensson et al. 2003;

Burk et al. 2005; Simonsson et al. 2006; Asimus et al. 2008; Elsherbiny et al. 2008). Induction of CYP2B6 is reported for Artemisinin, DHA, ARE, ARM and ART. Moreover, ARE and ARM induced CYP2B6 and CYP2C19 (Elsherbiny et al. 2008). In addition, Artemisinin activated the constitutive androstane receptor and pregnane X receptor (Burk et al. 2005), which may explain the up-regulation of CYP2B6 and CYP3A4. Elsewhere, Artemisinin is an activator of constitutive androstane receptor, but not pregnane X receptor that results in up-regulation of CYP2B (Simonsson et al. 2006). The data regarding CYP1A2 are contradictory (Bapiro et al. 2002, 2005; Asimus et al. 2007; He et al. 2007), whereas Artemisinin inhibits CYP2D6 (Asimus et al. 2007). Artemisinin leads to an auto-induction of drug metabolism, which reduces its own bioavailability (Gordi et al. 2005; Efferth et al. 2008).

9.4 Effects of Artemisinin and Artesunate In Vivo

Characterization and analysis of biomolecules in the context of intact organisms is crucial in understanding novel compounds effects. Here, we screen new findings concerning evidences that Artemisinin and ART are effective in vivo animal studies. The differential killing of tumour cells without affecting normal tissues is a highly desired beneficial feature in clinical oncology. In vivo studies pave the way for evaluation of bio-compounds' suitability to inhibit tumour cell growth in human beings. ART inhibits Kaposi's sarcoma xenograft growth in vivo with growth retardation in endothelial cells that accounts for the anti-angiogenic effect (Dell'Eva et al. 2004).

DHA inhibits human ovarian cancer cell growth in vivo when administered alone or in combination with carboplatin, presumably through the death receptor- and mitochondrion-mediated caspase-dependent apoptotic pathway (Chen et al. 2009).

ART significantly inhibits cell growth of human colorectal carcinoma cell line CLY, established from liver metastasis of a 64-year-old patient with colon adenocarcinoma. In vitro, ART strongly inhibits the hyperactive Wnt/β-catenin pathway and significantly promotes the apoptosis of CLY cells. In vivo, ART not only inhibited the volumetric development of tumour xenografts, but also delayed spontaneous liver metastasis (Li et al. 2007).

In human pancreatic cancer cells, DHA inhibits cell viability, down-regulated the expression of proliferating cell nuclear antigen and cyclin D1 and up-regulated p21 (WAF1/CIP1). Furthermore, DHA induces apoptosis by reducing the ratio of Bcl-2/Bax and increasing the activation of caspase-9 in a dose-dependent manner (Chen et al. 2009).

DHA and ART show strong cytotoxic effects on human papillomavirus-immortalized and transformed cervical cells in vitro through activation of the mitochondrial caspase pathway with resultant apoptosis. Topical application of DHA inhibits viral-induced tumour formation in vivo without preventing canine oral papilloma virus infection or replication in oral mucosa (Disbrow et al. 2005).

9.5 Toxicity

Toxicity studies in animals are necessary for any pharmaceutical intended for human use. The information obtained from these studies is useful in choosing doses for repeat-dose studies, providing preliminary identification of target organs of toxicity and occasionally revealing delayed toxicity. Acute toxicity studies may also aid in the selection of starting doses for Phase I human studies, and provide information relevant to acute overdosing in humans. Here, we reveal novel findings in the field of toxicity of Artemisinin and its derivatives, which are relevant for anticancer therapy in humans.

A discrepancy seems to prevail with regard to the toxicity and safety of the Artemisinin family of anti-malarials. While these compounds have been found to be virtually void of any serious side effects in humans, their neurotoxicity in animal models has raised concerns about their use. Mild and reversible hematological and electrocardiogram abnormalities, such as neutropenia and first-degree heart block have been infrequently observed (Toovey 2006). Various neurotoxic side effects represent the main aspects of toxicity of Artemisinin and its analogues in animal, in vitro and human clinical studies. A specific and consistent pattern of brainstem injuries that includes auditory processing centers has been reported from all laboratory animals studied. Neurotoxicity appears mediated in part through Artemisinin induced oxidative stress in exposed brainstems. In vitro studies suggested that Artemisinins neurotoxicity does not manifest immediately upon exposure, but that once commenced, it is inevitable and irreversible. Extrapolation from in vitro data suggests that 14 days may possibly be required for full development, casting doubt upon some animal safety studies and human necropsy studies. Uncertainty remains over the neurotoxicity of currently deployed Artemisinins, and their safety profile should be reviewed, especially in pediatric use (Toovey 2006).

In laboratory studies, Artemisinins can produce brainstem neurotoxicity. Selected nuclei in the medulla, pons and mesencephalon are usually found to be most vulnerable. Species-specific differences in the vulnerability of nuclei may also exist. While not yet completely understood, occurrence of the lesion seems to be dependent upon sustained rather than peak levels of circulating drug or metabolite. With daily administrations, the onset of signs of brainstem neurotoxicity frequently develops abruptly and sometimes is observable only at the end of, or after, a regimen of administration. Behavioral correlates of brainstem neurotoxicity in laboratory animals include ataxic symptoms such as tremor, gait impairment and balance disturbance (Genovese and Newman 2008).

In rats, dogs and monkeys ARM was associated with an unusual toxicity pattern in specific brain nuclei involving the auditory and vestibular pathways (Brewer et al. 1994b; Petras et al. 1997; Nontprasert et al. 2002). Although Artemisinin and its derivatives are tolerated well by malaria patients (Ribeiro and Olliaro 1998; Adjuik et al. 2004; Gordi and Lepist 2004), reports of toxicity studies are controversial. A report from Mozambique described a small but significant and irreversible hearing loss in patients exposed to ARM-lumefantrine (Toovey and Jamieson 2004). In contrast, in a case-control study from Thailand no irreversible and clinically significant neurophysiologic evidence of auditory brainstem toxicity could be attributed to ARM-lumefantrine in humans (Hutagalung et al. 2006). A recent prospective study came to the same result, in which neither audiometric nor auditory brainstem responses tests showed clinical evidence of auditory toxicity seven days after receiving oral ART and mefloquine (Carrara et al. 2008).

Affected areas in the brain stem were the reticular system with regard to autonomic control, the vestibular system, the auditory system (trapezoid nucleus), and the red nucleus, which is important for coordination (Brewer et al. 1994a, b; Kamchonwongpaisan et al. 1997; Genovese et al. 1998a, b; Petras et al. 1997, 2000; Panossian et al. 2005).

The main cause of the observed toxicity in animal studies seems to be the prolonged presence of Artemisinins upon slow release from oil-based intramuscular formulations. A longer exposure time to a lower peak blood concentration of an Artemisinin derivative was more neurotoxic than a shorter duration of exposure and a higher peak blood concentration (Li et al. 2002). In contrast, oral intake of these compounds, which is by far the most common formulation used for treatment of malaria patients, results in rapid clearance of these drugs and is, thus, unlikely to cause any toxicity in human subjects. Another plausible factor may be the relatively high doses of Artemisinin compounds used in animal studies. In conclusion, the observation of the toxicity of Artemisinin compounds in animals, but not in humans, is most likely due to different pharmacokinetic profiles after different routes of administrations (Gordi and Lepist 2004).

A clinical safety review of 108 clinical studies that enrolled 9,241 malaria patients provided substantial evidence that Artemisinins are safe and without serious adverse effects or significant severe toxicity, including neurotoxicity (Ribeiro and Olliaro 1998). Ataxia, slurred speech and hearing loss have been reported in few patients treated with Artemisinin (Davis et al. 2005). Although ART seems to be without toxicity, delayed coma recovery times in Gambian children with malaria, who were treated with *i.m.* ARM *versus i.v.* quinine was observed (van Hensbroek et al. 1996). Because of these conflicting results, a meta-analysis of 7 studies involving 1,919 patients with malaria was performed (Stepniewska et al. 2001). Applying a uniform coma recovery time definition, no significant difference in coma recovery time was found between patients treated with ARM and quinine. Additionally, no statistically significant difference was observed with regard to neurological sequelae. In another study, patients with malaria who were treated with ART were compared with patients treated with quinine (Dondorp et al. 2005). The authors did not find significant differences in terms of neurotoxic symptoms (i.e. times to speak, eat and sit) between treatment groups. Neurological sequelae did not occur after treatment. Interestingly, patients with malaria, who developed late onset hypoglycemia had a higher incidence of death than did patients treated with ART, who did not have hypoglycemia. This may be an issue that deserves additional investigation (Efferth et al. 2008).

In a clinical study, 60 out of 120 patients suffering from advanced non-small cell lung cancer were treated with ART combined with a standard chemotherapy regimen of vinorelbine and cisplatin versus standard chemotherapy alone. Toxicity observed included myelosuppression and digestion reactions without differences between ART-containing and non-containing treatment arms (Zhang et al. 2008). This indicates that ART did not further contribute to side effects other than those provoked by vinorelbine and cisplatin.

All in all, human based clinical studies with Artemisinin and its derivatives show advantageous effects in cancer treatment with less adverse reactions. Artemisinin seems eligible for adjuvant therapy against cancer. The development of non-neurotoxic Artemisinin-type drugs is possible and should be encouraged. However, phase I studies need to be conducted to pave the way for broader clinical implementation of this novel drug.

9.6 Clinical Oncology Cases

Application of Artemisinin and its derivatives in clinical oncology is still not common although the WHO officially recommends Artemisinin and its derivatives for the treatment of malaria in combination with other anti-malarial drugs. Here we deal with four clinical cases applying derivatives of Artemisinin for cancer therapy.

In a clinical case report, a 71-year-old male from India with laryngeal squamous cell carcinoma ($T_2N_1M_0$) was treated with ART over a period of nine months (60 mg ART *i.m.* per day for 16 days and 50 mg ART *p.o.* per day from day 16 onward). The tumour decreased by 70% to its original size after two months of treatment (Singh and Verma 2002).

Two patients with metastatic uveal melanoma were treated with 100 mg ART *p.o.* per day on a compassionate use basis in combination with standard chemotherapy, after standard chemotherapy alone was ineffective in stopping tumour growth. One patient experienced a temporary response after the addition of ART to fotemustine while the disease was progressing under therapy with fotemustine alone. The second patient first experienced a stabilization of the disease after the addition of ART to dacarbazine, followed by objective regressions of splenic and lung metastases. This patient was still alive 47 months after first diagnosis of stage IV uveal melanoma, a situation with a median survival of 2–5 months (Berger et al. 2005).

A 75 year-old male patient with pituitary macroadenoma was treated with ARM over a period of 12 months. ARM was administered *p.o.* to the patient over a period of 12 months. Although the tumour remained consistent in size, CT scan showed a reduction in its density, and clinically, the related symptoms such as vision, hearing and locomotion impairment considerable resolved. Overall, the ARM treatment was beneficial in improving the patient's quality of life (Singh and Panwar 2006).

In a Chinese clinical study, ART was applied in the treatment of 60 patients with advanced non-small cell lung cancer. ART (120 mg *i.v.* per day, from the 1st day to 8th day, for 8 days) combined with a chemotherapy regimen of vinorelbine and cisplatin elevated the short-term survival rate and prolonged the time to progression of patients compared to chemotherapy treatment alone (Zhang et al. 2008).

ART has the potential of augmenting the activity of established chemotherapies. More application of Artemisinin and its derivatives in clinical oncology is to be expected in the next years.

9.7 Biotechnological Production

Worldwide demand of Artemisinin has increased exponentially since the WHO officially recommends Artemisinin and its derivatives for the treatment of malaria, especially in ACT. As the raw material is extracted from plants with long growing seasons, Artemisinin is often in short supply. Chemical synthesis of Artemisinin is not practical due to its complexity and low yield (White 2008). Other possibilities for meeting the high demand for Artemisinin are found in the natural production of Artemisinin by phytotherapeutical, agricultural and biotechnological approaches.

The yield of Artemisinin in wild populations of sweet wormwood herb is low ($0.01 \pm 0.8\%$). Therefore, there is a considerable limitation to commercialization of the drug (Abdin et al. 2003; Van Geldre et al. 1997). Total synthesis of the product is feasible but time-consuming and expensive. Several synthesis routes with (–)-isopulegol, (+)-isolimenene or (R)-(+)-pulegone as starting molecules have been described (Efferth 2007). The semi-synthetic production of Artemisinin from its precursor artemisinic acid has also been shown. Artemisinic acid is present in 10-fold excess in the plants. Hence, the semi-synthetic Artemisinin yield is considerably higher than the isolation of Artemisinin from plants. To preserve the natural resources of sweet wormwood plants, Artemisinin-like endoperoxides, e.g. arteflene, have been synthesized chemically (Hofheinz et al. 1994).

Other possibilities for meeting the high demand for Artemisinin are found in the natural production of Artemisinin by phytotherapeutical, agricultural and biotechnological approaches.

Phytotherapeutical and agricultural approaches (Laughlin 1994; Delabays et al. 2001) allow:

- The cultivation of wild-type plants in fields and greenhouses.
- The breeding of high-yield cultivars. The Artemisinin contents vary between individual plants even under comparable cultivation conditions (temperature, humidity, characteristics of the soil, etc). Classical breeding techniques allow to cross high yield clones and to create synthetic variants of sweet wormwood herb.
- The cultivation of transgenic plants. Genetically modified plants deliver considerably higher amounts of Artemisinin than wild-type plants.

  Biotechnological approaches provide attractive possibilities for the large-scale production of Artemisinin:
- Hairy root cultures of sweet wormwood herb can be generated by infection of roots with *Agrobacterium rhizogens*. Hairy roots grow quickly, reach high

densities and can produce significant amounts of secondary metabolites such as Artemisinin (De Jesus-Gonzalez and Weathers 2003; Souret et al. 2003).

- The production of Artemisinin in cell cultures in vitro (Nair et al. 1986).
- The expression of the biosynthetic pathway for Artemisinin or related metabolites in genetically modified organisms, i.e. *Escherichia coli* and *Aspergillus flavipes* (Elmarakby et al. 1987; Martin et al. 2003; Hampton 2005) or *Saccharomyces cerevisiae* (Ro et al. 2006) has been reported. It is a pre-requisite that the biosynthetic pathways for Artemisinins in sweet wormwood herb are known. The biosynthesis of Artemisinin has been elucidated, and the corresponding genes have been cloned. In brief, starting from the cytosolic 3R-mevalonic acid pathway and 3-acetyl-CoA on one side and from the plasticidal 1-deoxy-D-xylulose 5-phosphate pathway, pyruvate and glyceraldehyde 3-phosphate as starting molecules on the other side, several enzymatic steps lead to the synthesis of farnesyl diphosphate. Several further enzymatic reactions result in the generation of dihydroartemisinic acid and Artemisinin (Bertea et al. 2005; Liu et al. 2006). If coding genes of these enzymes are transferred to microorganisms such as bacteria or yeast, it should be possible to reconstruct the biosynthetic pathway of Artemisinin in these organisms

Biotechnological approaches for the large-scale production of Artemisinin represent a technical challenge. The obtainable yields should exceed the ones obtained by classical breeding methods. The Artemisinin yield of one ton dry leaves of wild-type sweet wormwood herb is 6 kg/ha. Time to grow is 100 $\pm$ 120 days allowing three harvests per year under optimal conditions 18 kg Artemisinin/hectare and year. With the use of genetically engineered organisms, it should be possible to produce 25 kg Artemisinin within an 8-h working day. This calculation is based on the assumption that engineered yeast will produce 100 $\pm$ 150 mg Artemisinin per liter culture medium or 100 $\pm$ 150 g/1,000 l in an industrial set-up. The doubling time of yeast is about 1 h; hence, starting with 100 g Artemisinin at time point 0 will result in 25.6 kg Artemisinin after 8 h.

An alternative to total chemical synthesis of Artemisinin is the reconstruction of its biosynthetic pathway in microbes leading to the production of precursor molecules that can be converted to Artemisinin with relatively few chemical manipulations. Development of a semi-synthetic microbial process for the production of Artemisinin would allow for a consistent, second source of the drug to supplement cultivation of sweet wormwood herb. Heterologous production of Artemisinin precursors by fermentation is of active research interest, to ensure a consistent no-season supply of Artemisinin for ACT, the current WHO recommended treatment for malaria (see 9.1.3). Biosynthesis of amorpha-4,11-diene, the precursor of artemisinic acid has reached 0.5 g/l in *Escherichia coli* (Newman et al. 2006) and 150–600 mg/l in the yeast *Saccharomyces cerevisiae* (Lindahl et al. 2006; Shiba et al. 2007). Production of artemisinic acid in *Saccharomyces cerevisiae* has been reported at 100 mg/l (Ro et al. 2006). Artemisinic acid production was increased dramatically to 25-fold from a 100 mg/l flask process to a 2.5 g/l process in bioreactors by developing a high-density fed-batch fermentation process with a DO-stat algorithm that controlled carbon delivery and agitation simultaneously (Lenihan et al. 2008).

With the implementation of sophisticated biotechnological production techniques, it will be possible to meet the high demand for Artemisinin for malaria treatment and hopefully in the future for cancer chemotherapy as well.

References

Abdin MZ, Israr M, Rehman RU et al. Artemisinin, a novel antimalarial drug: biochemical and molecular approaches for enhanced production. Planta Med. 2003;69:289–99.

Achen MG, Jeltsch M, Kukk E et al. Vascular endothelial growth factor D (VEGF-D) is a ligand for the tyrosine kinases VEGF receptor 2 (Flk1) and VEGF receptor 3 (Flt4). Proc Natl Acad Sci U S A. 1998;95:548–53.

Adjuik M, Babiker A, Garner P et al. Artesunate combinations for treatment of malaria: meta-analysis. Lancet. 2004;363:9–17.

Anfosso L, Efferth T, Albini A et al. Microarray expression profiles of angiogenesis-related genes predict tumor cell response to Artemisinins. Pharmacogenomics J. 2006;6:269–78.

Asimus S, Elsherbiny D, Hai TN et al. Artemisinin antimalarials moderately affect cytochrome P450 enzyme activity in healthy subjects. Fundam Clin Pharmacol. 2007;21:307–16.

Asimus S, Hai TN, Van Huong N et al. Artemisinin and CYP2A6 activity in healthy subjects. Eur J Clin Pharmacol. 2008;64:283–92.

Bapiro TE, Andersson TB, Otter C et al. Cytochrome P450 1A1/2 induction by antiparasitic drugs: dose-dependent increase in ethoxyresorufin O-deethylase activity and mRNA caused by quinine, primaquine and albendazole in HepG2 cells. Eur J Clin Pharmacol. 2002;58:537–42.

Bapiro TE, Sayi J, Hasler JA et al. Artemisinin and thiabendazole are potent inhibitors of cytochrome P450 1A2 (CYP1A2) activity in humans. Eur J Clin Pharmacol. 2005;61:755–61.

Berger TG, Dieckmann D, Efferth T et al. Artesunate in the treatment of metastatic uveal melanoma – first experiences. Oncol Rep. 2005;14:1599–603.

Bertea CM, Freije JR, van der Woude H et al. Identification of intermediates and enzymes involved in the early steps of Artemisinin biosynthesis in *Artemisia annua*. Planta Med. 2005;71:40–7.

Boik J. Natural compounds in cancer therapy. Portland: Oregon Medical Press; 2001.

Brewer TG, Grate SJ, Peggins JO et al. Fatal neurotoxicity of arteether and artemether. Am J Trop Med Hyg. 1994a;51:251–9.

Brewer TG, Peggins JO, Grate SJ et al. Neurotoxicity in animals due to arteether and artemether. Trans R Soc Trop Med Hyg. 1994b;88 Suppl 1:S33–S36.

Broxterman HJ, Lankelma J, Hoekman K. Resistance to cytotoxic and anti-angiogenic anticancer agents: similarities and differences. Drug Resist Updat. 2003;6:111–27.

Burk O, Arnold KA, Nussler AK et al. Antimalarial Artemisinin drugs induce cytochrome P450 and MDR1 expression by activation of xenosensors pregnane X receptor and constitutive androstane receptor. Mol Pharmacol. 2005;67:1954–65.

Carrara VI, Phyo AP, Nwee P et al. Auditory assessment of patients with acute uncomplicated Plasmodium falciparum malaria treated with three-day mefloquine-artesunate on the north-western border of Thailand. Malar J. 2008;7:233.

Charles DJ, Simon JE, Wood KV et al. Germplasm variation in Artemisinin content of *Artemisia annua* L. using an alternative method of Artemisinin analysis from crude plant extracts. J Nat Prod. 1990;53:157–60.

Chen T, Li M, Zhang R et al. Dihydroartemisinin induces apoptosis and sensitizes human ovarian cancer cells to carboplatin therapy. J Cell Mol Med. 2009;13:1358–70.

Chen H, Sun B, Pan S et al. Dihydroartemisinin inhibits growth of pancreatic cancer cells in vitro and in vivo. Anticancer Drugs. 2009;20:131–40.

Chen HH, Zhou HJ, Fang X. Inhibition of human cancer cell line growth and human umbilical vein endothelial cell angiogenesis by Artemisinin derivatives in vitro. Pharmacol Res. 2003;48:231–6.

Chen HH, Zhou HJ, Wang WQ et al. Antimalarial dihydroartemisinin also inhibits angiogenesis. Cancer Chemother Pharmacol. 2004a;53:423–32.

Chen HH, Zhou HJ, Wu GD et al. Inhibitory effects of artesunate on angiogenesis and on expressions of vascular endothelial growth factor and VEGF receptor KDR/flk-1. Pharmacology. 2004b;71:1–9.

D'Alessandro S, Gelati M, Basilico N et al. Differential effects on angiogenesis of two antimalarial compounds, dihydroartemisinin and artemisone: implications for embryotoxicity. Toxicology. 2007;241:66–74.

Davis TM, Karunajeewa HA, Ilett KF. Artemisinin-based combination therapies for uncomplicated malaria. Med J Aust. 2005;182:181–5.

De Jesus-Gonzalez L, Weathers PJ. Tetraploid *Artemisia annua* hairy roots produce more Artemisinin than diploids. Plant Cell Rep. 2003;21:809–13.

Delabays N, Simonnet X, Gaudin M. The genetics of Artemisinin content in *Artemisia annua* L. and the breeding of high yielding cultivars. Curr Med Chem. 2001;8:1795–801.

Dell'Eva R, Pfeffer U, Vene R et al. Inhibition of angiogenesis in vivo and growth of Kaposi's sarcoma xenograft tumors by the anti-malarial artesunate. Biochem Pharmacol. 2004;68:2359–66.

Disbrow GL, Baege AC, Kierpiec KA et al. Dihydroartemisinin is cytotoxic to papillomavirus-expressing epithelial cells in vitro and in vivo. Cancer Res. 2005;65:10854–61.

Dondorp A, Nosten F, Stepniewska K et al. Artesunate versus quinine for treatment of severe falciparum malaria: a randomised trial. Lancet. 2005;366:717–25.

Efferth T. Willmar Schwabe Award 2006: antiplasmodial and antitumor activity of Artemisinin – from bench to bedside. Planta Med. 2007;73:299–309.

Efferth T, Benakis A, Romero MR et al. Enhancement of cytotoxicity of Artemisinins toward cancer cells by ferrous iron. Free Radic Biol Med. 2004;37:998–1009.

Efferth T, Briehl MM, Tome ME. Role of antioxidant genes for the activity of artesunate against tumor cells. Int J Oncol. 2003a;23:1231–5.

Efferth T, Davey M, Olbrich A et al. Activity of drugs from traditional Chinese medicine toward sensitive and MDR1- or MRP1-overexpressing multidrug-resistant human CCRF-CEM leukemia cells. Blood Cells Mol Dis. 2002c;28:160–8.

Efferth T, Dunstan H, Sauerbrey A et al. The anti-malarial artesunate is also active against cancer. Int J Oncol. 2001;18:767–73.

Efferth T, Fabry U, Osieka R. Apoptosis and resistance to daunorubicin in human leukemic cells. Leukemia. 1997;11:1180–6.

Efferth T, Fabry U, Osieka R. Interleukin-6 affects melphalan-induced DNA damage and repair in human multiple myeloma cells. Anticancer Res. 2002a;22:231–4.

Efferth T, Grassmann R. Impact of viral oncogenesis on responses to anti-cancer drugs and irradiation. Crit Rev Oncog. 2000;11:165–87.

Efferth T, Mattern J, Volm M. Immunohistochemical detection of P glycoprotein, glutathione S transferase and DNA topoisomerase II in human tumors. Oncology. 1992;49:368–75.

Efferth T, Oesch F. Oxidative stress response of tumor cells: microarray-based comparison between Artemisinins and anthracyclines. Biochem Pharmacol. 2004;68:3–10.

Efferth T, Olbrich A, Bauer R. mRNA expression profiles for the response of human tumor cell lines to the antimalarial drugs artesunate, arteether, and artemether. Biochem Pharmacol. 2002b;64:617–23.

Efferth T, Romero MR, Wolf DG et al. The antiviral activities of Artemisinin and artesunate. Clin Infect Dis. 2008;47:804–11.

Efferth T, Rucker G, Falkenberg M et al. Detection of apoptosis in KG-1a leukemic cells treated with investigational drugs. Arzneimittelforschung. 1996;46:196–200.
Efferth T, Sauerbrey A, Olbrich A et al. Molecular modes of action of artesunate in tumor cell lines. Mol Pharmacol. 2003b;64:382–94.
Efferth T, Volm M. Reversal of doxorubicin-resistance in sarcoma 180 tumor cells by inhibition of different resistance mechanisms. Cancer Lett. 1993;70:197–202.
Efferth T, Volm M. Pharmacogenetics for individualized cancer chemotherapy. Pharmacol Ther. 2005;107:155–76.
Elmarakby SA, el-Feraly FS, Elsohly HN et al. Microbial transformation studies on arteannuin B. J Nat Prod. 1987;50:903–9.
Elsherbiny DA, Asimus SA, Karlsson MO et al. A model based assessment of the CYP2B6 and CYP2C19 inductive properties by Artemisinin antimalarials: implications for combination regimens. J Pharmacokinet Pharmacodyn. 2008;35:203–17.
Folkman J. The role of angiogenesis in tumor growth. Semin Cancer Biol. 1992;3:65–71.
Fujita T, Felix K, Pinkaew D et al. Human fortilin is a molecular target of dihydroartemisinin. FEBS Lett. 2008;582:1055–60.
Gallo MA, Kaufman D. Antagonistic and agonistic effects of tamoxifen: significance in human cancer. Semin Oncol. 1997;24:71–80.
Genovese RF, Newman DB. Understanding Artemisinin-induced brainstem neurotoxicity. Arch Toxicol. 2008;82:379–85.
Genovese RF, Newman DB, Li Q et al. Dose-dependent brainstem neuropathology following repeated arteether administration in rats. Brain Res Bull. 1998b;45:199–202.
Genovese RF, Newman DB, Petras JM et al. Behavioral and neural toxicity of arteether in rats. Pharmacol Biochem Behav. 1998a;60:449–58.
Giao PT, de Vries PJ. Pharmacokinetic interactions of antimalarial agents. Clin Pharmacokinet. 2001;40:343–73.
Gordi T, Lepist EI. Artemisinin derivatives: toxic for laboratory animals, safe for humans? Toxicol Lett. 2004;147:99–107.
Gordi T, Xie R, Huong NV et al. A semiphysiological pharmacokinetic model for Artemisinin in healthy subjects incorporating autoinduction of metabolism and saturable first-pass hepatic extraction. Br J Clin Pharmacol. 2005;59:189–98.
Grant S, Qiao L, Dent P. Roles of ERBB family receptor tyrosine kinases, and downstream signaling pathways, in the control of cell growth and survival. Front Biosci. 2002;7:d376–89.
Hampton T. Collaboration hopes microbe factories can supply key antimalaria drug. JAMA. 2005;293:785–7.
Haynes RK. Artemisinin and derivatives: the future for malaria treatment? Curr Opin Infect Dis. 2001;14:719–26.
He F, Bi HC, Xie ZY et al. Rapid determination of six metabolites from multiple cytochrome P450 probe substrates in human liver microsome by liquid chromatography/mass spectrometry: application to high-throughput inhibition screening of terpenoids. Rapid Commun Mass Spectrom. 2007;21:635–43.
Hofheinz W, Burgin H, Gocke E et al. Ro 42-1611 (arteflene), a new effective antimalarial: chemical structure and biological activity. Trop Med Parasitol. 1994;45:261–5.
Hou J, Wang D, Zhang R et al. Experimental therapy of hepatoma with Artemisinin and its derivatives: in vitro and in vivo activity, chemosensitization, and mechanisms of action. Clin Cancer Res. 2008;14:5519–30.
Huan-huan C, Li-Li Y, Shang-Bin L. Artesunate reduces chicken chorioallantoic membrane neovascularisation and exhibits antiangiogenic and apoptotic activity on human microvascular dermal endothelial cell. Cancer Lett. 2004;211:163–73.
Huang XJ, Li CT, Zhang WP et al. Dihydroartemisinin potentiates the cytotoxic effect of temozolomide in rat C6 glioma cells. Pharmacology. 2008;82:1–9.
Huang XJ, Ma ZQ, Zhang WP et al. Dihydroartemisinin exerts cytotoxic effects and inhibits hypoxia inducible factor-1alpha activation in C6 glioma cells. J Pharm Pharmacol. 2007;59:849–56.

Hutagalung R, Htoo H, Nwee P et al. A case-control auditory evaluation of patients treated with artemether-lumefantrine. Am J Trop Med Hyg. 2006;74:211–4.
Jiao Y, Ge CM, Meng QH et al. Dihydroartemisinin is an inhibitor of ovarian cancer cell growth. Acta Pharmacol Sin. 2007;28:1045–56.
Joukov V, Pajusola K, Kaipainen A et al. A novel vascular endothelial growth factor, VEGF-C, is a ligand for the Flt4 (VEGFR-3) and KDR (VEGFR-2) receptor tyrosine kinases. EMBO J. 1996;15:290–8.
Kamchonwongpaisan S, McKeever P, Hossler P et al. Artemisinin neurotoxicity: neuropathology in rats and mechanistic studies in vitro. Am J Trop Med Hyg. 1997;56:7–12.
Kelter G, Steinbach D, Konkimalla VB et al. Role of transferrin receptor and the ABC transporters ABCB6 and ABCB7 for resistance and differentiation of tumor cells towards artesunate. PLoS ONE. 2007;2:e798.
Kerbel R, Folkman J. Clinical translation of angiogenesis inhibitors. Nat Rev Cancer. 2002;2:727–39.
Kim SJ, Kim MS, Lee JW et al. Dihydroartemisinin enhances radiosensitivity of human glioma cells in vitro. J Cancer Res Clin Oncol. 2006;132:129–35.
Klayman DL. Qinghaosu (Artemisinin): an antimalarial drug from China. Science. 1985;228: 1049–55.
Konkimalla VB, Blunder M, Korn B et al. Effect of Artemisinins and other endoperoxides on nitric oxide-related signaling pathway in RAW 264. 7 mouse macrophage cells. Nitric Oxide. 2008;19:184–91.
Konkimalla VB, McCubrey JA, Efferth T. The role of downstream signaling pathways of the epidermal growth factor receptor for Artesunate's activity in cancer cells. Curr Cancer Drug Targets. 2009;9:72–80.
Lai H, Sasaki T, Singh NP. Targeted treatment of cancer with Artemisinin and Artemisinin-tagged iron-carrying compounds. Expert Opin Ther Targets. 2005;9:995–1007.
Laughlin JC. Agricultural production of Artemisinin – a review. Trans R Soc Trop Med Hyg. 1994;88 Suppl 1:S.
Lee J, Zhou HJ, Wu XH. Dihydroartemisinin downregulates vascular endothelial growth factor expression and induces apoptosis in chronic myeloid leukemia K562 cells. Cancer Chemother Pharmacol. 2006;57:213–20.
Lenihan JR, Tsuruta H, Diola D et al. Developing an industrial artemisinic acid fermentation process to support the cost-effective production of antimalarial Artemisinin-based combination therapies. Biotechnol Prog. 2008;24:1026–32.
Li H, van Berlo D, Shi T et al. Curcumin protects against cytotoxic and inflammatory effects of quartz particles but causes oxidative DNA damage in a rat lung epithelial cell line. Toxicol Appl Pharmacol. 2008;227:115–24.
Li LN, Zhang HD, Yuan SJ et al. Artesunate attenuates the growth of human colorectal carcinoma and inhibits hyperactive Wnt/beta-catenin pathway. Int J Cancer. 2007;121:1360–5.
Li QG, Mog SR, Si YZ et al. Neurotoxicity and efficacy of arteether related to its exposure times and exposure levels in rodents. Am J Trop Med Hyg. 2002;66:516–25.
Li XQ, Bjorkman A, Andersson TB et al. Identification of human cytochrome P(450)s that metabolise anti-parasitic drugs and predictions of in vivo drug hepatic clearance from in vitro data. Eur J Clin Pharmacol. 2003;59:429–42.
Li Y, Wu YL. How Chinese scientists discovered Qinghaosu ngHaoSu (Artemisinin) and developed its derivatives? What are the future perspectives? Med Trop (Mars). 1998;58:9–12.
Lindahl AL, Olsson ME, Mercke P et al. Production of the Artemisinin precursor amorpha-4,11-diene by engineered Saccharomyces cerevisiae. Biotechnol Lett. 2006;28:571–80.
Liu C, Zhao Y, Wang Y. Artemisinin: current state and perspectives for biotechnological production of an antimalarial drug. Appl Microbiol Biotechnol. 2006;72:11–20.
Lotem J, Sachs L. Control of apoptosis in hematopoiesis and leukemia by cytokines, tumor suppressor and oncogenes. Leukemia. 1996;10:925–31.
Martin VJ, Pitera DJ, Withers ST et al. Engineering a mevalonate pathway in Escherichia coli for production of terpenoids. Nat Biotechnol. 2003;21:796–802.

McCarty MF. Turning an 'Achilles' Heel' into an asset – activation of HIF-1alpha during angiostatic therapy will increase tumor sensitivity to iron-catalyzed oxidative damage. Med Hypotheses. 2003;61:509–11.

McColl BK, Loughran SJ, Davydova N et al. Mechanisms of lymphangiogenesis: targets for blocking the metastatic spread of cancer. Curr Cancer Drug Targets. 2005;5:561–71.

McCubrey JA, Steelman LS, Chappell WH et al. Roles of the Raf/MEK/ERK pathway in cell growth, malignant transformation and drug resistance. Biochim Biophys Acta. 2007;1773:1263–84.

Mihara K, Svensson US, Tybring G et al. Stereospecific analysis of omeprazole supports Artemisinin as a potent inducer of CYP2C19. Fundam Clin Pharmacol. 1999;13:671–5.

Moore JC, Lai H, Li JR et al. Oral administration of dihydroartemisinin and ferrous sulfate retarded implanted fibrosarcoma growth in the rat. Cancer Lett. 1995;98:83–7.

Mu D, Chen W, Yu B et al. Calcium and survivin are involved in the induction of apoptosis by dihydroartemisinin in human lung cancer SPC-A-1 cells. Methods Find Exp Clin Pharmacol. 2007;29:33–8.

Mu D, Zhang W, Chu D et al. The role of calcium, P38 MAPK in dihydroartemisinin-induced apoptosis of lung cancer PC-14 cells. Cancer Chemother Pharmacol. 2008;61:639–45.

Nair MS, Acton N, Klayman DL et al. Production of Artemisinin in tissue cultures of *Artemisia annua*. J Nat Prod. 1986;49:504–07.

Nakase I, Gallis B, Takatani-Nakase T et al. Transferrin receptor-dependent cytotoxicity of Artemisinin-transferrin conjugates on prostate cancer cells and induction of apoptosis. Cancer Lett. 2009;274:290–8.

Nakase I, Lai H, Singh NP et al. Anticancer properties of Artemisinin derivatives and their targeted delivery by transferrin conjugation. Int J Pharm. 2008;354:28–33.

Nam W, Tak J, Ryu JK et al. Effects of Artemisinin and its derivatives on growth inhibition and apoptosis of oral cancer cells. Head Neck. 2007;29:335–40.

Navolanic PM, Steelman LS, McCubrey JA. EGFR family signaling and its association with breast cancer development and resistance to chemotherapy (Review. Int J Oncol. 2003;22:237–52.

Newman DJ, Cragg GM, Snader KM. Natural products as sources of new drugs over the period 1981–2002. J Nat Prod. 2003;66:1022–37.

Newman JD, Marshall J, Chang M et al. High-level production of amorpha-4,11-diene in a two-phase partitioning bioreactor of metabolically engineered Escherichia coli. Biotechnol Bioeng. 2006;95:684–91.

Nontprasert A, Pukrittayakamee S, Dondorp AM et al. Neuropathologic toxicity of Artemisinin derivatives in a mouse model. Am J Trop Med Hyg. 2002;67:423–9.

Oh S, Jeong IH, Ahn CM et al. Synthesis and antiangiogenic activity of thioacetal Artemisinin derivatives. Bioorg Med Chem. 2004;12:3783–90.

Oh S, Kim BJ, Singh NP et al. Synthesis and anti-cancer activity of covalent conjugates of Artemisinin and a transferrin-receptor targeting peptide. Cancer Lett. 2009;274:33–9.

Panossian LA, Garga NI, Pelletier D. Toxic brainstem encephalopathy after Artemisinin treatment for breast cancer. Ann Neurol. 2005;58:812–3.

Petras JM, Kyle DE, Gettayacamin M et al. Arteether: risks of two-week administration in Macaca mulatta. Am J Trop Med Hyg. 1997;56:390–6.

Petras JM, Young GD, Bauman RA et al. Arteether-induced brain injury in Macaca mulatta. I. The precerebellar nuclei: the lateral reticular nuclei, paramedian reticular nuclei, and perihypoglossal nuclei. Anat Embryol (Berl). 2000;201:383–97.

Pommier Y, Sordet O, Antony S et al. Apoptosis defects and chemotherapy resistance: molecular interaction maps and networks. Oncogene. 2004;23:2934–49.

Reizenstein P. Iron, free radicals and cancer. Med Oncol Tumor Pharmacother. 1991;8:229–33.

Relf M, LeJeune S, Scott PA et al. Expression of the angiogenic factors vascular endothelial cell growth factor, acidic and basic fibroblast growth factor, tumor growth factor beta-1, platelet-derived endothelial cell growth factor, placenta growth factor, and pleiotrophin in human primary breast cancer and its relation to angiogenesis. Cancer Res. 1997;57:963–9.

Reungpatthanaphong P, Mankhetkorn S. Modulation of multidrug resistance by Artemisinin, artesunate and dihydroartemisinin in K562/adr and GLC4/adr resistant cell lines. Biol Pharm Bull. 2002;25:1555–61.

Ribeiro IR, Olliaro P. Safety of Artemisinin and its derivatives. A review of published and unpublished clinical trials. Med Trop (Mars). 1998;58:50–3.

Ro DK, Paradise EM, Ouellet M et al. Production of the antimalarial drug precursor artemisinic acid in engineered yeast. Nature. 2006;440:940–3.

Segditsas S, Tomlinson I. Colorectal cancer and genetic alterations in the Wnt pathway. Oncogene. 2006;25:7531–7.

Shaul YD, Seger R. The MEK/ERK cascade: from signaling specificity to diverse functions. Biochim Biophys Acta. 2007;1773:1213–26.

Shiba Y, Paradise EM, Kirby J et al. Engineering of the pyruvate dehydrogenase bypass in Saccharomyces cerevisiae for high-level production of isoprenoids. Metab Eng. 2007;9:160–8.

Shimizu K, Oku N. Cancer anti-angiogenic therapy. Biol Pharm Bull. 2004;27:599–605.

Simonsson US, Lindell M, Raffalli-Mathieu F et al. In vivo and mechanistic evidence of nuclear receptor CAR induction by Artemisinin. Eur J Clin Invest. 2006;36:647–53.

Singh NP, Lai H. Selective toxicity of dihydroartemisinin and holotransferrin toward human breast cancer cells. Life Sci. 2001;70:49–56.

Singh NP, Lai HC. Artemisinin induces apoptosis in human cancer cells. Anticancer Res. 2004;24:2277–80.

Singh NP, Lai HC. Synergistic cytotoxicity of Artemisinin and sodium butyrate on human cancer cells. Anticancer Res. 2005;25:4325–31.

Singh NP, Panwar VK. Case report of a pituitary macroadenoma treated with artemether. Integr Cancer Ther. 2006;5:391–4.

Singh NP, Verma KB. Case report of a laryngeal squamous cell carcinoma treated with artesunate. Arch Oncol. 2002;10:279–80.

Souret FF, Kim Y, Wyslouzil BE et al. Scale-up of *Artemisia annua* L. hairy root cultures produces complex patterns of terpenoid gene expression. Biotechnol Bioeng. 2003;83:653–67.

Stepniewska K, Day N, Babiker A et al. A meta-analysis using individual patient data of trials comparing artemether with quinine in the treatment of severe falciparum malaria. Trans R Soc Trop Med Hyg. 2001;95:637–50.

Sukhija M, Medhi B, Pandhi P. Effects of Artemisinin, artemether, arteether on the pharmacokinetics of carbamazepine. Pharmacology. 2006;76:110–6.

Sundar SN, Marconett CN, Doan VB et al. Artemisinin selectively decreases functional levels of estrogen receptor-alpha and ablates estrogen-induced proliferation in human breast cancer cells. Carcinogenesis. 2008;29:2252–8.

Svensson US, Ashton M. Identification of the human cytochrome P450 enzymes involved in the in vitro metabolism of Artemisinin. Br J Clin Pharmacol. 1999;48:528–35.

Svensson US, Maki-Jouppila M, Hoffmann KJ et al. Characterisation of the human liver in vitro metabolic pattern of Artemisinin and auto-induction in the rat by use of nonlinear mixed effects modelling. Biopharm Drug Dispos. 2003;24:71–85.

Taketani S, Kakimoto K, Ueta H et al. Involvement of ABC7 in the biosynthesis of heme in erythroid cells: interaction of ABC7 with ferrochelatase. Blood. 2003;101:3274–80.

Tan RX, Zheng WF, Tang HQ. Biologically active substances from the genus Artemisia. Planta Med. 1998;64:295–302.

Tang W, Hemm I, Bertram B. Recent development of antitumor agents from Chinese herbal medicines. Part II. High molecular compounds(3). Planta Med. 2003a;69:193–201.

Tang W, Hemm I, Bertram B. Recent development of antitumor agents from Chinese herbal medicines; part I. Low molecular compounds. Planta Med. 2003b;69:97–108.

Toovey S. Are currently deployed Artemisinins neurotoxic? Toxicol Lett. 2006;166:95–104.

Toovey S, Jamieson A. Audiometric changes associated with the treatment of uncomplicated falciparum malaria with co-artemether. Trans R Soc Trop Med Hyg. 2004;98:261–9.

Tuttle TM. Technical advances in sentinel lymph node biopsy for breast cancer. Am Surg. 2004;70:407–13.
van Agtmael MA, Eggelte TA, van Boxtel CJ. Artemisinin drugs in the treatment of malaria: from medicinal herb to registered medication. Trends Pharmacol Sci. 1999;20:199–205.
van Geldre E, Vergauwe A, van den Eeckhout E. State of the art of the production of the antimalarial compound Artemisinin in plants. Plant Mol Biol. 1997;33:199–209.
van Hensbroek MB, Onyiorah E, Jaffar S et al. A trial of artemether or quinine in children with cerebral malaria. N Engl J Med. 1996;335:69–75.
Volm M, Kastel M, Mattern J et al. Expression of resistance factors (P-glycoprotein, glutathione S-transferase-pi, and topoisomerase II) and their interrelationship to proto-oncogene products in renal cell carcinomas. Cancer. 1993;71:3981–7.
Volm M, Koomagi R, Mattern J et al. Expression profile of genes in non-small cell lung carcinomas from long-term surviving patients. Clin Cancer Res. 2002a;8:1843–8.
Volm M, Koomagi R, Mattern J et al. Protein expression profiles indicative for drug resistance of non-small cell lung cancer. Br J Cancer. 2002b;87:251–7.
Wang J, Guo Y, Zhang BC et al. Induction of apoptosis and inhibition of cell migration and tube-like formation by dihydroartemisinin in murine lymphatic endothelial cells. Pharmacology. 2007a;80:207–18.
Wang J, Zhang B, Guo Y et al. Artemisinin inhibits tumor lymphangiogenesis by suppression of vascular endothelial growth factor C. Pharmacology. 2008;82:148–55.
Wang JX, Tang W, Shi LP et al. Investigation of the immunosuppressive activity of artemether on T-cell activation and proliferation. Br J Pharmacol. 2007b;150:652–61.
Wang JX, Tang W, Yang ZS et al. Suppressive effect of a novel water-soluble Artemisinin derivative SM905 on T cell activation and proliferation in vitro and in vivo. Eur J Pharmacol. 2007c;564:211–8.
Wartenberg M, Wolf S, Budde P et al. The antimalaria agent Artemisinin exerts antiangiogenic effects in mouse embryonic stem cell-derived embryoid bodies. Lab Invest. 2003;83:1647–55.
White NJ. Qinghaosu ngHaoSu (Artemisinin): the price of success. Science. 2008;320:330–4.
Willoughby JA, Sr, Sundar SN, Cheung M et al. Artemisinin blocks prostate cancer growth and cell cycle progression by disrupting Sp1 interactions with the cyclin-dependent kinase-4 (CDK4) promoter and inhibiting CDK4 gene expression. J Biol Chem. 2009;284:2203–13.
Woerdenbag HJ, Moskal TA, Pras N et al. Cytotoxicity of Artemisinin-related endoperoxides to Ehrlich ascites tumor cells. J Nat Prod. 1993;56:849–56.
Woodrow CJ, Haynes RK, Krishna S. Artemisinins. Postgrad Med J. 2005;81:71–8.
Wouters BG, van den Beucken T, Magagnin MG et al. Targeting hypoxia tolerance in cancer. Drug Resist Updat. 2004;7:25–40.
Wu XH, Zhou HJ, Lee J. Dihydroartemisinin inhibits angiogenesis induced by multiple myeloma RPMI8226 cells under hypoxic conditions via downregulation of vascular endothelial growth factor expression and suppression of vascular endothelial growth factor secretion. Anticancer Drugs. 2006;17:839–48.
Yamachika E, Habte T, Oda D. Artemisinin: an alternative treatment for oral squamous cell carcinoma. Anticancer Res. 2004;24:2153–60.
Yeung S, Pongtavornpinyo W, Hastings IM et al. Antimalarial drug resistance, Artemisinin-based combination therapy, and the contribution of modeling to elucidating policy choices. Am J Trop Med Hyg. 2004;71:179–86.
Yu JL, Coomber BL, Kerbel RS. A paradigm for therapy-induced microenvironmental changes in solid tumors leading to drug resistance. Differentiation. 2002;70:599–609.
Zhang ZY, Yu SQ, Miao LY et al. [Artesunate combined with vinorelbine plus cisplatin in treatment of advanced non-small cell lung cancer: a randomized controlled trial]. Zhong Xi Yi Jie He Xue Bao. 2008;6:134–8.

Zhou HJ, Wang WQ, Wu GD et al. Artesunate inhibits angiogenesis and downregulates vascular endothelial growth factor expression in chronic myeloid leukemia K562 cells. Vascul Pharmacol. 2007;47:131–8.
Zhou HJ, Wang Z, Li A. Dihydroartemisinin induces apoptosis in human leukemia cells HL60 via downregulation of transferrin receptor expression. Anticancer Drugs. 2008;19:247–55.

Chapter 10
Modern Cancer Research on Chinese Medicine: Acupuncture

Ruixin Zhang and Lixing Lao

Abstract Acupuncture, a popular modality of Chinese medicine, is commonly used to control cancer- or cancer therapy-caused symptoms, and accumulated evidence shows that it can play an important role in support care for cancer patients. The anti-emetic effects of acupuncture are well documented: studies consistently report that the modality significantly reduces the incidences of vomiting in patients receiving chemotherapy, and animal studies show that the combination of electroacupuncture (EA) and anti-emetic drugs produces more significant anti-emesis than either modality alone. Electroacupuncture on a bone cancer model significantly alleviated thermal and mechanic hyperalgesia compared to sham control, and studies have demonstrated the effectiveness of acupuncture on cancer pain in humans. Xerostomia studies show positive findings, with acupuncture increasing salivary flow, an effect that may be due to acupuncture-produced increase in blood flow in the tissues overlying the parotid gland. Patients with fatigue, hot flashes, depression, insomnia, and anxiety also may benefit from the use of acupuncture. Although the majority of these investigations showed positive results that demonstrate the effectiveness of acupuncture on symptom control, the findings of most have limited significance due to methodological weaknesses such as small sample size, absence of patient blinding to treatment, lack of standard outcome measurements, and inadequate randomization. Clearly, large-scale, placebo-controlled double-blind trials are needed to investigate the effect of acupuncture on these symptoms using rigorous, scientific methodology.

10.1 Introduction

Acupuncture has been used in China and other Asian countries for thousands of years for a variety of diseases and symptoms. In recent years cancer patients have begun to use it to control such cancer- or therapy-caused symptoms as emesis, pain,

R. Zhang (✉)
School of Medicine, Center for Integrative Medicine,
University of Maryland, Baltimore, MD, USA
e-mail: Rzhan001@umaryland.edu

W.C.S. Cho (ed.), *Supportive Cancer Care with Chinese Medicine*,
DOI 10.1007/978-90-481-3555-4_10,

xerostomia, and emotional disorders, among others. Growing evidence suggests that acupuncture is beneficial for chemotherapy-induced nausea, vomiting, and cancer pain, and may be beneficial for symptoms such as radiation therapy-induced xerostomia, fatigue, hot flashes, depression, anxiety, and insomnia (Table 10.1). The following paragraphs summarize the studies conducted on the effects of this modality on cancer symptoms and the side effects of cancer treatments, and the mechanisms by which acupuncture produces its effects.

Table 10.1 The effects of acupuncture for cancer related symptoms – RCTs and systematic reviews (SRs)

Symptoms	References	Findings
Nausea/vomiting	Ezzo et al. (2005) (SR 11 trials, $n = 1,247$)	EA alleviated acute vomiting within 24 h post-chemotherapy ($P = 0.01$) Acupressure alleviated acute nausea versus control ($P = 0.03$)
	Dibble et al. (2007) ($n = 160$)	Acupressure at PC6 alleviated delayed nausea/vomiting versus control ($P = 0.002$)
Pain	Alimi et al. (2003) ($n = 90$)	Auricular acupuncture decreased pain intensity versus control ($P < 0.0001$)
Xerostomia	Cho et al. (2008) ($n = 12$)	Acupuncture improved the score for dry mouth versus sham ($P < 0.05$) Acupuncture but not sham acupuncture significantly improved salivary flow rate versus baseline ($P < 0.05$)
	Blom et al. (1996) ($n = 38$)	Both acupuncture and superficial acupuncture increased salivary flow rates versus baseline ($P < 0.05$–0.01) without significant intergroup difference
Fatigue	Molassiotis et al. (2007b) ($n = 47$)	Acupuncture and acupressure significantly improved general fatigue ($P < 0.001$), physical fatigue ($P = 0.016$), activity ($P = 0.004$) and motivation ($P = 0.024$) versus sham acupressure
	Balk et al. (2009) ($n = 23$)	Both acupuncture and sham acupuncture improved fatigue, fatigue distress, quality of life and depression versus baseline without significant intergroup difference
Hot flashes	Deng et al. (2007) ($n = 72$)	Both acupuncture and sham acupuncture reduced hot flashes frequency versus baseline without significant intergroup difference
	Hervik and Mjåland (2009) ($n = 59$)	Acupuncture significantly reduced hot flash frequency ($P < 0.001$) versus sham

Table 10.1 (continued)

Symptoms	References	Findings
Depression	Leo and Ligot (2007) (SR 9 trials, $n = 666$)	Acupuncture treatment was often no different from placebo control
Insomnia	Yeung et al. (2009) (SR 20 trials, $n = 1{,}956$)	The data, while somewhat promising, allow no clear conclusion on the benefits of acupuncture for insomnia due to poor-quality research designs
Anxiety	Paraskeva et al. (2004) ($n = 50$)	Acupuncture and sham acupuncture alleviated anxiety equally versus baseline

10.2 Acupuncture Inhibition of Emesis

Nausea and vomiting remain problems for patients on cancer chemotherapy despite the availability of anti-emetics. Anti-emetic medications include serotonin ($5HT_3$) antagonists, glucocorticosteroids and phenothiazines. Combinations of these drugs show effectiveness but have unpleasant side effects such as drowsiness and mood disturbances. Furthermore, glucocorticosteroids may interfere with anti-tumoural effects of chemotherapeutic agents (Herr et al. 2003), and even with the best anti-emetic pharmacological agents, 60% of cancer patients continue to experience nausea and vomiting when undergoing chemotherapy (Collins and Thomas 2004). However, a variety of studies including clinical series, uncontrolled trials and randomized clinical trials (RCT) have consistently reported that acupuncture is effective for chemotherapy-induced nausea and vomiting (Table 10.1).

In an early study in 130 patients by Dundee et al. (1989), 10 Hz electroacupuncture (EA) at PC6 for 5 min before or shortly after cancer chemotherapy reduced the severity and frequency of nausea and vomiting, and 63% of the patients experienced complete relief for at least 8 h. And in an early pilot study of women being treated with the chemotherapy drug cisplatin, acupuncture was shown to decrease the intensity and duration of nausea and vomiting (Aglietti et al. 1990).

Dundee and Yang (1990) also reported that when, immediately following EA, an elasticized wrist band with a stud was placed over the acupoint PC6 and pressed regularly every 2 h (i.e. to apply acupressure, a modality related to acupuncture), anti-emesis lasted for 24 h in 95% of patients. In another study, emetic symptoms were reduced by acupressure at PC6 in 68 of 100 (68%) patients (Gardani et al. 2007). Furthermore, a high quality RCT with 160 breast cancer patients reported that acupressure at PC6 significantly decreased the amount of delayed (1 day post-chemotherapy) but not acute (within 24 h postchemotherapy) vomiting and the intensity of nausea over time compared with placebo acupressure at acupoint SI3 or usual care. This RCT clearly demonstrated that acupressure at the appropriate point alleviates chemotherapy-induced nausea and vomiting (Dibble et al. 2007).

The finding was confirmed by another RCT in the same year (Molassiotis et al. 2007a).

A recent case series evaluated the efficacy of EA in preventing anthracycline-based chemotherapy-related nausea and emesis refractory to a combination of a $5HT_3$-antagonist and dexamethasone. After the obtaining qi (De qi) sensation, usually experienced as heaviness or tingling at the site of insertion, was achieved at acupoints PC6 and ST36, the needles were stimulated 10 min before the start of bolus chemotherapy and then for a further 20 min at 10 Hz/10 mA/180 ms. Ninety-six percent of patients (26 of 27) reported significant reductions in both nausea and episodes of vomiting, and 37% reported no emetic episodes within the first 24 h after chemotherapy (Choo et al. 2006). These studies suggest that EA is an effective adjunct for reducing chemotherapy-related nausea and emesis and that it remains effective for at least 24 h.

In another case series 15 patients received 10 manual acupuncture treatments at PC6 over 3 weeks. The intensity of nausea before the last session and at the 1-week follow-up was significantly less than before treatment (Nystrom et al. 2008). The study demonstrated that multi-session acupuncture treatment produces even longer-term anti-emesis. And in addition to chemotherapy-induced nausea and vomiting, acupuncture has been shown to be effective for preventing postoperative nausea and vomiting (Gan et al. 2004).

A relatively large RCT compared a combination of EA and traditional anti-emetic therapy in 104 high-risk breast cancer patients receiving high-dosage chemotherapy. Once-daily EA of 2–10 Hz at PC6 and ST36 for 5 days significantly decreased episodes of emesis during the treatment period compared to a minimal needling group, in which needles were inserted subcutaneously with no manipulation, and to a group stimulated near acupoint LU7. The latter, however, had fewer episodes of emesis than did a group given anti-emetic pharmacotherapy alone. Differences among groups were not significant ($P = 0.18$) during the 9-day follow-up period (Shen et al. 2000). Another RCT of 142 cancer patients demonstrated that acupuncture (20 min, once every other day for 20 days) plus point injection of vitamin B6, which is commonly used to relieve nausea and vomiting, at PC6 (50 mg each side) significantly decreased episodes of emesis and increased the number of emesis-free days compared to acupuncture or vitamin B6 (50 mg, twice a day for 21 days) alone. The results suggest that this combination may be useful against emesis in cancer patients (You et al. 2009).

In an RCT in 11 children, acupuncture allowed a significant reduction in phenothiazine dosages and enabled patients to experience higher levels of alertness during chemotherapy. The acupuncture also reduced nausea and vomiting, although not significantly compared to control due to the small sample size (Reindl et al. 2006). These results were confirmed by a similar RCT in 23 children (Gottschling et al. 2008), in which 46 chemotherapy courses with and without acupuncture were compared. Acupuncture significantly decreased the need for anti-emetic medication and the per-course episodes of vomiting.

In 2005, a Cochrane review summarized eleven randomized trials ($n = 1{,}247$). The authors concluded that stimulation of acupoint PC6 with EA, but not manual acupuncture, reduced the incidence of acute vomiting but not acute nausea severity compared to control, while acupressure reduced mean acute nausea severity but not acute vomiting or delayed symptoms. Noninvasive electrostimulation showed no benefit (Ezzo et al. 2005). These trials only employed one (PC6) or two (PC6 and ST36) acupoints. Clinical trials that investigate the effects of acupuncture on additional anti-emetic acupoints in conjunction with modern pharmacological anti-emetic therapy are needed (Bao 2009).

An animal study characterized the effect of EA at PC6 on cyclophosphamide-induced emesis in ferrets. Combination therapy of EA with low dosage ondansetron, droperidol or metoclopramide significantly reduced the total number of emetic episodes by 52, 36 and 73%, respectively, as well as the number of emetic episodes in the first phase as compared to the sham acupuncture control. The combinations also significantly prevented emesis compared to EA or any of the drugs alone (Lao et al. 2003). These data indicate that EA and anti-emetic drugs interact positively, allowing drug dosage to be reduced while symptom control is maintained or improved. Ondansetron is a $5HT_3$ receptor antagonist, droperidol is a dopamine receptor 2 antagonist, and metoclopramide is a combination dopamine/$5HT_3$ antagonist, which suggests that EA may inhibit emesis by regulating the serotonin and dopamine systems. One study showed that EA at PC6 significantly reduces the number of episodes of vasopressin-induced retching and vomiting and that this anti-emetic effect could be abolished by naloxone pretreatment. This supports the implication that central opioid receptors are involved in acupuncture anti-emesis (Tatewaki et al. 2005).

The aforementioned studies support the effectiveness of acupuncture and acupressure for the treatment of chemotherapy-induced nausea and vomiting, and used in conjunction with current anti-emetic drugs, acupuncture and acupressure have been shown to be safe and effective for relief of nausea and vomiting caused by chemotherapy (Collins and Thomas 2004). Many patients suffer chemotherapy-related nausea and vomiting despite pharmacologic interventions. These non-pharmacological modalities may be used in such individuals to prevent emesis and to reduce their need for pharmaceuticals.

10.3 Acupuncture Alleviation of Cancer Pain

Pain is one of the most feared consequences of cancer. It has been reported that 30–50% of all patients in the early stages of cancer and 70–90% of patients with advanced cancer experience substantial and intractable pain (Foley 1999; Portenoy and Lesage 1999). Cancer pain is extremely disruptive, and its management is crucial to improving the quality of life of patients with cancer.

Opioids are the main pharmacological treatment for persistent cancer pain (World Health Organization 1986), but the frequency of their adverse effects markedly limit their use (McNicol et al. 2003; Pasternak 1988). Acupuncture offers an alternative and, importantly, an adjunct to conventional treatment (Table 10.1).

Acupuncture is commonly used to treat cancer pain (Sellick and Zaza 1997), and clinical series have demonstrated that the modality provides significant pain relief to cancer patients (Filshie and Redman 1985; Dang and Yang 1998; Guo et al. 1995; Xu et al. 1995). In an early report, 29 patients with malignant tumour-induced pain received EA treatment (Wen 1977). All experienced various degrees of pain relief and 25 out of 29 were able either to reduce or eliminate their analgesic requirements following multiple EA treatments. In 1985, a case series involving 183 cancer patients treated with acupuncture showed that 48% of patients reported relief of pain related to cancer or its treatment (Filshie and Redman 1985). A later case series showed that acupuncture decreased abdominal pain in all patients with mild or moderate pain and in 72% of those with severe pain (Xu et al. 1995). In another, 68–83% of patients with bone metastasis achieved pain relief after combined treatment of EA and an analgesic decoction of herbal drugs regardless of the location of the primary tumour (e.g. stomach, pancreas, uterine, esophagus, liver, and prostate) (Guo et al. 1995). In a fifth case series, five patients with cancer pain reported improvements after auricular EA treatment (Niemtzow and Niemtzow 2000). A more recent case series reported that acupuncture produced encouraging responses in patients with chemotherapy-induced, peripheral neuropathy (CIPN)-caused pain (Wong and Sagar 2006). Another study reported that the analgesic effect of acupuncture treatment is better than that of Three Step Administration, with a total effective rate of 94.1% in the acupuncture group versus 87.5% in the medication group (Chen et al. 2008).

A controlled study investigated the effect of acupuncture in postoperative pain management and arm movement in breast cancer patients after surgical excision of the cancer and axillary lymph node dissection (He et al. 1999). Forty-eight patients were treated with acupuncture on the third, fifth, and seventh days after surgery and on the day of discharge. Compared to a control group of 32 patients given the same surgery but not treated with acupuncture, the acupuncture group reported significant pain relief during arm movement on the fifth and seventh days following surgery and at discharge. The range of arm motion also increased significantly in the treatment group during the postoperative period compared to that of control. The authors concluded that acupuncture point selection based on the state of the patient and obtaining qi sensation was important to achieving effective treatment.

A randomized clinical trial reported equivalent analgesia in two groups given different acupuncture modalities and a conventional treatment group after 2 months of treatment, although the conventionally treated group experienced significantly superior analgesia compared to both acupuncture groups during the first 10 days of treatment. The researchers also reported that the patients in the acupuncture groups experienced improved quality of life and decreased side effects from the chemotherapy (Dang and Yang 1998).

A second double-blind RCT evaluated the effect of various combinations of auricular acupuncture, Chinese herbs, and epidural morphine on postoperative pain in 16 patients with liver cancer (Li et al. 1994). The study design was rather complicated and had a very small sample size ($n = 2$ per group). Based on the Visual

Analog Scale (VAS) 0–100 mm, all the combination treatment groups experienced better analgesia than that of a placebo-treated control group.

Alimi et al. (2000) performed both nonrandomized and randomized pain trials. Their nonrandomized, single-arm observational clinical study evaluated the effect of auricular acupuncture in 20 cancer patients who were still experiencing pain after treatment with analgesics. While patients continued their analgesic medication, auricular acupuncture needles were embedded in ear acupoints chosen according to clinical symptoms and electrodermal response and were left in place until they fell out. In some cases, the needles remained in place for 35 days, while in others they fell out after five. Pain intensity was measured by a nurse on the VAS 0–100 mm scale on days 0 and 60. Pain intensity decreased or remained stable after auricular acupuncture in all patients, with a significant average decrease of 33 mm. The same investigators reported a larger ($n = 90$) blinded controlled trial in which cancer pain intensity was significantly decreased in an auricular acupuncture treatment group in comparison with control groups (acupuncture or auricular seeds placed at placebo points) after 2 months of treatment (Alimi et al. 2003).

These studies suggest that acupuncture may be a valuable alternative modality within a comprehensive program of cancer pain management. Although most of the studies were positive and demonstrated the effectiveness of acupuncture on cancer pain control, the findings have limited significance due to methodological weaknesses such as small sample size, absence of patient blinding to treatment in most cases, lack of standard outcome measurements, and absence of adequate randomization. Further investigations into the effects of acupuncture on cancer pain using rigorous scientific methodology are warranted.

Although the clinical studies are ambiguous, studies using animal cancer pain models clearly show that acupuncture significantly alleviates cancer pain. Metastatic bone tumours are the most common cause of cancer-related pain (Reale et al. 2001). A rat model established by injecting AT-3.1 prostate cancer cells into the tibia of the adult male Copenhagen rat, which closely mimics bone cancer pain caused by prostate cancer-induced skeletal metastasis (Zhang et al. 2005), was treated with 10 Hz/2 mA/0.4 ms pulse EA for 30 min a day at the equivalent of human acupoint GB30 between days 14 and 18 after cancer-cell injection. For sham control, EA needles were inserted into GB30 without stimulation. Thermal hyperalgesia, a decrease in paw withdrawal latency to a noxious thermal stimulus, and mechanical hyperalgesia, a decrease in paw withdrawal pressure threshold, were measured at baseline and 20 min after EA. Electroacupuncture significantly attenuated the hyperalgesia (Fig. 10.1). Moreover, the EA inhibited up-regulation of preprodynorphin mRNA and dynorphin as well as interleukin-1 beta (IL-1β) and its mRNA compared to sham control (Fig. 10.2). Intrathecal injection of antiserum against dynorphin A (1–17) and IL-1 receptor antagonist (IL-1ra, 0.1 mg/rat) significantly inhibited the cancer-induced hyperalgesia, suggesting that EA alleviates bone cancer pain at least in part by suppressing spinal dynorphin and IL-1β expression (Zhang et al. 2008a, b). In another cancer pain model, B16-BL6 melanoma cells were injected into the plantar region of one hind paw of C57BL/6 mice. A single EA treatment on day 8

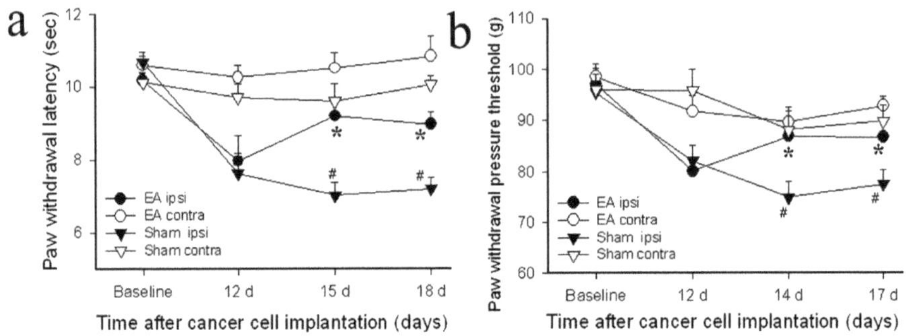

Fig. 10.1 Effects of electroacupuncture (EA) treatment on bone cancer-induced thermal (**a**) and mechanical (**b**) hyperalgesia ($n = 7$ per group). Baseline indicates hind paw withdrawal latency (**a**) and paw withdrawal pressure threshold (**b**) values before cancer cell inoculation. Electroacupuncture at 10 Hz, 2 mA and 30 min was given on days 14–18. Electroacupuncture significantly increased withdrawal latency and withdrawal pressure threshold of the hind paw ipsilateral to the inoculation compared to sham EA but induced no significant changes contralaterally. $^*P < 0.05$ compared to sham EA; $\#P < 0.05$ compared to contralateral values; ipsi: ipsilateral; contra: contralateral. Reprinted with permission from Elsevier Ltd, The European Journal of Pain 2008;12(7)

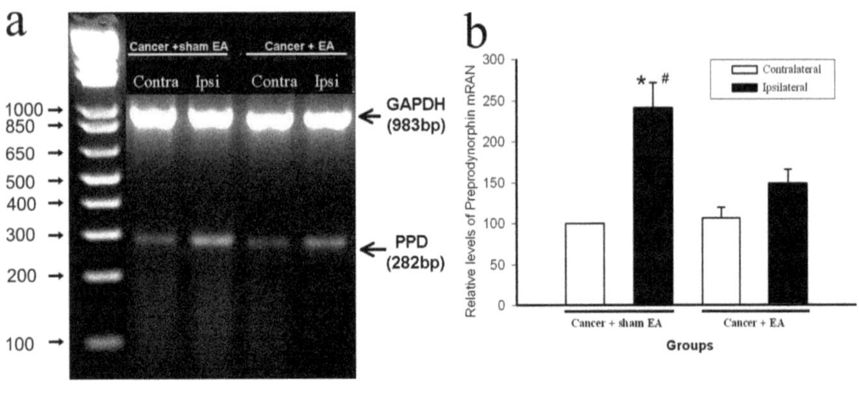

Fig. 10.2 Effect of electroacupuncture (EA) treatment on bone cancer-induced preprodynorphin mRNA up-regulation in the spinal cord ($n = 4$ per group). (**a**) An example of agarose gel electrophoresis of PCR products. GAPDH PCR (a specific 983-bp segment of cDNA) was used as an internal control. (**b**) Quantification of relative levels of spinal preprodynorphin mRNA expression. Each bar is expressed as a percentage (mean ± SEM) of levels in the contralateral spinal cords of cancer rats given sham EA, which was set arbitrarily as 100%. Preprodynorphin mRNA levels in the ipsilateral spinal cord were markedly higher than those in the contralateral spinal cord in rats with cancer plus sham EA. Electroacupuncture suppressed up-regulated preprodynorphin mRNA compared to sham EA. $\#P < 0.05$ compared to contralateral spinal cord; $^*P < 0.05$ compared to EA-treated cancer rats. Reprinted with permission from Elsevier Ltd, The European Journal of Pain 2008;12 (7)

after inoculation showed significant analgesia but not on day 20. Electroacupuncture treatments once every other day starting on day 8 showed analgesia at day 20, but EA starting on day 16 did not. The results demonstrate that EA exerts anti-hyperalgesic effects on early-stage but not late-stage cutaneous cancer pain (Mao-Ying et al. 2006). These animal studies support the clinical use of EA in the treatment of cancer pain.

10.4 Acupuncture Amelioration of Xerostomia

Xerostomia is caused by the dysfunction of parotid glands damaged by radiation therapy. Patients with xerostomia lose their taste and have difficulty speaking and swallowing. The use of parasympathomimetic drugs such as pilocarpine hydrochloride can stimulate salivary gland secretions and has been shown to be effective for patients with radiation therapy-caused xerostomia. However, such drugs may cause a number of unpleasant side effects that limit their efficacy (Johnson et al. 1993).

Studies show that acupuncture may be beneficial for these symptoms (Table 10.1). Several clinical series report that acupuncture may improve parotid gland function and alleviate speaking and swallowing symptoms (Johnstone et al. 2001; Morganstein 2005; Braga et al. 2008; Meidell and Holritz-Rasmussen 2009). For example, acupuncture was administered to eight patients at acupoints ST4, 5, 6, 7, LI3 and SP6. Once the patients experienced De qi, the needles were left without further stimulation for 20 min. A total of ten treatments, twice a week for 5 weeks, were given. The feeling of dryness of the mouth, assessed with VAS, decreased from 7.5 to 4.8 after five treatments ($P < 0.001$) and from 4.8 to 3.3 after five more ($P < 0.001$). Swallowing and speech function were also significantly improved after the acupuncture treatment, and both stimulated and unstimulated salivary flow rates improved compared to baseline although these results were not statistically significant (Meidell and Holritz-Rasmussen 2009). In another clinical series, seven xerostomia patients treated with acupuncture reported increase in salivary flow and ability to eat and speak (Morganstein 2005).

In an early controlled clinical trial by Blom et al. (1996), 20 of 38 patients with radiation-induced xerostomia were treated with classical acupuncture, and 18 were given superficial acupuncture as placebo. Acupuncture and placebo-acupuncture were given in two series, 6 weeks each, consisting of twelve 20-min treatments. Five to eight acupuncture points plus two to four auricular points were used for each patient. Significant differences in salivary flow rates were observed within each group, but there were no statistically significant differences between the groups during the year-long observation. The results suggest that acupuncture may be useful in the treatment of radiation-induced xerostomia and that superficial acupuncture should not be used as placebo acupuncture. The same group of researchers reported that patients receiving additional acupuncture treatments had consistently higher median salivary flow rates in both unstimulated and stimulated saliva compared to those who chose not to continue acupuncture during the 3-year observation (Blom and Lundeberg 2000).

In a recent controlled pilot study, 12 patients were randomized into real or sham acupuncture groups. Treatment was conducted twice weekly for 6 weeks in a single-blind setting. Acupuncture significantly improved unstimulated salivary flow rate at 6 weeks compared to baseline while sham control slightly improved it. Acupuncture also significantly improved the score for dry mouth by 2.33 points versus 0.33 for control according to the xerostomia questionnaire (Cho et al. 2008).

One group of researchers reported that the concentration of vasoactive intestinal polypeptide (VIP)-like immunoreactivity in chewing-stimulated saliva significantly increased after 24 20-min sessions of acupuncture in 17 xerostomia patients compared to baseline (Dawidson et al. 1998). Similarly, calcitonin gene-related peptide (CGRP) concentrations in the stimulated saliva of 14 xerostomia patients were significantly increased after treatment (Dawidson et al. 1999). Considering the influence of CGRP on salivary flow as well as VIP stimulation on salivary flow rate (Bobyock and Chernick 1989), it has been concluded that neuropeptide VIP and CGRP increase might be one mechanism behind this positive effect of acupuncture on salivary flow rates. It has also been shown that local blood flow in the skin overlying the parotid gland significantly increase during and after both manual acupuncture and low-frequency (2 Hz) electroacupuncture compared with superficial acupuncture in 21 patients with increased salivary flow after acupuncture treatment (Blom et al. 1993). And in a recent controlled trial in which 20 healthy volunteers received true or sham acupuncture, functional magnetic resonance imaging showed that unilateral manual acupuncture stimulation at LI2 was associated with bilateral activation of the insular and adjacent operculum accompanied by increased saliva production, while sham acupuncture at an adjacent site induced neither activation nor deactivation and was accompanied by less saliva production. This study suggests that changes in neuronal activity appear to be correlated to saliva production (Deng et al. 2008).

The results of these studies indicate that acupuncture may be a useful adjunct for the stimulation of salivary flow in some patients with xerostomia. Nevertheless, firm conclusions cannot be drawn due to insufficient evidence. Large-scale placebo-controlled double-blind trials are needed.

10.5 Effects of Acupuncture on Fatigue and Hot Flashes

Investigations conducted to determine the effects of acupuncture on other cancer-related symptoms and treatment-caused side effects such as fatigue, hot flashes, depression, anxiety, and insomnia show that acupuncture may be beneficial to these symptoms (Table 10.1).

Fatigue is a common symptom in patients with advanced cancer and an adverse effect of both chemotherapy and radiation therapy, but no effective treatment exists. Studies suggest that acupuncture has great potential in the management of cancer-related fatigue (Molassiotis et al. 2007b). A clinical series demonstrated that after acupuncture twice a week for 4 weeks (25 patients) or once a week for 6 weeks

(12 patients), Brief Fatigue Inventory scores improved 31.1% in patients who had completed cytotoxic chemotherapy but experienced persistent fatigue (Vickers et al. 2004). In a three-arm RCT, acupuncture ($n = 15$), acupressure ($n = 16$), and sham acupressure ($n = 16$), both acupuncture and acupressure for six 20-min sessions over 2 weeks significantly improved general fatigue, physical fatigue, activity, and motivation compared to sham acupressure. Fatigue improvement was 36, 19 and 0.6% in acupuncture, acupressure and control groups, respectively, after 2 weeks of treatment and was maintained at 22, 15 and 7% two weeks later. In contrast, a double-blind, randomized, placebo-controlled trial in cancer patients receiving external radiation therapy showed that both acupuncture and sham improved fatigue, fatigue distress, quality of life, and depression. Since the sample ($n = 23$) was small, no significance was found between two groups (Balk et al. 2009).

The immune system has been implicated in fatigue (Lorusso et al. 2009). A study showing that acupuncture significantly increases CD2(+), CD4(+), CD8(+), CD11b(+), CD16(+), CD19(+), CD56(+) cells as well as IL-4, IL-1β and IFN-γ levels in the peripheral blood cells (Yamaguchi et al. 2007) suggests that acupuncture may regulate the immune system to alleviate fatigue.

Hot flashes in menopausal women interfere with daily activities, sleep, and quality of life (Barton et al. 2001) and are more common, severe, and longer lasting in women with breast cancer than in healthy postmenopausal women (Harris et al. 2002). Estrogen remains the gold standard for treating these vasomotor symptoms (Shen and Stearns 2009). However, hormone therapy increases the risk of cardiovascular events in older women and in women with cardiovascular disease (Rossouw et al. 2002). After systematic review of six RCTs, the authors suggested that further research is required to determine whether acupuncture produces specific effects that alleviate hot flashes in patients with breast cancer (Lee et al. 2009). In a prospective, multicenter RCT in breast cancer patients of acupuncture versus hormone therapy, acupuncture significantly decreased the number of hot flashes in 24 h and the distress caused by hot flashes compared to baseline. The effect was maintained up to 24 months after 30-min EA treatments twice a week for the first 2 weeks and once a week for 10 weeks (Frisk et al. 2008). In another RCT in which 72 breast cancer patients were treated twice a week for 4 weeks, acupuncture needles were inserted into the skin at 19 designated acupuncture points, manipulated manually to obtain qi, retained for 20 min and then removed. Acupuncture reduced hot flash frequency but did not produce a significant effect compared to sham control (Deng et al. 2007). Similarly, Vincent et al. (2007) in their RCT found no significant effect from acupuncture compared to sham acupuncture administered in nonacupuncture, nonnmeridian areas, and whenever possible five centimeters or more away from an actual acupuncture point.

In contrast, a recent RCT of 59 postoperative female patients suffering from breast cancer found acupuncture to be effective for alleviating hot flashes. Needles were inserted unilaterally into eight acupuncture points and manipulated manually to obtain qi at the beginning and at the end of each 30-min treatment. Acupuncture or sham acupuncture was given twice weekly for the first 5 weeks, then once a week for five more. Hot flash frequency was reduced significantly ($P < 0.001$) in the acupuncture group compared to the sham group during treatment and during the following 12 weeks (Hervik and Mjåland 2009). This study suggests that getting De qi twice during a treatment is better than once and appropriate, multiple acupuncture sessions may be useful for treating hot flashes.

In most of the above RCTs, manual acupuncture was used. Since Ezzo et al. (2005) found that EA reduced the proportion of acute vomiting but manual acupuncture did not (RR = 0.76; 95% CI, 0.60–0.97; $P = 0.02$), EA with appropriate sham control should be conducted to determine the effect on hot flashes.

Although acupuncture needles are classically manipulated by hand, EA is now commonly used in Asian countries, particular in China, as well as in the West, and has become a regular part of modern practice. For instance, in Ezzo's eleven-RCT review of the effects of acupuncture on nausea and vomiting, only one reports the use of manual acupuncture (Ezzo et al. 2005). For research purposes, EA is easier to control, since using predetermined EA frequencies can reduce human bias that may result from variations in acupuncturists' skills.

10.6 Effects of Acupuncture on Depression, Insomnia and Anxiety

Depression is the most commonly reported psychological effect of cancer treatment (Maunsell et al. 1992; Mehnert and Koch 2008). Twenty-two percent of patients have moderate to high depression (Mehnert and Koch 2008), which is often linked with insomnia (Dow et al. 1996). Managing these burdensome side effects is critical for improving patient quality of life. Medicines for depression have unwanted side effects (Ferguson 2001).

Leo and Ligot (2007) summarized nine RCTs and suggested that acupuncture modalities were as effective as antidepressants for treating depression according to the limited studies available for comparison. They also reported that acupuncture is no different from placebo control. Another review of 14 RCTS reported that both acupuncture and medication are safe and effective. However, since the methodological quality of these trials is low, their conclusions need to be confirmed (Wang et al. 2008). Studies also demonstrate that EA exerts antidepressant effects in animal models of depression and that this effect is related, at least in part, to the serotonergic system (dos Santos et al. 2008).

Insomnia is serious problem for many cancer patients. A study in animals demonstrated that acupuncture at Sishencong (EX-HN1) significantly increased nitric oxide (NO) synthesis and NO content in the brain, suggesting that this compound may be involved in acupuncture's effects on insomnia (Gao et al. 2007).

Acupuncture effects on patients with insomnia have been investigated in both clinical series and RCTs (Kalavapalli and Singareddy 2007). In these studies, acupuncture consistently and significantly improved insomnia, but study quality was low. More RCTs with rigorous scientific methodology are needed to assess the usefulness of acupuncture for treating this condition. A Cochrane review by Yeung et al. (2009) summarizing 20 RCTs also found that the majority of evidence on acupuncture for insomnia is based on studies with poor research designs, so the data, while somewhat promising, do not allow clear conclusions on the benefits of acupuncture for insomnia. More RCTs with rigorous scientific methodology are needed to assess the usefulness of acupuncture for treating this condition; the positive results do support the need for large-scale placebo-controlled double-blind trials.

Another problem for cancer patients is anxiety. In animal studies, acupuncture at Shenmen (HT7) in rats significantly alleviated maternal separation-induced anxiety behavior and increased neuropeptide Y (NPY) in the basolateral amygdala (BLA) (Park et al. 2005). Since exogenous administration of NPY produces anti-anxiety actions in anxiety model (Heilig et al. 1993), these data suggest that acupuncture treatment might reduce anxiety-like behavior in adult rats by modulating the NPY system in the amygdala (Park et al. 2005).

A few RCTs demonstrate that acupuncture is beneficial to anxiety (Fanti et al. 2003; Kober et al. 2003; Paraskeva et al. 2004; Wang et al. 2001; Zhu et al. 2008). For example, 50 patients were randomly assigned to acupuncture or to sham acupuncture in which a needle is inserted into a control point located two centimeters lateral to the end of the right eyebrow. Anxiety was significantly decreased in both groups compared to baseline, but no difference was found between the two groups (Paraskeva et al. 2004). However, Fanti et al. (2003) found that acupuncture treatment ($n = 10$) significantly decreased patients' demand for sedative drugs compared to sham control ($n = 10$) by reducing both discomfort and anxiety during colonoscopy. Clearly, large-scale placebo-controlled double-blind trials are needed before acupuncture can be approved for treating anxiety.

10.7 Effects of Acupuncture on Other Cancer-Caused Symptoms

Limited studies show that acupuncture may be beneficial to other cancer-related symptoms such as leucopenia, weight loss, cough, thoracodynia, hemoptysis, fever, rectitis, dysphonia, esophageal obstruction, and postoperative lymphedema (Feng 1984; Xia et al. 1986; Zhang 1987; Niemtzow 2000; Yao 2000; Kanakura et al. 2002 Alem and Gurgel 2008). A review reported that although acupuncture use was associated with an increase in leukocytes in patients during chemotherapy or chemoradiotherapy, the methodological quality of these trials was poor. Thus no conclusions could be drawn regarding the effects of acupuncture on chemotherapy-induced leucopenia (Lu et al. 2007).

The emerging scientific evidence suggests that acupuncture can play an important role in the supportive care of cancer patients. As an adjunct to conventional care, acupuncture may lead to improvements in quality of life and alleviation of cancer-caused symptoms and the side effects of conventional treatment. Additionally, acupuncture and drug combinations interact positively to produce symptom control, thus allowing drug dosages to be decreased.

Acupuncture significantly alleviates chemotherapy-induced nausea and vomiting, is promising for cancer pain, and may be beneficial to xerostomia, fatigue, hot flashes, depression, anxiety, and insomnia, among other symptoms of cancer and cancer treatment. It should be noted that long-term treatment and treatment before chemotherapy is crucial when using acupuncture to control nausea and vomiting. Early acupuncture treatment is also beneficial in the control of cancer pain, and long-term treatment is also important in acupuncture control of xerostomia and hot flashes.

The evidence warrants large-scale, placebo-controlled double-blind trials to confirm these preliminary observations. Additionally, the mechanisms of acupuncture are not fully understood and warrant further studies in animal models and in humans.

References

Aglietti L, Roila F, Tonato M et al. A pilot study of metoclopramide, dexamethasone, diphenhydramine and acupuncture in women treated with cisplatin. Cancer Chemother Pharmacol. 1990;26:239–40.

Alem M, Gurgel M. Acupuncture in the rehabilitation of women after breast cancer surgery – a case series. Acupunct Med. 2008;26:87–93.

Alimi D, Rubino C, Leandri EP et al. Analgesic effects of auricular acupuncture for cancer pain. J Pain Symptom Manage. 2000;19:81–2.

Alimi D, Rubino C, Pichard-Leandri E et al. Analgesic effect of auricular acupuncture for cancer pain: a randomized, blinded, controlled trial. J Clin Oncol. 2003;21:4120–6.

Balk J, Day R, Rosenzweig M et al. Pilot, randomized, modified, double-blind, placebo-controlled trial of acupuncture for cancer-related fatigue. J Soc Integr Oncol. 2009;7:4–11.

Bao T. Use of acupuncture in the control of chemotherapy-induced nausea and vomiting. J Natl Compr Canc Netw. 2009;7:606–12.

Barton D, Loprinzi C, Wahner-Roedler D. Hot flashes: aetiology and management. Drugs Aging. 2001;18:597–606.

Blom M, Dawidson I, Fernberg JO et al. Acupuncture treatment of patients with radiation-induced xerostomia. Eur J Cancer B Oral Oncol. 1996;32B:182–90.

Blom M, Lundeberg T. Long-term follow-up of patients treated with acupuncture for xerostomia and the influence of additional treatment. Oral Dis. 2000;6:15–24.

Blom M, Lundeberg T, Dawidson I et al. Effects on local blood flux of acupuncture stimulation used to treat xerostomia in patients suffering from Sjögren's syndrome. J Oral Rehabil. 1993;20:541–8.

Bobyock E, Chernick W. Vasoactive intestinal peptide interacts with alpha-adrenergic-, cholinergic-, and substance-P-mediated responses in rat parotid and submandibular glands. J Dent Res. 1989;68:1489–94.

Braga FP, Sugaya NN, Hirota SK et al. The effect of acupuncture on salivary flow rates in patients with radiation-induced xerostomia. Minerva Stomatol. 2008;57:343–8.

Chen ZJ, Guo YP, Wu ZC. Observation on the therapeutic effect of acupuncture at pain points on cancer pain. Zhongguo Zhen Jiu. 2008;28:251–3.

Cho JH, Chung WK, Kang W et al. Manual acupuncture improved quality of life in cancer patients with radiation-induced xerostomia. J Altern Complement Med. 2008;14:23–6.

Choo SP, Kong KH, Lim WT et al. Electroacupuncture for refractory acute emesis caused by chemotherapy. J Altern Complement Med. 2006;12:963–9.

Collins KB, Thomas DJ. Acupuncture and acupressure for the management of chemotherapy-induced nausea and vomiting. J Am Acad Nurse Pract. 2004;16:76–80.

Dang W, Yang J. Clinical study on acupuncture treatment of stomach carcinoma pain. J Tradit Chin Med. 1998;18:31–8.
Dawidson I, Angmar-Mansson B, Blom M et al. Sensory stimulation (acupuncture) increases the release of vasoactive intestinal polypeptide in the saliva of xerostomia sufferers. Neuropeptides. 1998;32:543–8.
Dawidson I, Angmar-Månsson B, Blom M et al. Sensory stimulation (acupuncture) increases the release of calcitonin gene-related peptide in the saliva of xerostomia sufferers. Neuropeptides. 1999;33:244–50.
Deng G, Hou B, Holodny A et al. Functional magnetic resonance imaging (fMRI) changes and saliva production associated with acupuncture at LI-2 acupuncture point: a randomized controlled study. BMC Complement Altern Med. 2008;8:37.
Deng G, Vickers A, Yeung S et al. Randomized, controlled trial of acupuncture for the treatment of hot flashes in breast cancer patients. J Clin Oncol. 2007;25:5584–90.
Dibble SL, Luce J, Cooper BA et al. Acupressure for chemotherapy-induced nausea and vomiting: a randomized clinical trial. Oncol Nurs Forum Online. 2007;34:813–20.
dos Santos JG, Jr, Kawano F, Nishida MM et al. Antidepressive-like effects of electroacupuncture in rats. Physiol Behav. 2008;93:155–9.
Dow KH, Ferrell BR, Leigh S et al. An evaluation of the quality of life among long-term survivors of breast cancer. Breast Cancer Res Treat. 1996;39:261–73.
Dundee JW, Ghaly RG, Fitzpatrick KT et al. Acupuncture prophylaxis of cancer chemotherapy-induced sickness. J R Soc Med. 1989;82:268–71.
Dundee JW, Yang J. Prolongation of the antiemetic action of P6 acupuncture by acupressure in patients having cancer chemotherapy. J R Soc Med. 1990;83:360–2.
Ezzo J, Vickers A, Richardson MA et al. Acupuncture-point stimulation for chemotherapy-induced nausea and vomiting. J Clin Oncol. 2005;23:7188–98.
Fanti L, Gemma M, Passaretti S et al. Electroacupuncture analgesia for colonoscopy: a prospective, randomized, placebo-controlled study. Am J Gastroenterol. 2003;98:312–6.
Feng R. Relief of oesophageal carcinomatous obstruction by acupuncture. J Tradit Chin Med. 1984;4:3–4.
Ferguson J. SSRI antidepressant medications: adverse effects and tolerability. Prim Care Companion J Clin Psychiatry. 2001;3:22–7.
Filshie J, Redman D. Acupuncture and malignant pain problems. Eur J Surg Oncol. 1985;11: 389–94.
Foley KM. Advances in cancer pain. Arch Neurol. 1999;56:413–7.
Frisk J, Carlhall S, Kallstrom AC et al. Long-term follow-up of acupuncture and hormone therapy on hot flushes in women with breast cancer: a prospective, randomized, controlled multicenter trial. Climacteric. 2008;11:166–74.
Gan TJ, Jiao KR, Zenn M et al. A randomized controlled comparison of electro-acupoint stimulation or ondansetron versus placebo for the prevention of postoperative nausea and vomiting. Anesth Analg. 2004;99:1070–5.
Gao XY, Ma QL, Hu B. Effects of acupuncture at "Sishencong" (EX-HN 1) on physiological functions in the sleep disorder model mouse. Zhongguo Zhen Jiu. 2007;27:681–3.
Gardani G, Cerrone R, Biella C et al. A progress study of 100 cancer patients treated by acupressure for chemotherapy-induced vomiting after failure with the pharmacological approach. Minerva Med. 2007;98:665–8.
Gottschling S, Reindl T, Meyer S et al. Acupuncture to alleviate chemotherapy-induced nausea and vomiting in pediatric oncology – a randomized multicenter crossover pilot trial. Klin Padiatr. 2008;220:365–70.
Guo R, Zhang L, Gong Y et al. The treatment of pain in bone metastasis of cancer with the analgesic decoction of cancer and the acupoint therapeutic apparatus. J Tradit Chin Med. 1995;15:262–4.
Harris PF, Remington PL, Trentham-Dietz A et al. Prevalence and treatment of menopausal symptoms among breast cancer survivors. J Pain Symptom Manage. 2002;23:501–9.

He JP, Friedrich M, Ertan AK et al. Pain-relief and movement improvement by acupuncture after ablation and axillary lymphadenectomy in patients with mammary cancer. Clin Exp Obstet Gynecol. 1999;26:81–4.

Heilig M, McLeod S, Brot M et al. Anxiolytic-like action of neuropeptide Y: mediation by Y1 receptors in amygdala, and dissociation from food intake effects. Neuropsychopharmacology. 1993;8:357–63.

Herr I, Ucur E, Herzer K et al. Glucocorticoid cotreatment induces apoptosis resistance toward cancer therapy in carcinomas. Cancer Res. 2003;63:3112–20.

Hervik J, Mjåland O. Acupuncture for the treatment of hot flashes in breast cancer patients, a randomized, controlled trial. Breast Cancer Res Treat. 2009;116:311–6.

Johnson JT, Ferretti GA, Nethery WJ et al. Oral pilocarpine for post-irradiation xerostomia in patients with head and neck cancer. N Engl J Med. 1993;329:390–5.

Johnstone PA, Peng YP, May BC et al. Acupuncture for pilocarpine-resistant xerostomia following radiotherapy for head and neck malignancies. Int J Radiat Oncol Biol Phys. 2001;50:353–7.

Kalavapalli R, Singareddy R. Role of acupuncture in the treatment of insomnia: a comprehensive review. Complement Ther Clin Pract. 2007;13:184–93.

Kanakura Y, Niwa K, Kometani K et al. Effectiveness of acupuncture and moxibustion treatment for lymphedema following intrapelvic lymph node dissection: a preliminary report. Am J Chin Med. 2002;30:37–43.

Kober A, Scheck T, Schubert B et al. Auricular acupressure as a treatment for anxiety in prehospital transport settings. Anesthesiology. 2003;98:1328–32.

Lao L, Zhang G, Wong RH et al. The effect of electroacupuncture as an adjunct on cyclophosphamide-induced emesis in ferrets. Pharmacol Biochem Behav. 2003;74:691–9.

Lee M, Kim K, Choi S et al. Acupuncture for treating hot flashes in breast cancer patients: a systematic review. Breast Cancer Res Treat. 2009;115:497–503.

Leo RJ, Ligot JJ. A systematic review of randomized controlled trials of acupuncture in the treatment of depression. J Affect Disord. 2007;97:13–22.

Li QS, Cao SH, Xie GM et al. Combined traditional Chinese medicine and Western medicine. Relieving effects of Chinese herbs, ear-acupuncture and epidural morphine on postoperative pain in liver cancer. Chin Med J. 1994;107:289–94.

Lorusso L, Mikhaylova SV, Capelli E et al. Immunological aspects of chronic fatigue syndrome. Autoimmun Rev. 2009;8:287–91.

Lu W, Hu D, Dean-Clower E et al. Acupuncture for chemotherapy-induced leukopenia: exploratory meta-analysis of randomized controlled trials. J Soc Integr Oncol. 2007;5:1–10.

Mao-Ying QL, Cui KM, Liu Q et al. Stage-dependent analgesia of electro-acupuncture in a mouse model of cutaneous cancer pain. Eur J Pain. 2006;10:689–94.

Maunsell E, Brisson J, Deschenes L. Psychological distress after initial treatment of breast cancer. Assessment of potential risk factors. Cancer. 1992;70:120–5.

McNicol E, Horowicz-Mehler N, Fisk RA et al. Management of opioid side effects in cancer-related and chronic noncancer pain: a systematic review. J Pain. 2003;4:231–56.

Mehnert A, Koch U. Psychological comorbidity and health-related quality of life and its association with awareness, utilization, and need for psychosocial support in a cancer register-based sample of long-term breast cancer survivors. J Psychosom Res. 2008;64:383–91.

Meidell L, Holritz-Rasmussen B. Acupuncture as an optional treatment for hospice patients with xerostomia: an intervention study. Int J Palliat Nurs. 2009;15:12–20.

Molassiotis A, Helin AM, Dabbour R et al. The effects of P6 acupressure in the prophylaxis of chemotherapy-related nausea and vomiting in breast cancer patients. Complement Ther Med. 2007a;15:3–12.

Molassiotis A, Sylt P, Diggins H. The management of cancer-related fatigue after chemotherapy with acupuncture and acupressure: a randomised controlled trial. Complement Ther Med. 2007b;15:228–37.

Morganstein WM. Acupuncture in the treatment of xerostomia: clinical report. Gen Dent. 2005;53:223–6.

Niemtzow RC. Integration of complementary disciplines into the oncology clinic. Part I. Acupuncture. Curr Probl Cancer. 2000;24:184–93.

Niemtzow RC, Niemtzow RC. Integration of complementary disciplines into the oncology clinic. Part I. Acupuncture. Curr Probl Cancer. 2000;24:184–93.

Nystrom E, Ridderstrom G, Leffler AS. Manual acupuncture as an adjunctive treatment of nausea in patients with cancer in palliative care – a prospective, observational pilot study. Acupunct Med. 2008;26:27–32.

Paraskeva A, Melemeni A, Petropoulos G et al. Needling of the extra 1 point decreases BIS values and preoperative anxiety. Am J Chin Med. 2004;32:789–94.

Park HJ, Chae Y, Jang J et al. The effect of acupuncture on anxiety and neuropeptide Y expression in the basolateral amygdala of maternally separated rats. Neurosci Lett. 2005;377:179–84.

Pasternak GW. Multiple morphine and enkephalin receptors and the relief of pain. JAMA. 1988;259:1362–7.

Portenoy RK, Lesage P. Management of cancer pain. Lancet. 1999;353:1695–700.

Reale C, Turkiewicz AM, Reale CA. Antalgic treatment of pain associated with bone metastases. Crit Rev Oncol Hematol. 2001;37:1–11.

Reindl TK, Geilen W, Hartmann R et al. Acupuncture against chemotherapy-induced nausea and vomiting in pediatric oncology. Interim results of a multicenter crossover study. Support Care Cancer. 2006;14:172–6.

Rossouw JE, Anderson GL, Prentice RL et al. Risks and benefits of estrogen plus progestin in healthy postmenopausal women: principal results from the women's health initiative randomized controlled trial. JAMA. 2002;288:321–33.

Sellick S, Zaza C. Critical review of 5 nonpharmacologic strategies for managing cancer pain. Cancer Prev Control. 1997;2:7–14.

Shen W, Stearns V. Treatment strategies for hot flushes. Expert Opin Pharmacother. 2009;10:1133–44.

Shen J, Wenger N, Glaspy J et al. Electroacupuncture for control of myeloablative chemotherapy-induced emesis: a randomized controlled trial. JAMA. 2000;284:2755–61.

Tatewaki M, Strickland C, Fukuda H et al. Effects of acupuncture on vasopressin-induced emesis in conscious dogs. Am J Physiol Regul Integr Comp Physiol. 2005;288:R401–8.

Vickers AJ, Straus DJ, Fearon B et al. Acupuncture for postchemotherapy fatigue: a phase II study. J Clin Oncol. 2004;22:1731–5.

Vincent A, Barton DL, Mandrekar JN et al. Acupuncture for hot flashes: a randomized, sham-controlled clinical study. Menopause. 2007;14:45–52.

Wang SM, Peloquin C, Kain ZN. The use of auricular acupuncture to reduce preoperative anxiety. Anesth Analg. 2001;93:1178–80.

Wang L, Sun D, Zou W et al. Systematic evaluation of therapeutic effect and safety of acupuncture for treatment of depression. Zhongguo Zhen Jiu. 2008;28:381–6.

Wen H. Cancer pain treated with acupuncture and electrical stimulation. Mod Med Asia. 1977;13:12–6.

Wong R, Sagar S. Acupuncture treatment for chemotherapy-induced peripheral neuropathy – a case series. Acupunct Med. 2006;24:87–91.

World Health Organization. Cancer pain relieve. Geneva: WHO 1986;18–9.

Xia YQ, Zhang D, Yang CX et al. An approach to the effect on tumors of acupuncture in combination with radiotherapy or chemotherapy. J Tradit Chin Med. 1986;6:23–6.

Xu S, Liu Z, Xu M. Treatment of cancerous abdominal pain by acupuncture on zusanli (ST 36) – a report of 92 cases. J Tradit Chin Med. 1995;15:189–91.

Yamaguchi N, Takahashi T, Sakuma M et al. Acupuncture regulates leukocyte subpopulations in human peripheral blood. Evid Based Complement Alternat Med. 2007;4:447–53.

Yao W. Prof Sheng Canruo's experience in acupuncture treatment of throat diseases with yan si xue. J Tradit Chin Med. 2000;20:122–5.

Yeung W, Chung K, Leung Y et al. Traditional needle acupuncture treatment for insomnia: a systematic review of randomized controlled trials. Sleep Med. 2009;10:694–704.

You Q, Yu H, Wu D et al. Vitamin B6 points PC6 injection during acupuncture can relieve nausea and vomiting in patients with ovarian cancer. Int J Gynecol Cancer. 2009;19:567–71.

Zhang RX, Li A, Liu B et al. Electroacupuncture attenuates bone cancer pain and inhibits spinal interleukin-1β expression in a rat model. Anesth Analg. 2008a;105:1482–8.

Zhang RX, Li A, Liu B et al. Electroacupuncture attenuates bone-cancer-induced hyperalgesia and inhibits spinal preprodynorphin expression in a rat model. Eur J Pain. 2008b;12:870–8.

Zhang RX, Liu B, Wang L et al. Spinal glial activation in a new rat model of bone cancer pain produced by prostate cancer cell inoculation of the tibia. Pain. 2005;18:125–36.

Zhang Z. Effect of acupuncture on 44 cases of radiation rectitis following radiation therapy for carcinoma of the cervix uteri. J Tradit Chin Med. 1987;7:139–0.

Zhu T, Jin R, Zhong X et al. Effects of electroacupuncture combined with psychologic interference on anxiety state and serum NE content in the patient of internet addiction disorder. Zhongguo Zhen Jiu. 2008;28:561–4.

Chapter 11
Clinical Trials of Chinese Medicine for the Treatment of Cancer

Henry L. M. Liang and Dennis H. T. Chang

Abstract Despite the rapid improvement in cancer diagnosis and treatment, conventional anti-cancer therapies still have significant limitations. Complementary medicine, including Chinese medicine (CM), has been used for cancer treatments for centuries and may offer safe and effective therapeutic options. Indeed, there is increasing recognition of the use of CM in cancer treatment. We have reviewed clinical studies of CM for cancer and found that there has been a substantial increase in randomized controlled trials (RCTs) in the past two decades. The most common forms of CM interventions for cancer care are Chinese herbal medicine and acupuncture. The majority of studies have demonstrated beneficial effects of CM on the survival rates/time, quality of life and immune function of cancer patients when used alone or in conjunction with conventional therapies. Chinese medicine has also been shown to increase tumour responsiveness to conventional therapies and to alleviate chemotherapy-induced leucopoenia, nausea and vomiting, and radiation-induced xerostomia. Some studies have demonstrated that CM is beneficial for relieving cancer-related symptoms such as pain, and may offer an alternative approach to standard care for advanced cancer. There is also evidence to suggest that CM may be therapeutically useful for cancer prevention. However serious methodological deficiencies exist in many of these clinical trials. Further research on CM using robust RCT design is needed, to determine the efficacy, safety, cost effectiveness and mechanisms of action of the CM interventions used in cancer treatment.

11.1 Introduction

Cancer is overtaking heart disease as the leading cause of mortality worldwide (Jemal et al. 2009). Conventional treatments for cancer include surgery, chemotherapy and radiotherapy. Despite the rapid improvement in cancer diagnosis and

D.H.T. Chang (✉)
Centre for Complementary Medicine Research, College of Health and Science, Penrith South DC, NSW 1797, Australia
e-mail: D.Chang@uws.edu.au

W.C.S. Cho (ed.), *Supportive Cancer Care with Chinese Medicine*,
DOI 10.1007/978-90-481-3555-4_11,

treatment, therapeutic outcomes of the conventional interventions remain unsatisfactory (Chalkiadakis and Ziogas 2009; De Schutter and Nuyts 2009; Marin et al. 2009). In addition, many of the conventional interventions can cause traumatic side effects. These limitations, at least partially, explain the growing popularity of complementary and alternative medicine (CAM) including Chinese medicine (CM) in cancer care. In 2005, surveys in Japan and 14 European countries revealed that 44.6% and 35.9% of cancer patients respectively used CAM therapies (Hyodo et al. 2005; Molassiotis et al. 2005). These results are consistent with similar surveys conducted in other regions of the world (Cassileth and Vickers 2005).

The use of CM for the management of cancers can be traced back to Shang Dynasty 3,500 year ago (Zhou 2003). Over the centuries, various CM therapeutic interventions such as Chinese herbal medicine (CHM), acupuncture, moxibustion and qigong have been developed and employed in cancer treatment (Zhou 2003). Although there has been a substantial increase in randomized controlled trials (RCTs) over the past two decades, conclusive evidence to support the use of these interventions is still generally lacking. In this chapter, we have reviewed the relevant clinical trials published after 1990 with the aim to provide an overview of the current status of clinical research on CM for cancer management. Six areas are discussed including CM used as adjuvant treatment, CM for controlling adverse effects of chemotherapy and radiotherapy, CM for improving quality of life and immune functions, CM for relieving cancer related symptoms, and CM for palliative care.

11.2 Adjuvant Treatment with Chinese Medicine for Cancers

Chinese medicine has been widely used in conjunction with conventional chemo- or radio-therapies as a sensitizer to these interventions to achieve additional therapeutic benefits. There have been numerous RCTs conducted to evaluate the clinical efficacy of the combined therapies in patients with various types of cancers.

11.2.1 Lung Cancer

In a multi-centre clinical trial designed to evaluate the effectiveness of CHMs combined with conventional chemotherapy, 294 patients with stages III and IV non-small cell lung cancer (NSCLC) were prospectively randomized to receive chemotherapy alone (cisplatin + navelbine, or cisplatin + vindesine) ($n = 92$), CHMs alone (Hechan Tablet (Table 11.1), Shenyi Capsule (ginsenoside Rg3) or individualised herbal decoctions) ($n = 99$) or the CHMs combined with the chemotherapy ($n = 103$) for 9 weeks (Zhou et al. 2005). The results demonstrated that overall tumour response rate in the combination therapy group (26.2%) was significantly higher than that of either CHMs (4.0%) or chemotherapy groups (14.1%)

($P < 0.05$). In addition, a significant improvement in quality of life (QoL) and a reduction of the chemotherapy induced adverse drug reactions were also observed in the combination therapy group. A similar study ($n = 40$) by Li et al. (2003) demonstrated that the median and 1-year survival in NSCLC patients receiving chemotherapy (cisplatin + cyclophosphamide, or cisplatin + etoposide, or paclitexal + carboplatin) combined with one of the four CHM injections (359 ± 7 days; 42.7%) were all significantly higher than those receiving the chemotherapy (265 ± 1.8 days; 20.6%) or the CHM preparations alone (285 ± 17.92 days; 18.1%). The CHM injections used in this study include Kanglaite Injection, *Coix lacryma-jobi* (coix seed) extract, Aidi Injection (Table 11.1), Cinobufacini Injection, *Bufo bufo gargarizans* (toad venom) extract, and Elemene Injection, *Curcuma zedoaria* (zedoary) extract. These results are consistent with another randomized, multi-centre clinical trial in which a combination of CHMs and chemotherapy produced a greater median survival in patients with stages III and IV of NSCLC (Xu et al. 2007).

11.2.2 Colorectal and Gastric Cancers

These cancers represent the most common malignancies in the digestive system. A clinical trial by Guo evaluated the effectiveness of 5-fluorouracil (5-FU) plus a CHM, Fuzheng Yiai Decoction (Table 11.1), in colorectal cancer patients. Sixty-nine patients were randomized to receive the combination therapy ($n = 31$) and 5-FU treatment alone ($n = 38$). In the combination therapy group, the median (31.4 months), 1-year (100%), 3-year (82.4%) and 5-year (65.7%) survival were all significantly higher ($P < 0.05$) than those receiving the chemotherapy alone (18 months; 89.9%; 61.3% and 41.3% respectively). In addition, the combination therapy group also had a significantly lower 3-year recurrence rate (21.05% vs 48.38%, $P < 0.05$) (Guo, 1999). A similar trial assessing the benefits of a combined treatment of 5-FU with Quxie Capsule (Table 11.1) for advanced colorectal cancer also revealed a greater median survival time when compared to 5-FU alone (17 months vs 13 months, $P < 0.05$) (Yang et al. 2008b). In another study by Zhu et al. (2006) a combination therapy of super selective intra-arterial chemotherapy (etoposide + epirubicin + carboplatin) and Fuzheng Kang'ai Granule (Table 11.1) was compared to chemotherapy alone in gastric cancer patients ($n = 40{:}40$). The results demonstrated a significant difference in tumour response rates (82.5% vs 57.5%, $P < 0.01$), median survival (24.9 ± 1.36 months vs 13.7 ± 0.72 months, $P < 0.01$), and 1-year survival (70% vs 35%, $P < 0.01$) between the combination therapy and the chemotherapy groups. Wang et al. (2007a) compared a combination treatment of chemotherapeutic agents (docetaxel + cisplatin + fluorouracil) and Fuzheng Hewei Decoction ($n = 34$) and the chemotherapy treatment alone ($n = 32$) in patients with stage IV gastric cancer (Table 11.1) and reported a significantly higher one year survival rate (52.9% vs 25.0%, $P < 0.05$) in the combination therapy group. The tumour response rate, however, was comparable between the two treatment groups.

11.2.3 Liver cancer

A number of systematic reviews and meta-analyses have demonstrated the potential value of combinations of CHMs with chemotherapy/transcatheter arterial chemoembolization (TACE) for the treatment of liver cancer (Shu et al. 2005; Meng et al. 2008; Cho and Chen 2009b). For example, in a study by Lin et al. (2005) a combined treatment of a complex Chinese herbal formula, Shen Tao Ruan Gan pill (Table 11.1) with hepatic artery infusion of hydroxycamptothecin (HCPT) was evaluated in 85 patients with stage II-III liver cancer (tumour $\geq$ 5 cm in diameter). The patients were randomized to receive an 8-week treatment of the CHM combined with HCPT ($n = 52$) or HCPT alone ($n = 33$). The results showed that the median (326 days vs 262 days), 6-month (80.95% vs 64.29%), 1-year (41.39% vs 25.00%) and 2-year (12.42% vs 8.33%) survival of patients in the combination therapy group were all significantly greater than those receiving TACE treatment alone ($P < 0.05$). A similar study by Shao et al. (2001) showed that a 6–10 month combination treatment of Gan'ai I Decoction (oral) + Gan'ai II plaster (external use) (Table 11.1) with TACE ($n = 30$) significantly increased the 0.5-, 1- and 2-year survival (76.7% vs 50.0%; 56.7% vs 33.3%; 30.0% vs 16.7% respectively; $P < 0.05$), as well as reduced 1- and 2-year recurrence rates (43.3% vs 66.7%; 66.7% vs 90.0%; $P < 0.05$) in patients with stage II-III liver cancer when compared to those receiving TACE treatment alone ($n = 30$). Most recently, a meta-analysis performed to evaluate the efficacy of Chinese herbal therapy in hepatocellular cancer patients receiving TACE, suggests that the combination of TACE and CHMs may increase the complete or partial tumour response to TACE, prolong the patients' survival and improve their QoL (Cho and Chen 2009b). The Chinese herbal therapy was also associated with a significant enhancement of the immune effects. The authors concluded that the existing evidence support the use of CHMs to enhance the efficacy of TACE in hepatocellular carcinoma patients.

11.2.4 Breast Cancer

Breast cancer is the second most common type of cancer after lung cancer worldwide. In a clinical trial by Huang et al. (2008) 60 advanced breast cancer patients were randomly allocated to receive either conventional chemotherapy (cyclophosphamide, pirarubicin and 5-FU) ($n = 30$) or the chemotherapy plus Shenqi Fuzheng Injection (Table 11.1) ($n = 30$) over 6 weeks. The results showed that the combined therapy possessed significant benefits in improving QoL and cancer-related symptoms of the cancer patients. Furthermore, the combined therapy prevented the leucopoenia and the decreased lymphocyte subsets (CD3, CD4 and CD4/CD8) caused by the chemotherapeutical agents. However, there was no statistical difference in tumour response between the two treatment groups. In another trial in breast cancer patients by Wen et al. (2006) the combination of the modified Xiaoyao Decoction (Table 11.1) and conventional chemotherapy (cyclophosphamide-based or epirubicin-docetaxel regimens) also produced a significant improvement in QoL and prevented the leucopoenia and thrombopenia associated with the chemotherapy. As cancer prognosis is closely correlated with the body immunity, these findings provide evidence to support immunological enhancement and protective effects of CHMs for breast cancer.

11.2.5 Other Cancers

Radiotherapy is widely used to treat head and neck tumours as well as bone metastasis. Over the past two decades, the radiosensitization and radioprotection effects of CHMs have been increasingly recognised (Konkimalla and Efferth 2008). A recent systematic review suggested that CHMs combined with radiotherapy might enhance the therapeutic outcomes and improve the performance status of patients with nasopharyngeal cancer (Cho and Chen 2009a). Su et al. (2005) compared the effectiveness of Guliu Capsule (Table 11.1) combined with Strontium 89 (^{89}Sr) therapy ($n = 50$) vs ^{89}Sr therapy alone ($n = 50$) in patients with metastatic bone tumour and found that the combined therapy significantly reduced bone metastatic foci based on radionuclide bone imaging ($P < 0.05$) and relieved the ostalgia associated with bone metastasis ($P < 0.05$). In a study by Quan et al. (1999) a combination therapy of individualised CHMs (based on CM diagnosis) with radiotherapy (^{60}Co 4,000–5,000 Gy) also demonstrated a greater tumour response rate, as well as 1-, 2-, 3- and 4-year survival in patients with metastatic brain tumour when compared to the conventional radiotherapies alone.

11.3 Chinese Medicine for Controlling Adverse Effects of Cancer Therapies

Reduced blood cell production (in particular white blood cells) by cytotoxic chemotherapy is a potentially life-threatening condition in cancer patients. Accumulated evidence exists to support the potential benefits of CHM and acupuncture in the management of this complication (Wu et al. 2005b). A Chinese herbal formulation, Shengbaikuai Decoction (Table 11.1) was evaluated for treating chemotherapy induced leucopoenia in patients with hematogenic malignancies including leukaemia, lymphoma and multiple myeloma (Tan et al. 1998). Ninety patients were randomly allocated to receive Shengbaikuai Decoction ($n = 30$), a patent herbal preparation ($n = 30$) or placebo ($n = 30$). The results showed that the number of complete responders (WBC > 4,000/μL) at the 5th (10/30 vs 1/30 vs 0/30, $P < 0.01$) and the 14th (18/30 vs 8/30 vs 5/30, $P < 0.01$) days after the commencement of the treatment were significantly higher in the Shengbaikuai Decoction treatment group. In another trial reported by Wu et al. (2002) a 14-day treatment of Jisui Shengbai Decoction (Table 11.1) ($n = 32$) was compared with conventional medication (batilol and leucogen) ($n = 30$) for chemotherapy induced leucopoenia in patients with solid cancers (breast, stomach and lung cancers). The data showed that the number of complete responders was significantly higher in the CHM decoction group (25/32 vs 10/30, $P < 0.01$). In contrast, however, Mok et al. (2007) reported a negative outcome in a double-blind placebo-controlled randomized trial assessing the effect of CHMs (based on CM diagnosis) on the hematologic toxicity associated with chemotherapy in patients with breast or colon cancer. More recently an exploratory meta-analysis which assessed the therapeutic benefits of acupuncture for chemotherapy-induced leukopenia in seven individual clinical trials suggested that acupuncture treatment might be associated with an increase in leukocytes in patients during chemotherapy or chemoradiotherapy (Lu et al. 2007).

Nausea and vomiting are the most common adverse drug reactions of chemotherapy and can significantly impact on patients' QoL and treatment compliance. There have been numerous controlled clinical trials on acupuncture for chemotherapy-induced nausea and vomiting (CINV). A Cochrane review of 11 clinical studies suggests that electroacupuncture may confer therapeutic benefits for chemotherapy induced acute vomiting (Ezzo et al. 2006). In another recent systematic review, acupressure, as a non invasive intervention, in combination with antiemetics for CINV control is strongly recommended (Lee et al. 2008). However, the benefit of acupuncture for CINV control has not been confirmed by some other studies. In a clinical trial conducted by Streitberger et al. (2003) needle acupuncture in combination with intravenous injection of ondansetron failed to demonstrate a greater therapeutic benefit for acute CINV control compared to the placebo (nonskin-penetrating acupuncture). In a pilot study by Melchart et al. (2006) there was no difference in CINV control between acupuncture at PC6 and a close sham point in combination with conventional antiemetics. Another clinical trial also did not support acu-stimulation as an adjuvant approach to pharmacological antiemetics for control of CINV in female breast cancer patients (Roscoe et al. 2005). Given the inconsistent outcomes to date, further research is required to evaluate the efficacy and effectiveness of acupuncture for CINV control.

Hot flashes are common in breast cancer patients receiving antiestrogen treatment and prostate cancer patients receiving antiandrogens or castration therapy. Several recent clinical trials on acupuncture for hot flashes during hormone therapies have demonstrated somewhat conflicting outcomes. In a controlled trial, 59 women suffering from hot flashes following breast cancer surgery and antiestrogen medication were randomized to receive traditional acupuncture (TA) or sham acupuncture (SA) for 10 weeks. The results showed that the TA treatment produced 35% and 30% respective reductions in the mean number of hot flashes during and 12 weeks after the treatment when compared to the SA group indicating a potential benefit of acupuncture treatment for relieving hot flashes in breast cancer patients (Hervik and Mjaland 2009). In another controlled trial in breast cancer patients, however, statistical significance in the control of hot flashes between the TA and SA groups was not found ($P = 0.3$) (Deng et al. 2007). In prostate cancer patients, a recent clinical study demonstrated that electro-stimulation and traditional acupuncture produced 78% and 73% reductions in hot flash scores respectively. However, due to the lack of placebo control, the results remain inconclusive (Frisk et al. 2008). More research is required in this area.

Several clinical studies of CHMs and acupuncture were undertaken to evaluate their effectiveness in relieving acute radiation-induced mucositis (RIM) and xerostomia (RIX) in patients with head and neck cancer. In a clinical trial by Wu et al. (2007) 60 patients with RIM associated with ongoing conventional radiotherapy for head and neck cancers were randomized to receive Qingre Liyan Decoction (Table 11.1) ($n = 30$) or Dobell's Solution ($n = 30$). The results showed that the Qingre Liyan Decoction treatment significantly lowered the severity of RIM when compared to the Dobell's Solution group ($P < 0.05$). The epidermal growth factor in saliva and lymphocyte subsets counts (CD4 and CD8) was also higher in the CHM treated group ($P < 0.05$). A similar clinical trial also demonstrated that another CHM formula, Zou's Formulation (Table 11.1), significantly reduced the incidence and severity of RIM in patients with nasopharyngeal cancer with ongoing conventional radiotherapy (Zou et al. 2005). A recent acupuncture trial in cancer patients with RIX in a randomized, sham acupuncture controlled, subject blinded design demonstrated that acupuncture at LI2 induced a significantly greater saliva production (2.72 g vs 2.38 g, $P = 0.02$) and bilateral activation of the insula and adjacent operculum based on functional magnetic resonance imaging when compared to the sham acupuncture group (Deng et al. 2008).

11.4 Chinese Medicine for Improving QoL of Cancer Patients

QoL has been shown to be directly associated with the long term survival of cancer patients and the strategies for improving patients' QoL and well-being have been significantly emphasised and enhanced over the past two decades (Cella and Patel 2008). Several QoL outcome measures such as the European Organization for Research and Treatment of Cancer 30-item core QoL questionnaire (EORTC QLQ C-30) and Karnofsky Performance Status (KPS) have been widely employed in cancer clinical trials on CM. Accumulated evidence exists to support the use of CHMs for improving QoL in cancer patients. For example, Fei Ji Recipe (Table 11.1) combined with chemotherapy has shown to significantly improve patients' QoL measured by EORTC QLQ C-30 and KPS in NSCLC patients (You et al. 2006). In addition, this combined therapy also significantly improved the cancer-related symptoms and chemotherapy-induced adverse drug reactions when compared to the chemotherapy treatment alone ($P < 0.05$). Pan et al. (2005) reported that a 6-week combination treatment of another CHM, Fuzheng Yiliu Decoction (Table 11.1) and conventional chemotherapy significantly enhanced the KPS in 60 patients with intermediate and advanced gastrointestinal cancer. In a trial by Meng et al. (2003) modified Decoction of Four Noble Drugs (Sijunzi Decoction) (Table 11.1) combined with TACE was also shown to significantly enhance EORTC QLQ C-30 scores in patients with colon cancer accompanied by liver metastasis. Other Chinese herbal extracts and/or injections which demonstrated positive effects on QoL scores include mistletoe extract for breast cancer, ovarian cancer and NSCLC (Piao et al. 2004), Yanshu Injection, *Sophora flavescens* (lightyellow sophora root) extract, for advanced cancers in nasopharynx, lung, breast, ovary, esophageus, colon and pancreas (Wang et al. 2006) and Shenqi Fuzheng Injection (Table 11.1) for advanced breast cancer (Huang et al. 2008).

Acupuncture and moxibustion have also been widely used for improving QoL in cancer patients. Yang et al. (2008a) reported that a combination treatment of acupuncture (at RN12, ST36 and PC6), patent herbal medicine and standard supportive care in patients with stage IV gastric cancer ($n = 31$) produced a greater KPS score (60.2 ± 20.3 vs 42.8 ± 1.14, $P < 0.05$) than the standard supportive care group ($n = 30$). In another trial conducted by Liu et al. (2001) 81 patients with advanced lung, breast and digestive system cancers and non-Hodgkin's lymphomas were randomized to receive conventional chemotherapy (Group I, $n = 16$), chemotherapy plus a CHM, Gu Ben Yi Liu III (Table 11.1) (Group II, $n = 35$), or chemotherapy plus Gu Ben Yi Liu III plus moxibustion (at DU14, BL17 and ST36) (Group III, $n = 30$). The results showed that the KPS score in Group III was significantly higher than those in Group I (72 ± 11 vs 60 ± 11, $P < 0.01$) and Group II (72 ± 11 vs 65 ± 12, $P < 0.05$). Early evidence also exists to support the use of taichi and medical qigong to improve QoL in breast cancer patients (Mustian et al. 2008; Oh et al. 2008). These interventions, however, need to be further validated in future clinical trials.

11.5 Chinese Medicine for Enhancing Immune Function of Cancer Patients

Immunological deficiency is commonly associated with cancer development. Some conventional anticancer interventions such as chemotherapy and radiotherapy can further weaken the already vulnerable immunity in cancer patients (Bao et al. 2006; Chaudhuri et al. 2009). Chinese medicine has been suggested to possess immunoprotective and immune modulatory properties and can be useful for enhancing immune functions of cancer patients. In a clinical trial by Jiang et al. (2001) 101 patients with advanced lymphomas, lung, breast and stomach cancers were randomly allocated to receive chemotherapy combined with Jian Pi Yi Sheng formulation (Table 11.1) ($n = 54$) or chemotherapy alone ($n = 47$) over a period of 2 months. The results showed that the patients' immune functions measured by lymphocyte subsets (CD3, CD4 and CD4/CD8) and natural killer (NK) cells were significantly enhanced by the combined therapy. Fan et al. (2000) reported that the treatment with 9-herb Fuzheng Kang'ai Formulation (Table 11.1) combined with conventional chemotherapy for 2 months significantly enhanced interleukin-2 (IL-2) and T cells functions in lung cancer patients. In another randomized, double-blind and placebo-controlled trial, *Coriolus versicolor* (multicolored polypore) and *Salvia miltiorrhiza* (red sage root) combination was shown to alleviate lymphopenia associated with radiotherapy in patients with nasopharyngeal cancer

(Bao et al. 2006). Wu et al. (1994) demonstrated in a randomized, double-blind and placebo-controlled trial that needle acupuncture at ST36, LI11 and RN6 significantly enhanced IL-2 and NK cell activities in patients with lung and oesophagus cancers. Furthermore, needle acupuncture at PC6, LI4, ST36 and RN4 successfully prevented the deficiencies in lymphocyte subsets (CD3, CD4 and CD4/CD8) and β-endorphin in a similar cancer patient cohort (Wu et al. 1996).

11.6 Chinese Medicine for Relieving Cancer-Related Symptoms

Cancer pain significantly impacts on patients' QoL and remains as a major challenge in cancer care. There have been numerous controlled clinical trials to evaluate the effectiveness of CHMs (*via* external application, oral administration and/or intravenous injection) for relieving cancer induced pain. The majority of these studies suggested that CHMs are not only useful for alleviating cancer related pain, but also effective in reducing adverse drug reactions of conventional analgesics (Huang et al. 2004; Zhang et al. 2006; Wang et al. 2007b). Some commonly used herbs in these studies for relieving cancer pain include *Corydalis turtschaninovii* (corydalis tuber), *Ligusticum chuanxiong* (chuanxiong rhizome), *Boswellia carterii* (frankincense), *Commiphora molmol* (myrrh), *Cynanchum paniculatum* (panicled swallowwort root), *Aconitum carmichaeli* (prepared aconite root), *Aconitum kusnezoffii* (kusnezoff monkshood root), toad venom, *Buthus martensii* (scorplon), *Scolopendra subspinipes mutilans* (centipede), *Eupolyphaga sinensis* (wingless cockroach), *Dryobalanops aromatica* (borneol) and realgar. Acupuncture is another popular intervention for relieving cancer related pain and is trialed widely in cancer patients. In a RCT by Chen et al. (2008) the effects of acupuncture at the pain-points were compared to oral conventional analgesic agents in 66 advanced cancer patients with different intensities of pain. The results showed that the overall pain control rate in the acupuncture group was significantly higher than that in the conventional analgesics group (94.1% vs 87.5%, $P < 0.05$). In another RCT for chronic pain arising after cancer treatments, auricular acupuncture treatment produced a 36% reduction in pain intensity as opposed to 2% in the controlled group. The difference between the two groups was statistically significant ($P < 0.0001$) (Alimi et al. 2003). Scalp acupuncture at MS4 and MS8 in combination with epidural morphine analgesia also demonstrated significant therapeutic benefits evidenced by improvement in the Visual Analog Scale and Bruggemann Comfort Scale in postoperative pain control in colon cancer patients (He et al. 2007).

Weight loss and cachexia (common cancer related malnutrition) highly impinge on the life expectancy of cancer patients. Current standard nutritional support is ineffective (Bosaeus 2008). Some preliminary evidence exists to support the use of CHMs for the management of cachexia. A clinical trial in cancer patients with cachexia by Zhang (2000) showed that a 30 day treatment with a 13-herb formulation, Zhang's Recipe (Table 11.1), substantially increased the patients' food intake and performance status when compared to the megestrol (a hormone therapeutic agent used for anorexia and cachexia) treated group. Another clinical trial showed that Lactone-I, an active component from a CHM, *Atractylodes macrocephala* (bighead atractylodes rhizome) significantly increased the food intake, body weight, and mid-arm muscle circumference in advanced cancer patients with cachexia when compared to the patients receiving fish oil enriched nutritional supplementation (Liu et al. 2005).

Malignant ascites, usually caused by ovary or liver cancers, is associated with a poor prognosis in cancer patients. Wang et al. (1999) conducted a clinical trial where 94 patients with ovarian cancer-induced ascites were randomly allocated to three treatment groups receiving Elemene, zedoary extract, cisplatin, and Elemene plus cisplatin respectively *via* intraperitoneal injection. The data demonstrated that the combined treatment of Elemene and cisplatin significantly reduced the rate of ascites formation (82.3%) when compared to the cisplatin (53.3%) or Elemene (50.0%) treatment alone. In another RCT in 61 patients with ascites caused by primary liver cancer, a combination therapy of Xiaoshui Decoction (Table 11.1) and cisplatin *via* intraperitoneal injection significantly reduced the rate of ascites formation (29/33 vs 21/28) and increased 1-year survival (33.3% vs 14.3%) when compared to cisplatin treatment alone. In addition, the patients receiving the combination therapy also had a significantly greater improvement in QoL and presented less symptoms related to cancer (Wu et al. 2005a).

11.7 Palliative Care for Patients with Advanced Cancers

Numerous clinical trials conducted to date demonstrate potential therapeutic benefits of CHMs and acupuncture in palliative cancer care (Standish et al. 2008; Molassiotis et al. 2009). In a prospective, RCT by Tian et al. (2008) 97 patients with advanced primary hepatocarcinoma were randomly treated with either CHMs, including injection of *Brucea javanica* (brucea fruit) acid, TACE, Ganji Recipe and Ailitong (Table 11.1) or conventional TACE. Although there was no difference in tumour response between the two groups, the median (8.9 months vs 5.3 months), 6-month (31/47 vs 20/47), and 1-year (17/44 vs 8/44) survival times were all significantly greater in the CHM treated group. Moreover, the CHM treatment produced better pain control, improved QoL and lowered therapeutic toxicity in these patients. Li and Wei (2001) studied the effectiveness of Jinlongshe Oral Liquid (Table 11.1) in stage III and IV gastric cancer patients and reported that the herbal treatment significantly relieved the cancer related symptoms and improved patients' QoL. When used together with conventional chemotherapy, the CHM treatment also increased patients' survival rate. Similarly, Changfukang Capsule (Table 11.1) was found to be safe and clinically beneficial for improving QoL of patients with advanced colorectal cancer (Xiong et al. 2003). Clinical trials also suggest that Cinobufacini and Elemene Injections are clinically effective to be used as an alternative intervention for advanced cancers in palliative care (Jia et al. 2002; Hu et al. 2004).

Table 11.1 Chinese herbal formulations used in clinical trials for the treatment of cancer

Name of formulation	Composition of formulation	Details of studies	References
Aidi injection	*Mylabris phalerata, Panax ginseng, Astragalus membranaceus and Acanthopanax senticosus*	RCT ($n = 120$); Used alone or combined with chemotherapy for NSCLC	Li et al. (2003)
Ailitong	*Bufo bufo gargarizans, Strychnos nux-vomica preparata, Cynanchum paniculatum, Adenosma glutionosum, Dryobalanops aromarica,* etc	Prospective RCT ($n = 97$); Combined with Ganji Recipe (internal use) for patients with advanced primary liver cancer	Tian et al. (2008)
Changfukang capsule	*Brucea javanica, Camptotheca acuminata, Sargentodoxa cuneata, Codonopsis pilosula,* etc	RCT ($n = 120$); Used alone for patients with colorectal cancer	Xiong et al. (2003)
Feiji Recipe	*Astragalus membranaceus, Atractylodes macrocephala, Glehnia littoralis, Selaginella doederleinii, Paris polyphylla, Pleione bulbocodioides, Cornus officinalis, Epimedium grandiflorum*	RCT ($n = 120$); Combined with chemotherapy for QoL of NSCLC patients	You et al. (2006)
Fuzheng Hewei decoction	*Codonopsis pilosula, Astragalus membranaceus, Ophiopogon japonicus, Panax quinquefolium, Atractylodes macrocephala, Poria cocos, Pinellia ternata, Citrus reticulata, Citrus reticulata, Angelica sinensis, Coix lacryma-jobi, Akebia quinata, Actinidia chinensis, Bletilla striata, Citrus aurantium, Curcuma aromatica, Bambusa tuldoides, Coptis chinensis, Typha angustifolia and Trogopterus xanthipes*	RCT ($n = 66$); Combined with chemotherapy for advanced gastric cancer	Wang et al. (2007a)

Table 11.1 (continued)

Name of formulation	Composition of formulation	Details of studies	References
Fuzheng Kang'ai formulation	*Rehmannia glutinosa, Rehmannia glutinosa preparata, Asparagus cochinchinensis, Ophiopogon japonicus, Astragalus membranaceus, Codonopsis pilosula, Houttuynia cordata, Cimicifuga foetida and Scrophularia ningpoensis*	RCT ($n = 48$); Combined with chemotherapy for patients with lung cancer	Fan et al. (2000)
Fuzheng Kang'ai granule	*Codonopsis pilosula, Atractylodes macrocephala, Astragalus membranaceus, Coix lacryma-jobi, Solanum lyratum, Paris polyphylla, Oldenlandia diffusa, Psoralea corylifolia, Salvia chinensis and Glycyrrhiza uralensis*	RCT ($n = 80$); Combined with super selective intra-arterial chemotherapy for gastric cancer	Zhu et al. (2006)
Fuzheng Yiai decoction	*Coix lacryma-jobi, Panax ginseng, Ganoderma lucidum, Panax notoginseng, Astragalus membranaceus, Atractylodes macrocephala, Ficus carica, Fagopyrum tataricum, Polyporus umbellatus, Cremastra appendiculata, Sophora tonkinensis, Salvia miltiorrhiza and Patrinia villosa*	RCT ($n = 69$); Combined with chemotherapy for colorectal cancer	Guo (1999)
Fuzheng Yiliu Decoction	*Astragalus membranaceus, Atractylodes macrocephala, Curcuma phaeocaulis, Oldenlandia diffusa and Selaginella doederleinii*	RCT ($n = 60$); Combined with chemotherapy for QoL of patients with advanced gastrointestinal cancer	Pan et al. (2005)

Table 11.1 (continued)

Name of formulation	Composition of formulation	Details of studies	References
Gan'ai I	*Astragalus membranaceus, Codonopsis pilosula, Poria cocos, Ganoderma lucidum, Stephania tetrandra, Rehmannia glutinosa, Ligustrum lucidum, Eclipta prostrata, Salvia miltiorrhiza, Ligusticum chuanxiong, Buthus martensii, Curcuma phaeocaulis, Dioscorea opposita, Cremastra appendiculata, Coix lacryma-jobi, Bupleurum chinense, Oldenlandia diffusa, Scutellaria barbata, Paris polyphylla, Akebia quinata, Curcuma aromatica, Hordeum vulgare, Crataegus pinnatifida and Massa fermentata*	RCT ($n = 60$); Combined with Gan'ai II (external use), and TACE for stage II-III liver cancer	Shao et al. (2001)
Gan'ai II	*Realgar, Aluminum potassium, Daemonorops draco, Eupolyphaga sinensis, Boswellia carterii, Commiphora myrrha, Paris polyphylla, Dryobalanops aromarica, Phellodendron chinense, Selaginella moellendorffii, Solanum nigrum, Mentha haplocalyx, Bufo bufo gargarizans, Polistes olivaceous, Gekko swinhonis,* etc	RCT ($n = 60$); Combined with Gan'ai I (internal use), and TACE for stage II-III liver cancer	Shao et al. (2001)
Ganji Recipe	*Codonopsis pilosula, Atractylodes macrocephala, Bupleurum chinense, Glycyrrhiza uralensis, Paeonia lactiflora, Smilax glabra, Eupolyphaga sinensis, Curcuma phaeocaulis, Hirudo nipponica, Scutellaria barbata, Oldenlandia diffusa,* etc	Prospective RCT ($n = 97$); Combined with Ailitong (external use) for patients with advanced primary liver cancer	Tian et al. (2008)

Table 11.1 (continued)

Name of formulation	Composition of formulation	Details of studies	References
Guben Yiliu III	*Astragalus membranaceus, Pseudostellaria heterophylla, Atractylodes macrocephala, Poria cocos, Ligustrum lucidum, Lycium barbarum, Cornus officinalis, Gallus gallus domesticus, Hordeum vulgare, Crataegus pinnatifida, Massa fermentata, Solanum lyratum, Solanum nigrum and Spatholobus suberectus*	RCT ($n = 81$); Combined with moxibustion and chemotherapy for advanced cancers in lung, breast and digestive system, and non-Hodgkin's lymphomas	Liu et al. (2001)
Guliu capsule	Herbal ingredients were not provided	RCT ($n = 100$); Combined with ^{89}Sr therapy for metastatic bone tumour	Su et al. (2005)
Hechan tablet	*Agrimonia pilosa, Houttuynia cordata, Panax ginseng, Bufo bufo gargarizans, Fritillaria thunbergii, Pinellia ternata, Asparagus cochinchinensis, Lepidium apetalum and Ranunculus ternatus*	Multi centre, prospective RCT ($n = 294$); Used alone or combined with chemotherapy for NSCLC	Zhou et al. (2005)
Jianpi Yisheng formulation	*Astragalus membranaceus, Salvia miltiorrhiza, Polyporus umbellatus, Poria cocos, Lycium barbarum, Ligustrum lucidum, Epimedium grandiflorum, Scutellaria barbata, Trionyx sinensis, Coix lacryma-jobi and Ziziphus jujuba*	RCT ($n = 101$); Combined with chemotherapy for patients with advanced malignancies	Jiang et al. (2001)
Jinlongshe Oral liquid	*Arisaema erubescens preparata, Pinellia ternata, Citrus reticulata, Citrus aurantium, Fritillaria cirrhosa, Sinapis alba, Buthus martensii, Gallus gallus domesticus, Glycyrrhiza uralensis,* etc	RCT ($n = 104$); Used alone or combined with chemotherapy for patients with stage III-IV gastric cancer	Li and Wei (2001)

Table 11.1 (continued)

Name of formulation	Composition of formulation	Details of studies	References
Jisui Shengbai decoction	*Astragalus membranaceus, Codonopsis pilosula, Atractylodes macrocephala, Epimedium grandiflorum, Cuscuta chinensis, Ligustrum lucidum, Lycium barbarum, Angelica sinensis, Paeonia lactiflora, Spatholobus suberectus, Equus africanus asinus, Citrus reticulata, Glycyrrhiza uralensis and Pig marrow (cooked separately)*	RCT ($n = 62$); Used alone for chemotherapy induced leukopenia in patients with solid cancers	Wu et al. (2002)
Modified Sijunzi decoction	*Codonopsis pilosula, Atractylodes macrocephala, Poria cocos and Glycyrrhiza uralensis preparata*	RCT ($n = 39$); Combined with TACE for QoL of patients with colon cancer accompanied by liver metastasis	Meng et al. (2003)
Modified Xiaoyao decoction	*Bupleurum chinense, Angelica sinensis, Paeonia lactiflora, Atractylodes macrocephala, Poria cocos and Glycyrrhiza uralensis*	RCT ($n = 65$); Combined with chemotherapy for breast cancer	Wen et al. (2006)
Qingre Liyan decoction	*Lonicera japonica, Belamcanda chinensis, Lasiosphara fenzlii, Astragalus membranaceus, Glehnia littoralis, Ophiopogon japonicus, Trichosanthes kirilowii, Scrophularia ningpoensis, Ligusticum chuanxiong, Agrimonia pilosa, Imperata cylindrica and Glycyrrhiza uralensis*	RCT ($n = 60$); Used alone for radiation induced mucositis in patients with head and neck cancers	Wu et al. (2007)
Quxie capsule	*Croton tiglium, Evodia rutaecarpa, Zingiber officinale, Cinnamomum cassia, Aconitum carmichaeli, Pinellia ternata, Citrus reticulata,* etc	RCT ($n = 40$); Combined with chemotherapy for advanced colorectal cancer	Yang et al. (2008b)

Table 11.1 (continued)

Name of formulation	Composition of formulation	Details of studies	References
Shengbaikuai decoction	*Astragalus membranaceus, Cinnamomum cassia, Paeonia lactiflora, Saposhnikovia divaricata, Atractylodes macrocephala, Glycyrrhiza uralensis, Zingiber officinale, Ziziphus jujuba, Angelica sinensis and Spatholobus suberectus*	RCT ($n = 115$); Used alone for chemotherapy-induced leukopenia in patients with hematogenic malignancies	Tan et al. (1998)
Shenqi Fuzheng injection	*Panax ginseng and Astragalus membranaceus*	RCT ($n = 60$); Combined with chemotherapy for advanced breast cancer	Huang et al. (2008)
Shentao Ruangan Pill	*Artemisia capillaris, Oldenlandia diffusa, Scutellaria barbata, Curcuma phaeocaulis, Prunus persica, Angelica sinensis, Salvia miltiorrhiza, Panax ginseng, Poria cocos, Cordyceps sinensis,* etc	RCT ($n = 85$); Combined with hepatic artery infusion with hydroxycamptothecin for liver cancer (II-III stages; tumour $\geq$ 5 cm in diameter)	Lin et al. (2005)
Xiaoshui decoction	*Astragalus membranaceus, Polygonum orientale, Lindera aggregata, Polyporus umbellatus, Sarcandra glabra, Angelica sinensis, Lycium barbarum, Curcuma phaeocaulis, Oldenlandia diffusa, Sophora flavescens,* etc	RCT ($n = 61$); Combined with cisplatin intraperitoneal injection for patients with ascites related to primary liver cancer	Wu et al. (2005a)
Zhang's Recipe	*Astragalus membranaceus, Spatholobus suberectus, Coix lacryma-jobi, Codonopsis pilosula, Angelica sinensis, Poria cocos, Paeonia lactiflora, Dioscorea opposita, Lycium barbarum, Citrus reticulata, Massa fermentata, Hordeum vulgare and Crataegus pinnatifida*	Controlled trial ($n =$ 52); Used alone for cancer patients with cachexia	Zhang (2000)

Table 11.1 (continued)

Name of formulation	Composition of formulation	Details of studies	References
Zou's formulation	*Salvia miltiorrhiza, Paeonia veitchii, Rehmannia glutinosa, Scrophularia ningpoensis, Ophiopogon japonicus, Imperata cylindrica, Scutellaria baicalensis, Glehnia littoralis, Oldenlandia diffusa and Pseudostellaria heterophylla*	RCT ($n = 120$); Used alone for radiation induced mucositis in patients with nasopharyngeal cancer	Zou et al. (2005)

Abbreviations: RCT: randomized controlled trial; NSCLC: non-small cell lung cancer; TACE: transcatheter arterial chemoembolization; QoL: quality of life

11.8 Conclusions

The majority of clinical trials reviewed have demonstrated beneficial effects of CM on the survival, QoL and immune functions of cancer patients when used alone or in conjunction with conventional therapies. Some of these interventions also increased the tumour responsiveness to conventional therapies and alleviated chemotherapy-induced adverse drug reactions. Evidence also exists to support the use of CM as an alternative approach in relieving cancer related symptoms such as pain and cachexia in standard palliative care for advanced cancer patients.

However, some serious methodological issues such as small sample size, lack of adequate placebo control, and inappropriate randomization and statistical analysis, were identified in these studies. It is worth noting that some Chinese herbal formulations used in the clinical trials contain potentially toxic herbs such as *Cremastra variabilis* (bulb of Chinese tulip), prepared aconite root, scorplon, *Whitmania acranulata* (feech) and toad venom. Although minor CHM-related adverse events (*e.g.* nausea and diarrhea) were reported in some individual trials, no studies have appropriately evaluated and graded the adverse events using the Common Toxicity Criteria. It is, therefore, somewhat premature to draw definitive conclusions on the effectiveness and safety of CM for cancer care. Nevertheless, the existing data provide a good insight into the role CM plays in cancer care and shed light on the approaches for future research in this field.

The areas that warrant further investigations include the efficacy of the CM interventions using rigorous RCT design, cost effectiveness, interactions between CHMs and conventional chemotherapeutic agents and potential adverse events of the CHMs used in the cancer treatment. The individualised treatment protocols and standardised assessment outcome measures should also be carefully considered in future study design. More research is also required to validate the integrative approach in cancer care using CM in conjunction with conventional therapies. Further preclinical studies are also needed to establish safety profiles and mechanisms of action of CM interventions used in cancer treatments.

References

Alimi D, Rubino C, Pichard-Leandri E et al. Analgesic effect of auricular acupuncture for cancer pain: a randomized, blinded, controlled trial. J Clin Oncol. 2003;21:4120–6.

Bao YX, Wong CK, Leung SF et al. Clinical studies of immunomodulatory activities of Yunzhi-Danshen in patients with nasopharyngeal carcinoma. J Altern Complement Med. 2006;12: 771–6.

Bosaeus I. Nutritional support in multimodal therapy for cancer cachexia. Support Care Cancer. 2008;16:447–51.

Cassileth BR, Vickers AJ. High prevalence of complementary and alternative medicine use among cancer patients: implications for research and clinical care. J Clin Oncol. 2005;23(12): 2590–2.

Cella DF, Patel JD. Improving health-related quality of life in non-small-cell lung cancer with current treatment options. Clin Lung Cancer. 2008;9:206–12.

Chalkiadakis GE, Ziogas D. Progress and limitations of surgery in improving outcomes of esophagogastric junction cancer. Ann Surg Oncol. 2009;16:2074–5.

Chaudhuri D, Suriano R, Mittelman A et al. Targeting the immune system in cancer. Curr Pharm Biotechnol. 2009;10:166–84.

Chen ZJ, Guo YP, Wu ZC. Observation on the therapeutic effect of acupuncture at pain points on cancer pain. Zhongguo Zhen Jiu. 2008;28:251–3.

Cho WC, Chen HY. Clinical efficacy of traditional Chinese medicine as a concomitant therapy for nasopharyngeal carcinoma: a systematic review and meta-analysis. Cancer Invest. 2009a;27:334–44.

Cho WC, Chen HY. Transcatheter arterial chemoembolization combined with or without Chinese herbal therapy for hepatocellular carcinoma: meta-analysis. Expert Opin Investig Drugs. 2009b;18:617–35.

De Schutter H, Nuyts S. Radiosensitizing potential of epigenetic anticancer drugs. Anticancer Agents Med Chem. 2009;9:99–108.

Deng G, Hou BL, Holodny AI et al. Functional magnetic resonance imaging (fMRI) changes and saliva production associated with acupuncture at LI-2 acupuncture point: a randomized controlled study. BMC Complement Altern Med. 2008;8:37.

Deng G, Vickers A, Yeung S et al. Randomized, controlled trial of acupuncture for the treatment of hot flashes in breast cancer patients. J Clin Oncol. 2007;25:5584–90.

Ezzo J, Streitberger K, Schneider A. Cochrane systematic reviews examine P6 acupuncture-point stimulation for nausea and vomiting. J Altern Complement Med. 2006;12:489–95.

Fan G, Zong W, Zuo J. Dynamic observation and clinical significance of integrated traditional Chinese and Western medicine on interleukin-2 system, T cell and erythrocyte immune system in patients of lung cancer. Zhongguo Zhong Xi Yi Jie He Za Zhi. 2000;20:586–8.

Frisk J, Spetz AC, Hjertberg H et al. Two modes of acupuncture as a treatment for hot flushes in men with prostate cancer – a prospective multicenter study with long-term follow-up. Eur Urol. 2008;55:156–63.

Guo Z. Clinical observation on treatment of 38 cases of postoperational large intestinal cancer by Fuzheng Yiai Decoction combined with chemotherapy. Zhongguo Zhong Xi Yi Jie He Za Zhi. 1999;19:20–2.

He BM, Li WS, Li WY. Effect of previous analgesia of scalp acupuncture on post-operative epidural morphine analgesia in the patient of intestinal cancer. Zhongguo Zhen Jiu. 2007;27: 369–71.

Hervik J, Mjaland O. Acupuncture for the treatment of hot flashes in breast cancer patients, a randomized, controlled trial. Breast Cancer Res Treat. 2009;116:311–6.
Hu ZB, Xiong J, Rong Z et al. Cinobufacini injection for advanced cancers. Liaoning J Tradit Chin Med. 2004;31:836–7.
Huang LZ, Zhang XM, He X. Analgesic effects of Wenyang Zhitong capsule on bone metastatic carcinoma. Chin Inf J Tradit Chin Med. 2004;11:197–8.
Huang ZF, Wei JS, Li HZ et al. Effect of Shenqi Fuzheng injection combined with chemotherapy on thirty patients with advanced breast cancer. Zhongguo Zhong Xi Yi Jie He Za Zhi. 2008;28:152–4.
Hyodo I, Amano N, Eguchi K et al. Nationwide survey on complementary and alternative medicine in cancer patients in Japan. J Clin Oncol. 2005;23:2645–54.
Jemal A, Siegel R, Ward E et al. Cancer statistics, 2009. CA Cancer J Clin. 2009;59:225–49.
Jia BZ, Li JF, Gu CS. Elemene injection for bladder cancer. Guizhou Med J. 2002;26:810–1.
Jiang CM, Pang MR, Gong LY. Clinical observation on effect of chemotherapy combined with Chinese medicine in treating advanced tumour patients and on immunologic parameters. Zhongguo Zhong Xi Yi Jie He Za Zhi. 2001;21:885–7.
Konkimalla VB, Efferth T. Evidence-based Chinese medicine for cancer therapy. J Ethnopharmacol. 2008;116:207–10.
Lee J, Dodd M, Dibble S et al. Review of acupressure studies for chemotherapy-induced nausea and vomiting control. J Pain Symptom Manage. 2008;36:529–44.
Li LN, Liu WS, Xu K. Effect of combination of syndrome differentiation depending treatment and chemotherapy on prognostic factors in treating mid-late patients with non-small call lung cancer. Zhongguo Zhong Xi Yi Jie He Za Zhi. 2003;23:575–9.
Li XY, Wei PK. Jinlongshe Oral Liquid for advanced gastric cancer. Hubei J Tradit Chin Med. 2001;23:3–5.
Lin LZ, Zhou DH, Liu K et al. Analysis on the prognostic factors in patients with large hepatocarcinoma treated by Shentao Ruangan Pill and hydroxycamptothecine. Zhongguo Zhong Xi Yi Jie He Za Zhi. 2005;25:8–11.
Liu J, Yu RC, Rao XQ. Study on effect of moxibustion and Guben Yiliu III combined with chemotherapy in treating middle-late stage malignant tumour. Zhongguo Zhong Xi Yi Jie He Za Zhi. 2001;21:262–4.
Liu Y, Ye F, Qiu GQ et al. Effects of lactone I from *Atractylodes macrocephala* Koidz on cytokines and proteolysis-inducing factors in cachectic cancer patients. Di Yi Jun Yi Da Xue Xue Bao. 2005;25:1308–11.
Lu W, Hu D, Dean-Clower E et al. Acupuncture for chemotherapy-induced leucopoenia: exploratory meta-analysis of randomized controlled trials. J Soc Integr Oncol. 2007;5:1–10.
Marin JJ, Romero MR, Blazquez AG et al. Importance and limitations of chemotherapy among the available treatments for gastrointestinal tumours. Anticancer Agents Med Chem. 2009;9: 162–84.
Melchart D, Ihbe-Heffinger A, Leps B et al. Acupuncture and acupressure for the prevention of chemotherapy-induced nausea – a randomised cross-over pilot study. Support Care Cancer. 2006;14:878–82.
Meng MB, Cui YL, Guan YS et al. Traditional Chinese medicine plus transcatheter arterial chemoembolization for unresectable hepatocellular carcinoma. J Altern Complement Med. 2008;14:1027–42.
Meng ZQ, Xu YY, Liu LM et al. Clinical evaluation of integration of transcatheter arterial chemoembolization and traditional Chinese medicine in treating metastatic liver cancer. Zhong Xi Yi Jie He Xue Bao. 2003;1:187–8, 233.
Mok TS, Yeo W, Johnson PJ et al. A double-blind placebo-controlled randomized study of Chinese herbal medicine as complementary therapy for reduction of chemotherapy-induced toxicity. Ann Oncol. 2007;18:768–74.
Molassiotis A, Fernadez-Ortega P, Pud D et al. Use of complementary and alternative medicine in cancer patients: a European survey. Ann Oncol. 2005;16:655–63.

Molassiotis A, Potrata B, Cheng KK. A systematic review of the effectiveness of Chinese herbal medication in symptom management and improvement of quality of life in adult cancer patients. Complement Ther Med. 2009;17:92–120.

Mustian KM, Palesh OG, Flecksteiner SA. Tai chi chuan for breast cancer survivors. Med Sport Sci. 2008;52:209–17.

Oh B, Butow P, Mullan B et al. Medical qigong for cancer patients: pilot study of impact on quality of life, side effects of treatment and inflammation. Am J Chin Med. 2008;36:459–72.

Pan B, Cheng T, Nan KJ et al. Effect of Fuzheng Yiliu decoction combined with chemotherapy on patients with intermediate and late stage gastrointestinal cancer. World J Gastroenterol. 2005;11:439–42.

Piao BK, Wang YX, Xie GR et al. Impact of complementary mistletoe extract treatment on quality of life in breast, ovarian and non-small cell lung cancer patients. A prospective randomized controlled clinical trial. Anticancer Res. 2004;24:303–9.

Quan D, Lu Y, Li Z. Clinical observation on radio- or chemotherapy plus traditional Chinese medicine in treating brain metastatic tumour. Zhongguo Zhong Xi Yi Jie He Za Zhi. 1999;19:392–4.

Roscoe JA, Matteson SE, Morrow GR et al. Acustimulation wrist bands are not effective for the control of chemotherapy-induced nausea in women with breast cancer. J Pain Symptom Manage. 2005;29:376–84.

Shao ZX, Cheng ZG, Yin X. Clinical study on treatment of middle-advanced stage liver cancer by combined treatment of hepatic artery chemoembolization with Gan'ai No. I and No. II. Zhongguo Zhong Xi Yi Jie He Za Zhi. 2001;21:168–70.

Shu X, McCulloch M, Xiao H et al. Chinese herbal medicine and chemotherapy in the treatment of hepatocellular carcinoma: a meta-analysis of randomized controlled trials. Integr Cancer Ther. 2005;4:219–29.

Standish LJ, Kozak L, Congdon S. Acupuncture is underutilized in hospice and palliative medicine. Am J Hosp Palliat Care. 2008;25:298–308.

Streitberger K, Friedrich-Rust M, Bardenheuer H et al. Effect of acupuncture compared with placebo-acupuncture at P6 as additional antiemetic prophylaxis in high-dose chemotherapy and autologous peripheral blood stem cell transplantation: a randomized controlled single-blind trial. Clin Cancer Res. 2003;9:2538–44.

Su XC, Wang YL, Yang XY et al. Effect of Guliu capsule combined with 89Sr therapy on metastatic bone tumour. Di Yi Jun Yi Da Xue Xue Bao. 2005;25:1164–5, 77.

Tan D, Xie Z, Zhong M. A clinical observation on the leucopoenia treated with Shengbaikuai Decoction. Zhongguo Zhong Xi Yi Jie He Za Zhi. 1998;18:408–10.

Tian HQ, Liang GW, Huang XQ et al. Prospective randomized controlled study on complex treatments of traditional Chinese medicine for advanced primary hepatocarcinoma. China Med Her. 2008;5:17–21.

Wang HZ, Wang HB, Gao H. Clinical observation on treatment of 34 advanced gastric carcinoma patients by chemotherapy of DCF regimen combined with Fuzheng Hewei Decoction. Zhongguo Zhong Xi Yi Jie He Za Zhi. 2007a;27:927–9.

Wang J, Sui LH, Lou G et al. Elemene injection for ovarian cancer-induced ascites. ACTA Chin Med Pharmacol. 1999;1:35–6.

Wang JP, Ge XG, Wang Y et al. High intensity focused ultrasound combined with Chinese herbal medicine for controlling pain in pancreas cancer. Liaoning J Tradit Chin Med. 2007b;34: 1607–8.

Wang ZY, Li GS, Huang HX. Clinical observation on treatment of 75 mid-late stage cancer patients with Yanshu Injection. Zhongguo Zhong Xi Yi Jie He Za Zhi. 2006;26:681–4.

Wen LB, Yang LP, Huang HS. Modified Xiaoyao decoction for controlling toxicity of chemotherapy in postoperative breast cancer. J Tradit Chin Med Univ Hum. 2006;26:38–40.

Wu B, Zhou RX, Zhou MS. Effect of acupuncture on interleukin-2 level and NK cell immunoactivity of peripheral blood of malignant tumour patients. Zhongguo Zhong Xi Yi Jie He Za Zhi. 1994;14:537–9.

Wu B, Zhou RX, Zhou MS. Effect of acupuncture on immunomodulation in patients with malignant tumours. Zhongguo Zhong Xi Yi Jie He Za Zhi. 1996;16:139–41.

Wu D, Bao WG, Ding YH. Clinical and experimental study of Xiaoshui decoction in the treatment of primary liver cancer caused ascites. Zhongguo Zhong Xi Yi Jie He Za Zhi. 2005a;25:1066–9.

Wu MH, Yuan B, Liu QF et al. Study of Qingre Liyan decoction in treating and preventing acute radioactive oral mucositis. Chin J Integr Med. 2007;13:280–4.

Wu TX, Munro AJ, Guanjian L. Chinese medical herbs for chemotherapy side effects in colorectal cancer patients. Cochrane Database Syst Rev. 2005b;1:CD004540.

Wu XG, Ma TX, Liu XT et al. Jisui Shengbai decoction for chemotherapy-induced leucopoenia in malignant tumours. Zhong Liu Fang Zhi Za Zhi. 2002;9:336–7.

Xiong SQ, Liu BQ, Wang BD et al. Changfukang capsule for colon cancer. Pharmacol Clin Appl Chin Herb Med. 2003;19:45–6.

Xu ZY, Jin CJ, Shen DY. Clinical study on treatment of advanced non-small-cell lung cancer with Chinese herbal medicine in different stages combined with chemotherapy. Zhongguo Zhong Xi Yi Jie He Za Zhi. 2007;27:874–8.

Yang HM, Zhen YJ, Wan Q et al. Effects of traditional Chinese medicine on improvement of quality of life in elderly patients with IV stage stomach cancer. Pract Geriatr. 2008a;22:54–6.

Yang YF, Chen ZX, Xu Y et al. Randomized controlled study on effect of Quxie capsule on survival time and quality of life in patients with advanced colorectal carcinoma. Zhongguo Zhong Xi Yi Jie He Za Zhi. 2008b;28:111–4.

You J, Shi ZM, Han BH. Evaluation on effect of Feiji Recipe on quality of life of patients with non-small cell lung cancer by adopting international questionnaire of QoL. Zhongguo Zhong Xi Yi Jie He Za Zhi. 2006;26(1):33–7.

Zhang J. Effect of Chinese herbal medicine on cancer-associated cachexia. Zhongguo Zhong Xi Yi Jie He Za Zhi. 2000;20:871.

Zhang T, Ma SL, Xie GR et al. Clinical research on nourishing yin and unblocking meridians Recipe combined with opioid analgesics in cancer pain management. Chin J Integr Med. 2006;12:180–4.

Zhou DH. Clinical oncology of Chinese medicine. Beijing: People's Health Publishing House; 2003.

Zhou DH, Lin LZ, Zhou YQ. Analysis of short-term therapeutic efficacy of integrated traditional and Western medicine in treating non-small cell lung cancer. Zhongguo Zhong Xi Yi Jie He Za Zhi. 2005;25:1061–5.

Zhu JS, Song MQ, Wang L et al. Immunoregulation and short-term therapeutic effects of super-selective intra-arterial chemotherapy combined with traditional Chinese drugs on gastric cancer patients. Zhong Xi Yi Jie He Xue Bao. 2006;4:478–81.

Zou YH, Liu XM, Tan LR. Chinese herbal medicine for treatment of 60 cases of acute radiation-induced mucositis in nasopharyngeal carcinoma. J Tradit Chin Med. 2005;46:520–2.

Chapter 12
Toxicology, Safety and Herb–drug Interactions in Cancer Therapy

Shu-Feng Zhou

Abstract Cancer patients always seek alternative approaches without advising the oncologists about their use of herbal/dietary supplements. There are increased reports on the interaction of herbal medicines and anticancer drugs that is becoming a safety concern. For example, a clinical study in cancer patients reported that treatment of *Hypericum perforatum* (St John's wort) at 900 mg/day orally for 18 days decreased the plasma levels of the active metabolite of irinotecan, SN-38, by 42%. In healthy subjects, 2 weeks of treatment with St John's wort at 900 mg/day significantly decreased the systemic exposure of imatinib by 32%. In women with advanced breast cancer, coadministration of garlic supplement reduced the clearance of docetaxol by 23.1–35.1%, although the difference did not achieve statistical significance. A recent clinical trial in patients with resected breast or colon cancer has revealed that Chinese herbal medicines did not alleviate chemotherapy-induced haematological toxicity, but significantly reduced drug-induced nausea. Most anticancer drugs undergo Phase I and/or II metabolism and are substrates of P-glycoprotein, breast cancer resistance protein, multidrug resistance associated proteins, and/or other transporters. Induction and inhibition of these enzymes and transporters is considered an important mechanism for herb–anticancer drug interactions. Timely identification of the herbal medicines involved and victim anticancer drugs is important to remind both oncologists and cancer patients of the possible safety concerns arising from combined use of herbs with any anticancer drugs. Monitoring plasma concentrations of concurrently administered anticancer drugs and observing for possible signs of clinical toxicity are necessary when herbal remedies is used concurrently.

S.-F. Zhou (✉)
Discipline of Chinese Medicine, School of Health Sciences, RMIT University, Bundoora, VIC 3083, Australia
e-mail: shufeng.zhou@rmit.edu.au

W.C.S. Cho (ed.), *Supportive Cancer Care with Chinese Medicine*,
DOI 10.1007/978-90-481-3555-4_12, © Springer Science+Business Media B.V. 2010

12.1 Introduction

The major modules of cancer treatment are surgery, radiation, chemotherapy and immunotherapy (Gatenby 2009). However, these therapies are only successful when the cancer is detected at an early stage, or limited to certain types of cancer (e.g. leukemia). Due to limited diagnostic means for detecting pro-carcinoma status and cancers at early stages, most patients present in the advanced stage of cancer or with extensive local infiltration. For advanced tumours, in particular those tumours developed from epithelial tissues such as lung, colon, breast, prostate and pancreas, these therapies are less successful.

Chemotherapy represents one of the major means for cancer treatment, which aims to kill or disable tumour cells while preserving the normal cells in the body (Gatenby 2009). Chemotherapeutic agents generally have a narrow margin of safety, and are used in combination usually given at a maximum tolerated dose to achieve maximum cancer cell killing (Chabner and Roberts 2005). They kill tumour cells by direct cytotoxicity, or activating host immune response, inhibiting the proliferation processes of tumour cells, and inducing apoptosis (Cotter 2009). For most anticancer drugs, there is a large interindividual variability in their pharmacokinetics and this can result in unpredictable toxicity and variable antitumour effects (Undevia et al. 2005). However, most patients do not respond to these drugs and they often experience severe side effects such as severe diarrhea and loss of hairs. The primary reason for this is because the drug kills both normal and tumour cells and drug levels within tumour cells are too low. Drug resistance and dose-limiting toxicities are the major problems for the success of cancer chemotherapy (Yague and Raguz 2005).

Since the response rate of cancer patients to chemotherapy is low and patients often experience significant drug-induced toxicities, they always seek alternative approaches for treating the cancer and/or reducing the toxicities of chemotherapeutic drugs. Reports indicate that between 7 and 64% of adult cancer patients use at least one kind of complementary and alternative medicine (Ernst and Cassileth 1998), and 13–63% of these patients have reported the use of herbal products (Sparreboom et al. 2004a). It was reported that ~50% of patients with breast or gynecologic malignancies use complementary and alternative medicine, and as much as 5% of this population takes the herbal supplement, garlic (Warshafsky et al. 1993). The combined use of herbs with anticancer drugs will raise the potential of pharmacokinetic and/or pharmacodynamic herb–anticancer drug interactions (Fugh-Berman 2000; Hu et al. 2005b; Izzo 2005).

This chapter highlights our current knowledge on the safety concerns when herbal medicines are used in combination with oncological drugs and the clinical implications. To retrieve relevant data, the author has searched through computer-based literatures by full text search in MEDLINE (via PubMed), ScienceDirect, Current Contents Connect (ISI), Cochrane Library, CINAHL (EBSCO), CrossRef Search and EMBASE (all from inception to 10 July 2009). Keyword search terms used included cancer, tumour, chemotherapy, drug interaction, herb, herbal medicine, botanic drug and plant drug together with combination terms including pharmacokinetics, clearance, toxicity, response, drug monitoring, oncology and human (patient).

12.2 Reported Clinical Herb–Anticancer Drug Interactions

12.2.1 Irinotecan + Hypericum perforatum (St John's Wort)

Irinotecan (CPT-11; Camptosar) is a potent DNA topoisomerase I inhibitor used in the treatment of advanced colorectal and lung cancer, giving an objective response in about 20% treated patients (Canal et al. 1996; Gupta et al. 1997; Kudoh et al. 1998). As a prodrug, irinotecan is converted to its active metabolite 7-ethyl-10-hydroxy-camptothecin (SN-38) by two isoforms of human liver and intestinal carboxylestesterases (hCE1 and hCE2) (Fig. 12.1) (Rivory et al. 1996a; Humerickhouse et al. 2000; Bencharit et al. 2002). SN-38 is further converted to its inactive glucuronide by uridine diphosphate glucuronosyltransferases (UGT1A1, 1A7 and 1A9) (Santos et al. 2000; Hanioka et al. 2001; Mathijssen et al. 2001). SN-38 glucuronide can be converted back to SN-38 by bacterial β-glucuronidase in the gut and both SN-38 and CPT-11 can be reabsorbed into the enterohepatic circulation (Takasuna et al. 1996; Chu et al. 1997b). A second major metabolism pathway of CPT-11 is cytochrome P-450 (CYP3A4 and CYP3A5)–mediated bipiperidine side chain oxidation to form 7-ethyl-10[4-N(5-aminopentanoic-acid)-1-piperidino] carbonyloxycamptothecin (APC) and 7-ethyl-10- (4-amino-1-piperidino) carbonyloxycamptothecin (NPC) (Fig. 12.1) (Rivory et al. 1996b; 1997; Haaz et al. 1998; Santos et al. 2000). NPC, but not APC, can undergo hydrolysis to SN-38 by human hepatic and plasma carboxylesterases (Dodds et al. 1998; Kehrer et al. 2000; Rivory 2000). Both APC and NPC lack cytotoxicity (Rivory 2000). The major dose-limiting toxicities of CPT-11 are myelosuppression and gastrointestinal toxicity, in particular unpredictable severe diarrhea (Gupta et al. 1994; Sugiyama et al. 1998; Rothenberg et al. 2001) (Fig. 12.1).

Several drug transporters have been implicated in the active efflux of CPT-11 when multidrug resistance was studied. P-gp and multidrug resistance associated protein-2 (MRP2; cMOAT, canalicular multispecific organic anion transporter) conferred resistance to CPT-11 by effluxing the drug out of the tumour cells (Sugiyama et al. 1998). In drug-resistant tumour cells overexpressing P-gp, the cellular accumulation of CPT-11 and SN-38 are decreased (Yang et al. 1995). CPT-11 and SN-38 in unconjugated and conjugated forms are also actively effluxed out of cells by MRP1 (Chu et al. 1999). Moreover, breast cancer resistance protein (BCRP) can transport CPT-11 and SN-38 and confers resistance to the two compounds (Schellens et al. 2000; Maliepaard et al. 2001). The high-level expression of these transporters for CPT-11 and SN-38 in tumour cells has been implicated in tumour resistance to CPT-11.

In an unblinded, randomized crossover study involving 5 cancer patients, it was found that treatment of St John's wort at 900 mg/day orally for 18 days decreased the plasma levels of the active metabolite of irinotecan, SN-38 by 42% (Mathijssen et al. 2002). This was accompanied by a decreased myelosuppression. These findings indicate that patients on irinotecan treatment should refrain from taking St John's wort.

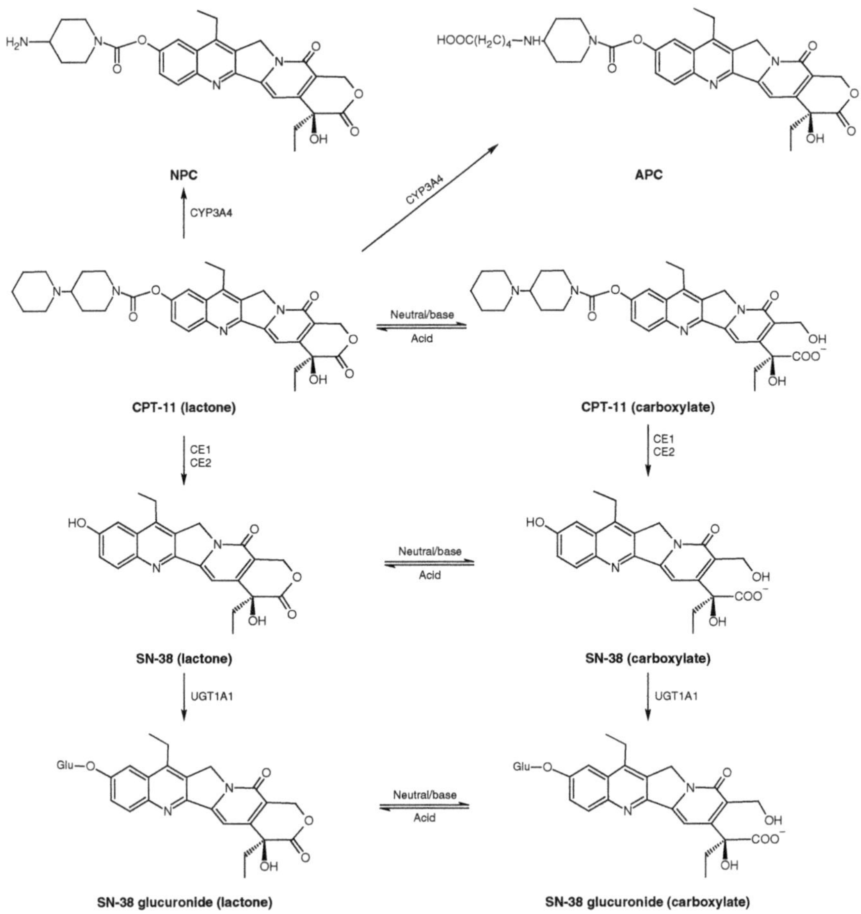

Fig. 12.1 Metabolic scheme of irinotecan in humans. Irinotecan is converted to its active metabolite SN-38 by hCE1 and hCE2. SN-38 is further converted to its inactive glucuronide by UGT1A1, 1A7 and 1A9

The mechanism for reduced SN-38 exposure level by St John's wort is unknown, but in vitro and in vivo studies in rats at our laboratory demonstrated that St John's wort accelerated SN-38 glucuronidation and modulated the transport of CPT-11 and SN-38 (Hu et al. 2007). Notably, our studies in rats indicate that St John's wort treatment also significantly attenuated the blood and gastrointestinal toxicity of CPT-11, probably due to reduced exposure to SN-38, and antiinflammatory and apoptosis inhibitory effect of St John's wort components (Hu et al. 2005a; 2006). Since SN-38 is the primary contributor for killing cancer cells, cancer patients on CPT-11 chemotherapy should avoid consumption of St John's wort products.

St John's wort is a very popular herbal antidepressant (Di Carlo et al. 2001; Nathan 2001; Linde et al. 2005). St John's wort contains over two dozens of constituents, among which the naphthodianthrones (e.g. hypericin and pseudohypericin), the phloroglucinols (e.g. hyperforin and adhyperforin), and a broad range of flavonoids are the major active components (Fig. 12.2). It is well-known that St John's wort extract is a potent inducer of CYP3A4 and 2B6, and the responsible component was hyperforin (Moore et al. 2000; Wentworth et al. 2000; Goodwin et al. 2001). However, using cDNA-expressed enzymes, St John's wort extracts and several of its major components have been found to inhibit the activities of CYP1A2, 2C9, 2C19, 2D6 and 3A4 (Obach 2000). The flavonoid I3,II8-biapigenin is a potent competitive inhibitor of CYP3A4, 2C9, and 1A2 with K_i of 0.038, 0.32, and 0.95 μM, respectively; whereas hyperforin is a competitive inhibitor of CYP2C9 and 3A4 activities with K_i of 1.8 and 0.48 μM, respectively (Obach 2000). However, St John's wort does not alter the CYP2C9, 1A2, or 2D6 activities in vivo in humans (Roby et al. 2000; Wang et al. 2001) (Fig. 12.2).

12.2.2 Irinotecan + *Silybum marianum* (Milk Thistle)

van Erp et al. (2005) investigated the effect of milk thistle 200 mg, thrice a day, for 4 or 12 days, on the pharmacokinetics of irinotecan in 6 cancer patients. Short-term (4 days) or more prolonged intake of milk thistle (12 days) had no significant effect on irinotecan clearance. The AUC ratio of SN-38 and irinotecan was slightly decreased by milk thistle (2.58% vs 2.23% vs 2.17%; $P = 0.047$), whereas the relative extent of glucuronidation of SN-38 was similar. The maximum plasma concentrations of silybin ranged between 0.0249 and 0.257 μM/L, which were too low to inhibit CYP3A4- and UGT1A1-mediated metabolism of irinotecan in vivo. Silybin (also known as silybinin) is one of the major active components of milk thistle, which significantly inhibits CYP3A4 and UGT1A1 in vitro (Sridar et al. 2004; Zuber et al. 2002). Silybin inactivated CYP3A4 and 2C9 in a mechanism-based manner (Sridar et al. 2004). The inactivation was time-, concentration- and NADPH-dependent.

In a clinical study, treatment of milk thistle for 28 days did not significantly affect CYP1A2, 2D6, 2E1 or 3A4 activity (Gurley et al. 2004), when probe drug cocktails of midazolam and caffeine were used, followed 24 h later by chlorzoxazone and debrisoquin. Extracts of milk thistle are well-known to prevent or reverse hepatotoxicity of reactive drug metabolites or naturally occurring toxins (Kroll et al. 2007). Silibinin has hepatoprotective properties that protect liver cells against toxins (Vogel et al. 1984; Das and Vasudevan 2006; Pradhan and Girish 2006).

However, modulation of P-gp by milk thistle may cause drug interactions and alter the response to anticancer drugs that are P-gp substrates. In vitro studies indicated that silymarin significantly modulated P-gp. It increased daunomycin accumulation in P-gp-positive cells, but not P-gp-negative cells, in a drug concentration- and P-gp expression level-dependent manner (Zhang and Morris 2003). Silymarin potentiated doxorubicin cytotoxicity in P-gp-positive cells, while it inhibited P-gp ATPase activity and azidopine photoaffinity labeling of P-gp, suggesting a direct interaction with P-gp substrate binding (Zhang and Morris 2003). These findings indicated that silymarin and its metabolite(s) inhibited P-gp-mediated cellular efflux, raising a potential for significant drug interactions with P-gp substrates.

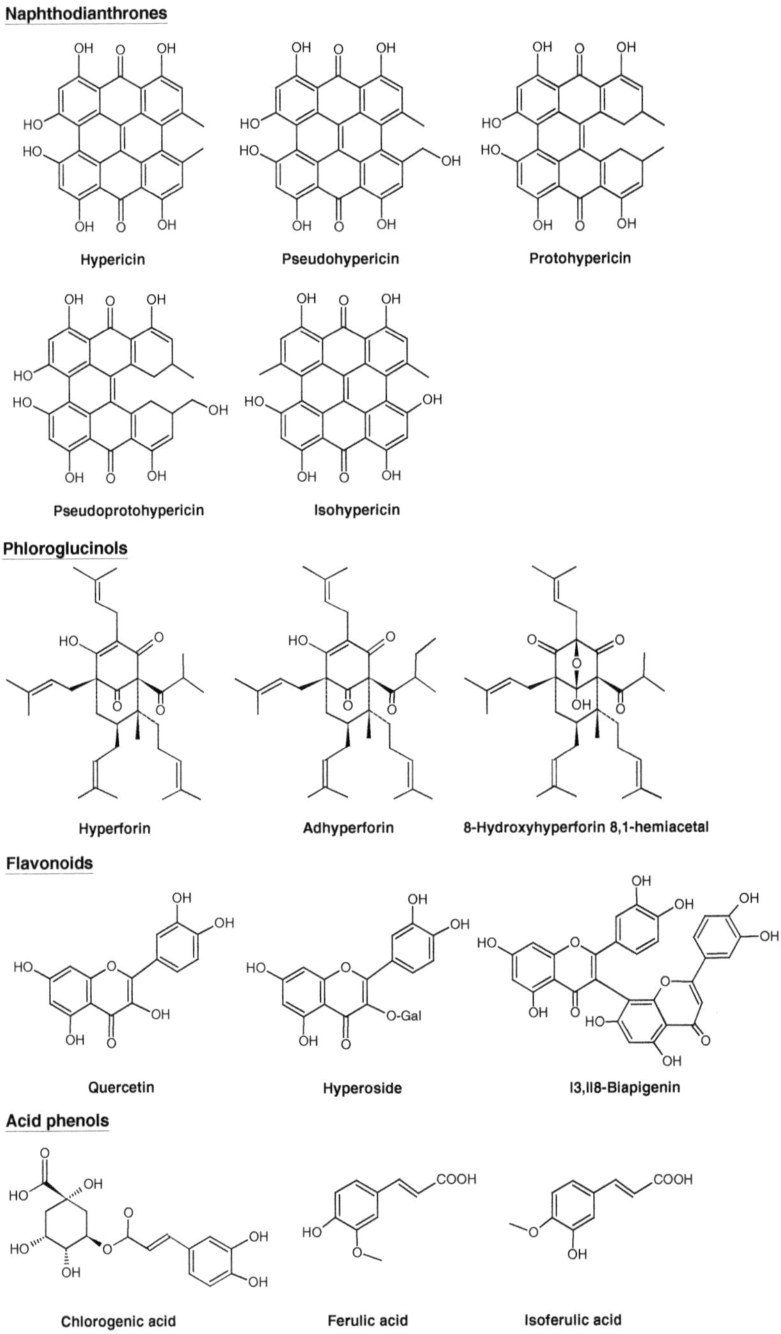

Fig. 12.2 Major active ingredients in St John's wort. St John's wort mainly contains naphthodianthrones, the phloroglucinols, and a broad range of flavonoids

12.2.3 Imatinib + St John's Wort

Imatinib (Gleevec; STI571) is a selective and potent inhibitor of the Bcr-Abl and c-kit tyrosine kinases and is approved by FDA for the treatment of Philadelphia chromosome-positive chronic myelogenous leukemia and gastrointestinal stromal tumours (Cohen et al. 2002, 2005b; Johnson et al. 2003). The metabolism of imatinib is complicated. Its Phase I metabolism pathways included *N*-demethylation (e.g. formation of its main metabolite CGP74588), piperazine ring oxidation with lactam formation (APG049, APG050, M29.6 and M28.8), piperazine-*N*-4 oxidation (CGP71422), pyridine *N*-oxidation (CGP72383) and benzylic hydroxylation (AFN911) (Fig. 12.3) (Gschwind et al. 2005). Furthermore, the loss of the piperazine moiety by oxidative deamination and rapid further oxidation of the intermediate aldehyde to a carboxylic acid led to the formation of the metabolite M42.2. Phase II metabolic routes included direct conjugation of imatinib and the *N*-desmethyl metabolite (CGP74588), resulting in M21.0 and M20.0a, respectively, most probably at nitrogen, and glucuronidation of oxidative metabolites (Gschwind et al. 2005). Following oral administration in healthy volunteers, the $t_{1/2\beta}$ of imatinib and its major active metabolite, the *N*-demethyl derivative (CGP74588), are

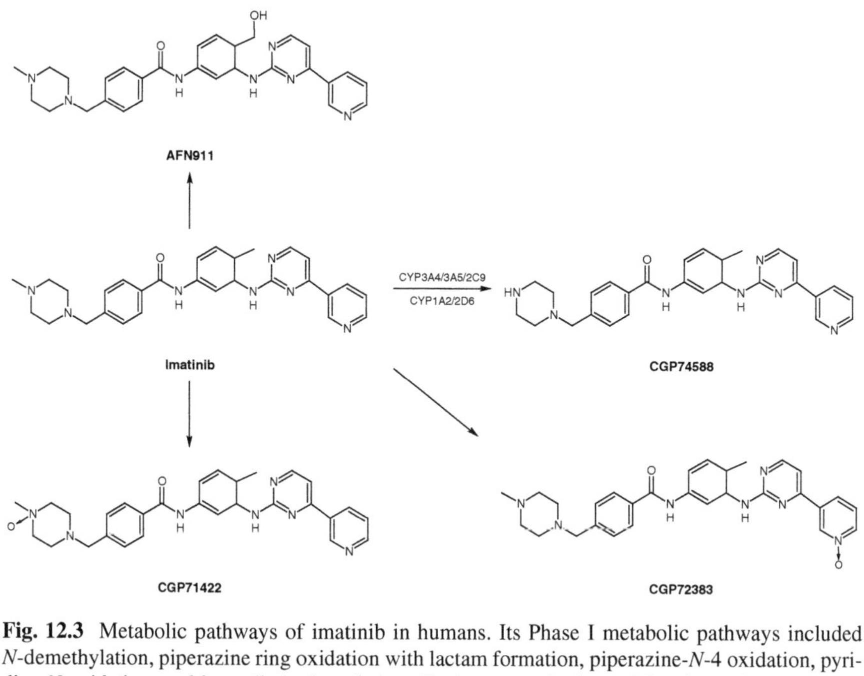

Fig. 12.3 Metabolic pathways of imatinib in humans. Its Phase I metabolic pathways included *N*-demethylation, piperazine ring oxidation with lactam formation, piperazine-*N*-4 oxidation, pyridine *N*-oxidation, and benzylic hydroxylation. Furthermore, the loss of the piperazine moiety by oxidative deamination and rapid further oxidation of the intermediate aldehyde to a carboxylic acid led to the formation of the metabolite M42.2. Phase II metabolic routes included direct conjugation of imatinib and the *N*-desmethyl metabolite, resulting in M21.0 and M20.0a, respectively

approximately 18 and 40 h, respectively (Gschwind et al. 2005). In vitro, imatinib was metabolized to the active CGP74588 by CYP3A4 and 3A5 and, to a lesser extent, by CYP2D6, 1A2 and 2C9 (van Erp et al. 2007). CGP74588 showed in vitro potency similar to the parent imatinib. The plasma AUC for this metabolite is about 15% of the AUC for imatinib (Gschwind et al. 2005). In addition, imatinib formed the major oxidative metabolite (M9) via *N*-oxidation on the piperazine ring (Ma et al. 2008, 2009). The apparent oral clearance of imatinib was potentially reduced in individuals with at least 1 *CYP2D6*4* allele (Gardner et al. 2006), suggesting an important role of CYP2D6 in imatinib metabolism in vivo (Fig. 12.3).

The C_{max} and AUC of imatinib were increased by 26 and 40%, respectively, when imatinib was coadministered with a single dose (400 mg) of ketoconazole (a CYP3A4 inhibitor) in healthy subjects (Dutreix et al. 2004). Caution is recommended when administering imatinib with potent CYP3A4 inhibitors such as ketoconazole, itraconazole, indinavir, nelfinavir, ritonavir, saquinavir, telithromycin, clarithromycin, atazanavir and voriconazole. Grapefruit juice may also increase plasma levels of imatinib and should be avoided. However, ritonavir 600 mg daily for 3 days did not alter the pharmacokinetics of imatinib at steady-state (van Erp et al. 2007). It appears that imatinib is insensitive to potent CYP3A4 inhibition at steady state and alternate elimination pathways contribute to its metabolism.

Imatinib is a potent competitive inhibitor of CYP2C9, 2D6, and 3A4/5 in vitro with K_i values of 27, 7.5 and 8 μM, respectively (van Erp et al. 2007). Imatinib increased the C_{max} and AUC of simvastatin (a CYP3A4 substrate) 2- and 3.5-fold, respectively, in patients with chronic myeloid leukemia (O'Brien et al. 2003). Particular caution is recommended when imatinib is concurrently used with CYP3A4 substrate drugs that have a narrow therapeutic window (e.g. alfentanil, cyclosporine, diergotamine, quinidine, sirolimus, ergotamine, fentanyl, pimozide and tacrolimus). Coadministration of imatinib at 400 mg twice daily increased the plasma AUC of metoprolol (a CYP2D6 substrate) by ~23% in Chinese patients with chronic myeloid leukaemia ($n = 20$), about 17% increase in CYP2D6 intermediate metabolizers ($n = 6$), 24% in extensive metabolizers ($n = 13$), and 28% for the subject with unknown CYP2D6 status ($n = 1$) (Wang et al. 2008). Imatinib has a weak to moderate inhibition on CYP2D6 in vivo.

Two clinical studies have been conducted to investigate the effect of St John's wort treatment on its pharmacokinetics of imatinib (Frye et al. 2004; Smith 2004). In an open-label, crossover, and fixed-sequence study with 10 healthy subjects, 2 weeks of treatment with St John's wort at 900 mg/day significantly decreased the AUC of imatinib by 32%, C_{max} by 29%, and elimination half-life by 21% (Smith 2004). The protein binding of imatinib was not altered by St John's wort (Smith 2004). Similar results were observed in another clinical study involving 12 healthy subjects (Frye et al. 2004). Administration of SJW at 900 mg/day for 14 days significantly increased clearance of imatinib by 43% (from 12.5 to 17.9 L/h). The AUC of imatinib was decreased by 30% (from 34.5 to 24.2 μg h/mL ($P < 0.001$). Imatinib elimination half-life and C_{max} were also significantly decreased (12.8 vs 9.0 h; 2.2 vs 1.8 μg/mL). In addition, the C_{max} of the active metabolite of imatinib, *N*-desmethyl-imatinib, was increased by 11.6%, but its AUC was not altered

(Frye et al. 2004). These results indicate that patients taking imatinib should avoid St John's wort administration and if concomitant use of St John's wort with imatinib is chosen, an increase in the imatinib dose becomes necessary to maintain clinical effectiveness.

Treatment of rifampin (a potent CYP3A4 inducer) at 600 mg once daily for 11 days significantly decreased the single dose C_{max} and AUC of imatinib by 54 and 74%, respectively (Bolton et al. 2004). The oral clearance of imatinib was increased by 3.8-fold. If alternative treatment cannot be administered, a dose adjustment of imatinib should be considered. Rifampin appears to be a more potent inducer of CYP3A4 than St John's wort. The magnitude of the effect of St John's wort on imatinib was generally similar to that reported for St John's wort on other CYP3A4 substrates such as cyclosporine [41–60% (Bauer et al. 2003)] and tacrolimus [57.8% (Mai et al. 2003)]. In patients on rifampicin or other CYP3A4 inducers, alternative therapeutic agents with less CYP3A induction potential should be selected when imatinib is administered.

Imatinib is a substrate of P-gp (Hamada et al. 2003), BCRP (Nakanishi et al. 2006; Ozvegy-Laczka et al. 2004), MRP4, organic anion transporting polypeptide 1A2 (OATP1A2), and organic cation transporter-1 (OCT1) (Hu et al. 2008). There is a possibility of herb–imatinib interaction through modulation of the expression and activity of these trasnporters. Both elacridar and pantoprazole (both P-gp and BCRP inhibitors) significantly increased the AUC of orally administered imatinib in wild-type but also in *P-gp/Bcrp* knockout mice (Oostendorp et al. 2009). The reduced clearance was not due to a reduction in biliary excretion. Fecal excretion of imatinib was significantly decreased in *P-gp* and *P-gp/Bcrp* knockout but not in *Bcrp* knockout mice, whereas the brain penetration was significantly higher in *P-gp/Bcrp* knockout mice compared to single *P-gp* or *Bcrp* knockout or wild-type mice (Oostendorp et al. 2009). It appears that both P-gp and BCRP have only a modest effect on the pharmacokinetics of imatinib in vivo.

12.2.4 Erlotinib + Dietary/Herbal Supplements

Erlotinib (CP-358774; OSI-774; Gefitinib) is an orally bioavailable synthetic anilinoquinazolines that selectively and reversibly bind to the intracellular ATP-binding site of the epidermal growth factor receptor (EGFR) tyrosine kinase (Dowell et al. 2005; Moyer et al. 1997). It has been approved in the United States for the treatment of refractory locally advanced or metastatic non-small cell lung cancer (Johnson et al. 2005). In 2005, the FDA also approved its use in combination with gemcitabine for treatment of locally advanced, unresectable, or metastatic pancreatic cancer (Moore et al. 2007; Saif 2008; Van Cutsem et al. 2009). Erlotinib has shown a survival benefit in the treatment of advanced lung cancer in Phase III trials (Gatzemeier et al. 2007; Gridelli et al. 2007, 2008). Although also being palliative, erlotinib lacks the normal tissue toxicity inherent to cytotoxic agents, e.g. hematologic suppression, vomiting, and mucocutaneous ulceration, but displayed presumed target effects, such as rash and diarrhea (Dowell et al. 2005; Herbst et al. 2005).

Erlotinib has an oral bioavailability of ~60% with a $t_{1/2\beta}$ of 8 h (Frohna et al. 2006) and undergoes extensive (>98% of a total dose) metabolism to form nine oxidative metabolites and four glucuronides, with ~80% of the administered dose excreted in feces (Ling et al. 2006). A number of metabolites of erlotinib have been identified in the rat and dog, with *O*-demethylation, oxidation of the acetylene moiety, and aromatic hydroxylation being the major metabolic routes. Following oral administration to healthy subjects, the pharmacologically active metabolite M14 (formed by *O*-demethylation) accounted for ~5% of the total circulating radioactivity, with a $t_{1/2\beta}$ of 7.7 h M6, M11 and M16 had an abundances at ~2, ~4 and ~1%, respectively, of circulating radioactivity (Fig. 12.4) (Ling et al. 2006). In urine, M11 represented the major metabolite (~2% of the dose) and all other urinary metabolites were minor (each <1% of the dose). In feces, 10 metabolites were radiochemically quantifiable, with M11, M6, and M16 being the major ones (27.2, 20.6, and 9.6% of dose, respectively) (Ling et al. 2006). The major metabolic pathways of erlotinib include *O*-demethylation of the side chains followed by oxidation to a carboxylic acid, M11 (29.4% of dose); oxidation of the acetylene moiety to a carboxylic acid, M6 (21.0%); hydroxylation of the aromatic ring to M16 (9.6%);

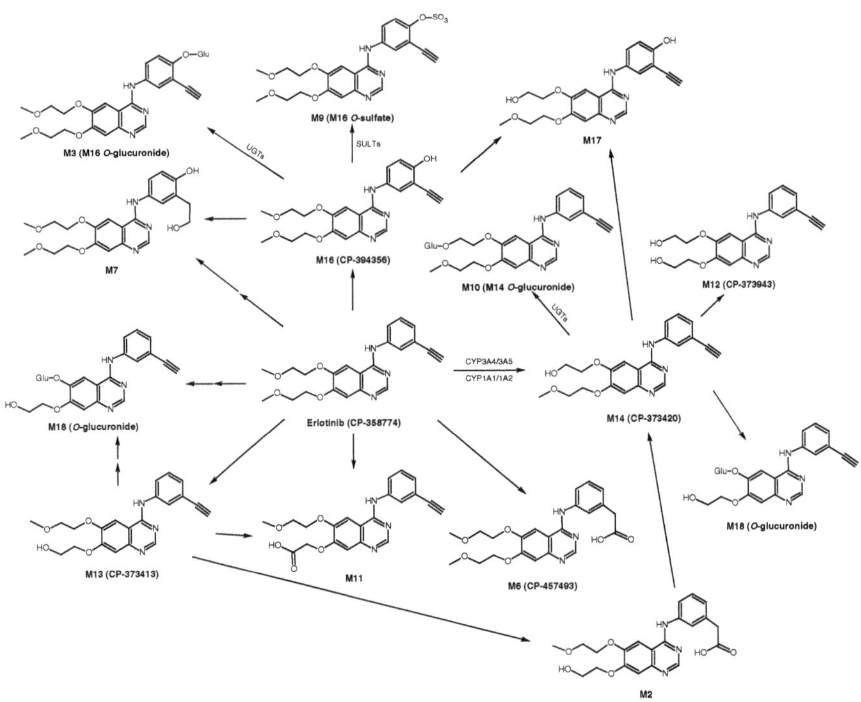

Fig. 12.4 Metabolic scheme of erlotinib in humans. The major metabolic pathways of erlotinib include *O*-demethylation of the side chains followed by oxidation to M11; oxidation of the acetylene moiety to M6; hydroxylation of M16; *O*-demethylation of M6 to M2; and *O*-demethylation of the side chains to M13 and M14. The oxidative metabolites of erlotinib underwent further conjugation with glucuronic acid and sulfuric acid. Erlotinib was metabolized to M14 primarily by CYP3A4, 3A5, and 1A1

O-demethylation of M6 to M2 (4.9%); and *O*-demethylation of the side chains to M13 and M14 (together 4.9%) (Fig. 12.4) (Ling et al. 2006). The oxidative metabolites of erlotinib underwent further conjugation with glucuronic acid (M3, M8, and M18) and sulfuric acid (M9) excreted into the feces and to a minor extent into the urine (Fig. 12.4).

The metabolism of erlotinib was mediated predominantly by hepatic CYP3A4 and 3A5, and, to a lesser extent, by CYP1A2 and 2C8, as well as by the pulmonary CYP1A1, and by CYP1B1 expressed in tumour tissue (Ling et al. 2006). Studies using recombinant enzymes have found that erlotinib was metabolized to M14 primarily by CYP3A4, 3A5, and 1A1, with a contribution from CYP1A2 (Li et al. 2007). A computer-based simulation model, SimCYP, predicted that CYP3A4 contributed to approximately 70% of the metabolic elimination of erlotinib, with CYP1A2 being responsible for the other ~30% (Rakhit et al. 2008).

Consistently, ketoconazole caused a ~2-fold increase in the AUC and maximum plasma concentration of erlotinib in healthy subjects (Rakhit et al. 2008). When gefitinib was coadministered with ciprofloxacin, an inhibitor of both CYP3A4 and 1A2 (Fuhr et al. 1992; Granfors et al. 2004), the erlotinib AUC and C_{max} increased by 39 and 17%, respectively. On the other hand, pre-treatment with the CYP3A4 inducer rifampicin for 7 days decreased erlotinib AUC by about 2/3–4/5 in patients with non-small cell lung cancer (Cohen et al. 2005a). In a separate study, treatment with rifampicin for 11 days decreased erlotinib AUC by 42.4%. Cigarette smoking has been shown to reduce erlotinib AUC and patients should be advised to stop smoking. There is a case in which a potential drug interaction resulted in increased phenytoin levels after initiation of erlotinib therapy in a patient on phenytoin therapy (Grenader et al. 2007). It appears erlotinib inhibits CYP2C9 which metabolizes phenytoin. Erlotinib is an inducer of CYP3A4 through activation of the nuclear receptor pregnane X receptor (Harmsen et al. 2009). Pretreatment of gefitinib decreased the AUC of midazolam (a CYP3A4 substrate) by 24%.

Drugs that alter the pH of the upper gastrointestinal tract may alter the solubility of erlotinib and decrease its bioavailability. Coadministration of erlotinib with omeprazole (a proton pump inhibitor) decreased the erlotinib AUC by 46% (Johnson et al. 2005). Increasing the dose of gefitinib when coadministered with such agents is not likely to compensate for the loss of drug exposure, since proton pump inhibitors increase pH of the upper gastrointestinal tract for an extended period. In this regard, the concomitant use of proton pump inhibitors or histamine 2 receptor blockers (e.g. ranitidine and cimetidine) with gefitinib should be avoided. The use of antacids may be considered in place of histamine 2 receptor blockers or proton pump inhibitors in patients receiving gefitinib (Johnson et al. 2005). However, there is no clinical study that has evaluated the effect of antacids on the pharmacokinetics of erlotinib. If an antacid is necessary, both drugs should be separated taken by at least several hours.

Due to the substantial role of CYP3A4 in the metabolic clearance of erlotinib, herbal and dietary supplements that modulate this enzyme may cause interactions with erlotinib. Administration of BAS 100, a novel mechanism-based CYP3A4 inhibitor isolated from grapefruit juice, resulted in a 2.1-fold increase in erlotinib systemic exposure following oral administration to wild-type and humanised CYP3A4 transgenic mice (Smith et al. 2008). This study demonstrates that grapefruit juice may increase the low and variable oral bioavailability of erlotinib in cancer patients. On the other hand, it can be expected that St John's wort would reduce its oral bioavailability and thus combined use of this antidepressant with erlotinib should be avoided.

12.2.5 Gefitinib + Dietary/Herbal Supplements

Gefitinib (Iressa; ZD1839) is an orally active inhibitor of the EGFR tyrosine kinase implicated in the proliferation, metastasis, angiogenesis and apoptosis inhibition of cancer cells (Albanell et al. 2001; Wakeling 2005). This drug is indicated as second- and third-line monotherapy for the treatment of patients with locally advanced or metastatic non-small cell lung cancer after failure of both platinum-based and docetaxel chemotherapies (Herbst and Kies 2003; Tanovic and Alfaro 2004). Several clinical studies have demonstrated that gefitinib as monotherapy resulted in clinically significant symptom relief, tumour response and was well tolerated (Albanell et al. 2002; Cappuzzo et al. 2003; Kris et al. 2003).

Gefitinib is absorbed slowly after oral administration with mean bioavailability of 60%, with an elimination half-life of about 48 h (Swaisland et al. 2005b). Elimination is eliminated by metabolism and excretion in feces (86% of a dose). Daily oral administration of gefitinib to cancer patients resulted in a 2-fold accumulation compared to single dose administration. Three sites of biotransformation have been identified in experimental animals and patients: metabolism (mainly dealkylation) of the *N*-propoxymorpholino-group (to yield M537194 and M608239), demethylation of the methoxy-substituent on the quinazoline (to form M523595), and oxidative defluorination of the halogenated phenyl group (to form M387783) (Fig. 12.5) (McKillop et al. 2004a, c). Morpholine ring oxidation was the predominant pathway in rats (McKillop et al. 2004c) and this pathway (yielding M608236 and M537194), together with *O*-demethylation of the quinazoline methoxy group (leading to M523595 formation), were the main metabolic routes of gefitinib in dogs and humans (McKillop et al. 2004a, c). Five metabolites were identified in human plasma with *O*-desmethylgefitinib (M523595) being the predominant metabolite which had plasma levels comparable to those of gefitinib (McKillop et al. 2004a). Although this metabolite showed similar EGFR tyrosine kinase activity to gefitinib in the isolated enzyme assay, it had only 1/14 of the potency of gefitinib and minimal antitumour activity (McKillop et al. 2006) (Fig. 12.5).

When gefitinib was incubated with human liver microsomes, at least 16 metabolites have been identified, and the metabolism of gefitinib involved three regions of the molecule like in vivo (McKillop et al. 2004b). The major pathway was morpholine ring-opening and step-wise removal of the morpholine ring and propoxy side chain. Metabolite I (M537194) was probably generated by *N*-dealkylation of metabolite N at the morpholine nitrogen and metabolite J by further *N*-dealkylation of metabolite I at the same site. Metabolite P could result from metabolite J by *O*-dealkylation of the propoxy side chain, although it could be yielded directly

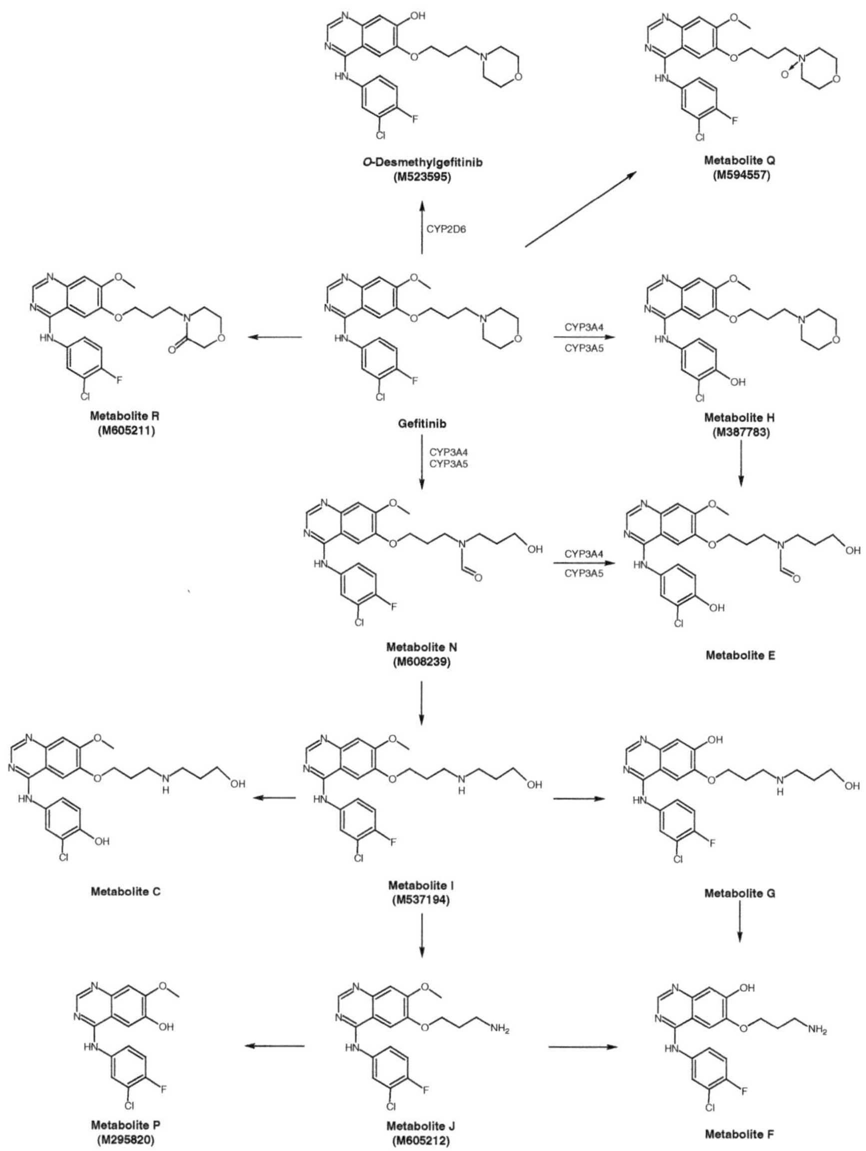

Fig. 12.5 Metabolic scheme of gefitinib in humans. The major metabolic routes of gefitinib include dealkylation of the *N*-propoxymorpholino-group, demethylation of the methoxy-substituent on the quinazoline, and oxidative defluorination of the halogenated phenyl group. CYP2D6 catalyzed rapid and extensive metabolism of gefitinib to M523595, while CYP3A4 and 3A5 catalyzed the formation of most other metabolites

from gefitinib by *O*-dealkylation of the intact morpholine ring propoxy side chain (McKillop et al. 2004b). Metabolite J (M605212) also appeared to be further metabolized to metabolite F by *O*-demethylation of the quinazoline methoxy group, while metabolite H was formed by oxidative defluorination of gefitinib (McKillop et al. 2004b). Metabolite E was probably formed either by *O*-dealkylation of metabolite H, or by oxidative defluorination of metabolite N. Metabolite Q (M594557) was an *N*-oxide of gefitinib, while the minor metabolite R (M605211) was formed by oxidation of the morpholine ring which could be a precursor for subsequent morpholine ring-opening (McKillop et al. 2004b).

When metabolite I (M537194) was incubated with human liver microsomes, at least four metabolites (C, F, G and P) were formed, two of which (metabolites F and P) had been generated during gefitinib metabolism (McKillop et al. 2004b). Metabolite G was yielded by *O*-demethylation of the quinazoline methoxy group of metabolite I (M537194). In addition, metabolite C was formed by oxidative defluorination in a manner similar to that with gefitinib.

Following incubation of M387783 (metabolite H) with human liver microsomes, four metabolites (B, C, D and E) were identified (McKillop et al. 2004b). Metabolite E had also been observed with gefitinib metabolism and metabolite C had been formed from metabolite I (M537194). Metabolite E was further metabolized to the secondary amine, metabolite C, and then to the primary amine, metabolite B by *N*-dealkylation.

Incubation of *O*-desmethylgefitinib (M523595) with human liver microsomes yielded several metabolites, including metabolites G, A, F and K, with metabolite G being the most abundant (McKillop et al. 2004b). M523595 was metabolized by similar routes to those seen with gefitinib, metabolite I (M537194) and metabolite H (M387783). Metabolite K was yielded by *O*-dealkylation of the morpholine ring. Metabolite G and metabolite F were probably formed by sequential *N*-dealkylation of metabolite K, although it was also likely that these products were formed by alternative pathways. Furthermore, M523595 underwent oxidative defluorination to form metabolite A, in a manner analogous to gefitinib and M537194 (McKillop et al. 2004b).

McKillop et al. (2005) further investigated the CYPs involved in the metabolism of gefitinib. The formation of most metabolites was significantly decreased by ketoconazole (a potent CYP3A4 inhibitor), but the formation of M523595 was inhibited by quinidine only which is a selective inhibitor of CYP2D6. In vitro, gefitinib was metabolized extensively by recombinant CYP3A4, yielding a similar metabolite profile to human liver microsomes, but M523595 was not generated. CYP1A2, 2C9 and 2C19 produced no measurable metabolism of gefitinib, while CYP3A5 produced a metabolite profile similar to CYP3A4, but to a much lower degree. In contrast, CYP2D6 catalysed rapid and extensive metabolism of gefitinib to M523595. Another study by Li et al. (2007) also found that CYP3A4, 3A5, 1A1 and 2D6 were involved in the metabolism of gefitinib. While M523595 formation was catalyzed by CYP2D6, the overall metabolism of gefitinib was primarily by CYP3A4, and this was not obviously diminished in liver microsomes from CYP2D6 poor metabolizers.

Rifampicin, an inducer of CYP3A4, decreased the plasma AUC of gefitinib by 85% in healthy volunteers (Swaisland et al. 2005a). Concomitant administration of itraconazole (200 mg daily for 12 days), an inhibitor of CYP3A4, with gefitinib (250 mg single dose) to healthy volunteers, increased gefitinib AUC by 88% (Swaisland et al. 2005a). Co-administration of high doses of ranitidine with sodium bicarbonate (to maintain the gastric pH above pH 5.0) reduced gefitinib AUC by 44% (Cohen et al. 2003). On the other hand, coadministration of metoprolol with gefitinib resulted in a 35% increase in the AUC of metoprolol which is a substrate of CYP2D6 (Johnson and Burlew 1996; Goryachkina et al. 2008; Rau et al. 2009), and this change was not statistically significant. These findings indicate that gefitinib is predominantly metabolized by CYP3A4 in vivo and it is a weak inhibitor of CYP2D6.

There are no clinical reports on the interactions of gefitinib with St John's wort or grapefruit juice although CYP3A4 is a major contributor to the metabolism of this drug. It can be expected that St John's wort would decrease the AUC of gefitinib while grapefruit juice could increase the AUC of gefitinib.

12.2.6 Docetaxel + *Allium sativum* (Garlic)

Docetaxel (Taxotere; RP 56976), a semisynthetic taxoid, is an antimitotic agent that acts by disrupting the microtubular network in cells that is essential for mitotic and interphase cellular functions (Cortes and Pazdur 1995; Fulton and Spencer 1996). It is approved for the management of early and advanced breast cancer, locally advanced and metastatic lung cancer and hormone refractory prostate cancer (Crown 2001; Beer et al. 2003; Blagden and Kaye 2005; Lyseng-Williamson and Fenton 2005; Ramaswamy and Puhalla 2006; Saloustros et al. 2008). Docetaxel has recently been approved for the treatment of advanced gastric cancer. The pharmacokinetics and metabolism of docetaxel have been investigated after intravenous infusion in mice, dogs and cancer patients (Bruno and Sanderink 1993). Multiphasic disposition profiles have been observed with rapid initial tissue uptake and large distribution volumes. Hepatobiliary extraction is the major route of elimination, with similar metabolic pathways in all the species.

In human liver microsomes, at least four metabolites are formed from successive oxidations of the *tert*-butyl group on the synthetic side chain (Marre et al. 1996). The major metabolite (VI) corresponded to the alcohol. Metabolites V and VII are two oxazolidine-type compounds, resulting from cyclization of an unstable inter mediate aldehyde. Metabolite IV corresponds to the carboxylic acid. Following cyclization, this compound may result in an oxazolidinedione derivative, the major docetaxel metabolite observed in human feces (Bruno and Sanderink 1993). Further in vitro studies have indicated that docetaxel is extensively metabolized by CYP3A4 and 3A5 to form metabolite VI (Marre et al. 1996). CYP2C8 is also involved in its metabolism, but the metabolites are unidentified. The metabolism of docetaxel can be inhibited by CYP3A4 inhibitors, such as ketoconazole, erythromycin, troleandomycin and nifedipine (Marre et al. 1996), and CYP3A4/5 inhibition by ketoconazole increased fecal parent drug excretion 2-fold in cancer patients (Engels et al. 2007). Docetaxol is a substrate of P-gp (Shirakawa et al. 1999; van Zuylen et al. 2000), MRP2 (Huisman et al. 2005), MRP7 (Chen et al. 2003a; Hopper-Borge et al. 2004) and OATP1B3 (Smith et al. 2005).

Cox et al. (2006) investigated the effect of garlic supplementation containing 3,600 μg allicin per tablet on the pharmacokinetics of docetaxel (a CYP3A4 substrate) in women with metastatic breast cancer treated with docetaxel 30 mg/m^2 given weekly for 3 of 4 weeks. Three days after the initial dose of docetaxel, patients took 600 mg of garlic twice daily for 12 days. In 10 evaluable patients, the mean baseline clearance of docetaxel was 30.8 L/h/m^2. Coadministration of garlic reduced mean clearance of docetaxel to 23.7 L/h/m^2 and 20.0 L/h/m^2 on days 8 and 15, respectively, but the difference did not achieve statistical significance (Cox et al. 2006). Peak concentration, AUC, volume of distribution, and elimination half-life, were also not statistically significantly different. However, the mean AUC ratio between day 15 and day 1 was 3.74 in three individuals with the *CYP3A5*1A/*1A* genotype compared with 1.02 in six individuals carrying the *CYP3A5*3C/*3C* genotype. It appears that garlic decreases the clearance of docetaxel in patients carrying a *CYP3A5*1A* allele.

Garlic, a widely used medicinal herb, is reported to have antimicrobial and immune-enhancing effects (Harris et al. 2001; Kyo et al. 2001). It is one of the herbal supplements most commonly used by HIV-infected patients to improve health and to treat some opportunistic infections (Standish et al. 2001). Garlic contains high-level sulfur-containing compounds (e.g. allicin and alliin, see Fig. 12.6), numerous uercetin/isoflavinoids (such as nobiletin, uercetin, rutin and tangeretin), polysaccharides, prostaglandins, saponins and terpenes (such as citral, geraniol, linalool,

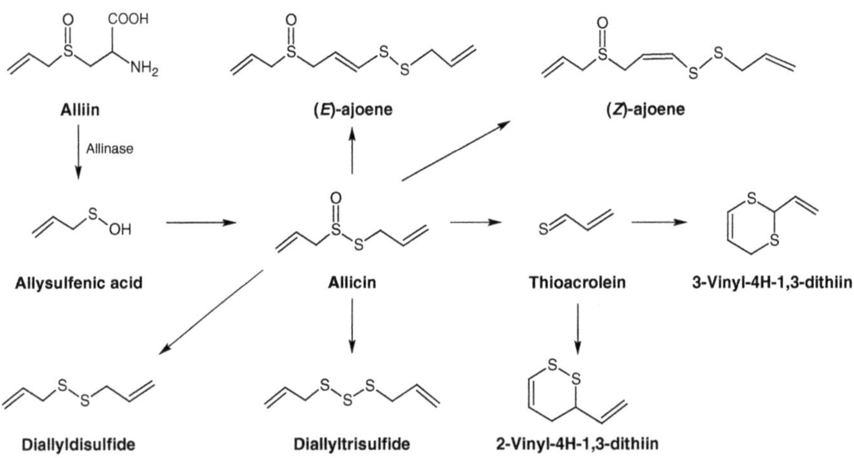

Fig. 12.6 Metabolic scheme of alliin. When crushed, *Allium sativum* yields allicin by the enzyme allinase. Allicin will break down to result in diallyl disulphide, diallyl trisulphide and thioacrolein. Allicin can be converted to ajoene

and α- and β-phellandrene) (Dausch and Nixon 1990; Singh et al. 2001). Allicin is not present in garlic unless tissue damage occurs, and is formed by the action of the enzyme alliinase on alliin. Allicin can in turn produce other sulfur compounds, including ajoene, allyl sulfides and vinyldithiins. Garlic has been shown to potentially modulate the activity of various CYPs, both in vitro and in vivo. The extracts from fresh and aged garlic inhibited CYP3A4 in human liver microsomes (Foster et al. 2001) (Fig. 12.6).

12.2.7 Etoposide + Grapefruit Juice

Etoposide (VP-16; VePesid), a semisynthetic derivative of podophyllotoxin, is used in combination with other approved chemotherapeutic agents as first-line treatment in patients with small cell lung cancer (Hande 1998). This drug induces DNA strand breaks by an interaction with DNA topoisomerase II or the formation of free radicals (Clark and Slevin 1987; Hande 1998). The elimination half-live of etoposide ranged between 5 and 10 h; the urinary excretion of unchanged etoposide ranged from 30 to 40% of the intravenous dose; and several metabolites were identified in plasma and urine such as *cis*-(picro) lactone, hydroxy acid derivatives, 4'-*O*-glucuronide of etoposide or agrycon, 3'-demethyletoposide (Clark and Slevin 1987). Biliary excretion of unchanged drug and/or metabolites is an important route of etoposide elimination as fecal recovery of radioactivity is 44% of the intravenous dose. The hydroxy acid metabolite, formed by opening of the lactone ring, is observed in the urine of adult and pediatric patients (Clark and Slevin 1987). It is also present in human plasma, presumably as the *trans* isomer. Glucuronide and/or sulfate conjugates of etoposide are also excreted in human urine. Only 8% or less of an intravenous dose is excreted in the urine as radiolabeled metabolites of ^{14}C-etoposide (Clark and Slevin 1987). In addition, *O*-demethylation (3'-demethylation) of the dimethoxyphenol ring was mainly catalyzed by CYP3A4 with minor contribution from CYP1A2 and 2E1 to form the corresponding catechol (3-OH-etoposide) (Relling et al. 1994; Kawashiro et al. 1998). The oral bioavailability of etoposide is approximately 50% (range: 25–75%). The bioavailability of etoposide capsules appears to be linear up to a dose of at least 250 mg/m^2.

The systemic exposure to etoposide is significantly affected by cyclosporine, a CYP3A4 substrate and inhibitor, in cancer patients. Coadministed cyclosporine gave a 38% decrease in renal and a 52% decrease in nonrenal clearance of etoposide. The AUC of etoposide was increased by 80% with a 38% decrease in total body clearance of etoposide by cyclosporine (Lum et al. 1992). In pediatric patients, cyclosporine almost doubled the clearance of etoposide (Bisogno et al. 1998) and thus dose reduction is needed. Ifosfamide coadministration increased the clearance by 28% ($P < 0.0005$) and reduced the AUC of etoposide by 23% in patients with small cell lung cancer (You et al. 2008). However, tamoxifen did not alter the pharmacokinetics of etoposide in patients with hepatocellular carcinoma (Corona et al. 1999). Cisplatin or carboplatin only had a minor effect on the pharmacokinetics of etoposide in cancer patients (Thomas et al. 2002).

Etoposide was mainly excreted as hydroxyl acid derivatives and glucuronides in humans after oral administration (Clark and Slevin 1987). Etoposide glucuronides accounted for the disposition of 15–35% of administered etoposide dose (Arbuck et al. 1986; D'Incalci et al. 1986). UGT1A1 was the enzyme for the alcoholic glucuronidation of etoposide (Watanabe et al. 2003; Wen et al. 2007). In human liver microsomes, one phenolic and two alcoholic glucuronides have been observed, with the predominant form of etoposide glucuronide being the phenolic glucuronide (Fig. 12.7) (Wen et al. 2007). In vitro studies using recombinant human UGTs demonstrated that etoposide glucuronidation was mainly catalyzed by UGT1A1 (Wen et al. 2007). UGT1A8 and 1A3 also catalyzed the glucuronidation of etoposide, but the activities were approximately 10 and 1% of UGT1A1 (Wen et al. 2007) (Fig. 12.7).

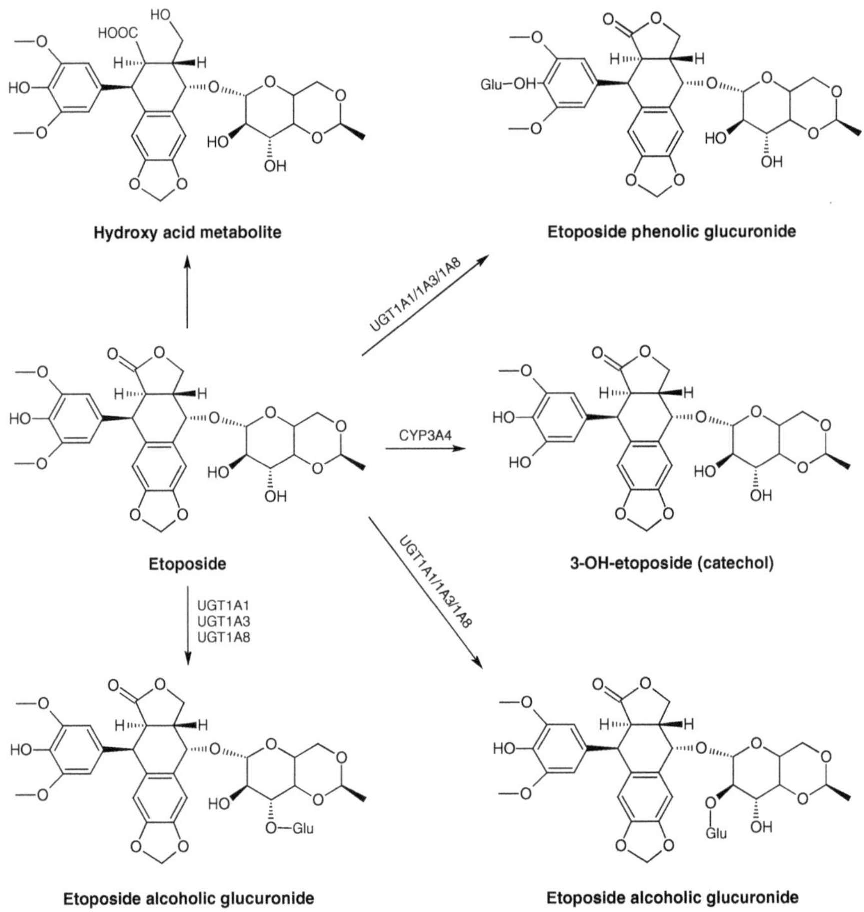

Fig. 12.7 Metabolism of etoposide. *O*-demethylation of the dimethoxyphenol ring of etoposide was mainly catalyzed by CYP3A4 with minor contribution from CYP1A2 and 2E1. In human liver microsomes, one phenolic and two alcoholic glucuronides have been observed, which was mainly formed by UGT1A1, with minor contributions from UGT1A8 and 1A3

In a randomized crossover study, six cancer patients were sequentially treated with 50 mg *i.v.* etoposide over 1 h, 50 mg orally, or 50 mg orally post grapefruit juice on day 1, day 4, and day 8 (Reif et al. 2002). Pretreatment with grapefruit juice resulted in an unexpected decrease of 26.2% in the AUC after oral treatment. Median absolute bioavailability with and without pretreatment with grapefruit juice was 52.4 and 73.2%, respectively (Reif et al. 2002). Grapefruit juice seems to reduce rather than increase oral bioavailability of etoposide.

The mechanisms for the above findings are unknown. Grapefruit juice has been found to significantly increase oral bioavailability of most dihydropyridines (e.g. felodipine), terfenadine, saquinavir, nicotine, cyclosporine, midazolam, triazolam and verapamil (Ducharme et al. 1995; Yee et al. 1995; He et al. 1998; Bailey et al. 1998, 1991, 2000; Kane and Lipsky 2000; Mohri and Uesawa 2001; Bressler 2006; Hukkanen et al. 2006). The plasma concentrations or AUC of lovastatin, cisapride and astemizole can also be markedly increased by grapefruit juice (Bailey et al. 1998, 2000). As the duration of effect of grapefruit juice can last 24 h, repeated consumption of grapefruit juice can lead to a cumulative increase in the AUC and C_{max} of coadministered drugs. The inhibition of CYP3A4 activity with no change of *CYP3A4* mRNA and P-gp is believed to be the primary mechanism (Bailey et al. 1998; Kane and Lipsky 2000). Similar to etoposide, the pharmacokinetics of many other drugs were not altered by grapefruit juice. For example, grapefruit juice did not alter the bioavailability of digoxin, diltiazem and amlodipine in human volunteers, and indinavir in HIV-positive patients (Sigusch et al. 1994; Vincent et al. 2000; Becquemont et al. 2001). Although these drugs undergo extensive presystemic metabolism, CYP3A4 is a minor contributor. It appears that somehow the grapefruit juice might induce the metabolism of etoposide or alter the biliary excretion of etoposide and its metabolites.

Bergamottin is a major furanocoumarin in grapefruit juice (Manthey and Buslig 2005). It has been demonstrated to be, in part, responsible for the increased bioavailability of certain drugs in what has become known as the grapefruit juice effect (Bailey et al. 2000). This compound reversibly inhibited the activities of CYP1A2, 2A6, 2C9, 2C19, 2D6, 2E1 and 3A4 in human liver microsomes (He et al. 1998; Baumgart et al. 2005). Bergamottin also inactivated CYP3A4 following metabolic activation in a time- and concentration-dependent manner (He et al. 1998; Lim et al. 2005). Its hydroxylated product, 6',7'-dihydroxy bergamottin, is also a mechanism-based inhibitor of CYP3A4 (He et al. 1998; Lim et al. 2005). Bergamottin also inactivated CYP3A5 and 2B6 (Bumpus et al. 2005; Lin et al. 2005). The ability of bergamottin and 6',7'-dihydroxy bergamottin to inactivate CYP3A4 and other CYPs is thought to be the major reason for the grapefruit juice-induced drug interactions that have been observed clinically (Bailey et al. 2000; Kakar et al. 2004; Bressler 2006). The loss of catalytic activity exhibited pseudo-first-order kinetics. During bergamottin-induced inactivation, CYP3A4 retained more than 90% of the heme, but 50% of the apoprotein in the inactivated CYP3A4 could not be recovered. This suggests that the inactivation may involve apoprotein modification in the active site of the enzyme instead of heme adduct formation or heme fragmentation (He et al. 1998). In addition, 6',7'-epoxy-bergamottin, a stable epoxide found in grapefruit peel, was shown to inhibit the activity of CYP3A4 (Wangensteen et al. 2003).

12.3 Do Chinese Herbal Medicines Reduce Chemotherapy-Induced Organ Toxicities?

In clinical practice, a number of standard supportive therapies such as growth factors and symptom-alleviating therapies (e.g. analgesics and anti-diarrhea agents) are available in cancer chemotherapy to protect the bone marrow and gastrointestinal tracts and alleviate organ-toxicity associated symptoms. However, several studies have found that a substantial number of cancer patients also use Chinese herbal medicines (CHM) in combination with anticancer drugs in an attempt to reduce drug toxicities and to consolidate the immune system (Block et al. 2004).

12.3.1 TJ-14

A randomized study in 44 previously untreated patients with advanced non-small-cell lung cancer revealed that oral TJ-14 (major component: *Scutellaria baicalensis* (baikal skullcap root) extract, 7.5 g/day) administration ameliorated irinotecan-induced diarrhea severity and reduced frequency of diarrhea grades 3 and 4 as well (Mori et al. 2003). Similarly, treatment of rats with baicalin (25 mg/kg orally twice daily) or Kampo medicines (TJ-14 and TJ-114; 125–1,000 mg/kg orally twice daily) from the day before to 4 or 10 days after the start of irinotecan administration resulted in significantly decreased diarrhea and histological injuries and accelerated healing of the intestinal tract (Takasuna et al. 1995; Kase et al. 1997a).

The mechanism for this may be multi-factorial. The rat study indicated TJ-14 suppressed significantly increased colonic prostaglandin E_2 by irinotecan which is closely related to the onset of diarrhea (Kase et al. 1997b). Baicalin is a β-glucuronidase inhibitor, and may reduce the deconjugation of SN-38 glucuronide to toxic SN-38 in the intestine (Narita et al. 1993). TJ-14 also increased colonic water absorption impaired by repeated dosing of irinotecan in rats (Kase et al. 1997b). In addition, baicalein, the major component in TJ-14, may modulate P-gp function and thus alter the disposition of CPT-11 and SN-38. Evidence has indicated that the biliary excretion of both irinotecan and SN-38 depend on the presence of drug-transporting proteins, notably P-gp and canalicular multispecific organic anion transporter that are present on the bile canalicular membrane (Chu et al. 1997a, 1998; Sugiyama et al. 1998).

12.3.2 Chinese Herbal Medicines

A recent double-blind, placebo-controlled and randomized clinical trial was conducted by Mok et al. (2007) to investigate the efficacy of toxicity reduction of CHM in 120 patients with early-stage resected breast or colon cancer. These patients were treated with adjuvant chemotherapy in combination with an herbal formula consisting of multiple CHMs for 14 days or with a placebo. The incidence of grade 3/4 anemia, leucopoenia, neutropenia, and thrombocytopenia in patients treated with CHM for 14 days is not significantly different from that in patients receiving placebo only (5.4%, 47.3%, 52.7% and 1.8% vs 1.8%, 32.2%, 44.7%, and 3.6%, respectively). However, the incidence of nausea is significantly decreased in the CHM-treated group compared to the control group (14.6% vs 35.7%). There were no significant differences in other non-hematologic toxicities between the CHM and placebo groups. The change in the score for each domain in the European Organization for Research and Treatment of Cancer (EORTC) QLQC30 between each cycle of chemotherapy and baseline was compared and there was no significant difference between the CHM and placebo groups.

The findings from the above study indicate that CHM does not alleviate chemotherapy-induced hematological toxicity, but significantly reduces cytotoxic drug-induced nausea. The results are encouraging and suggest that CHM may play a role in the management of chemotherapy-induced toxicities. However, the current study has several intrinsic limitations, which compromise its scientific significance. For example, the authors did not conduct well-designed stratification analysis and the placebo used in this study contains medicinal tea (e.g. *Camellia amellia*), so the conclusion appears unconvincing. A stratification analysis will check for the effects of other potential covariables such as age, gender, performance status, and tumour type and chemotherapy regimen on toxicity profiles. In particular, the choice of a placebo containing medicinal herbal components is unacceptable. In addition, the herbal treatment regimen was 14 days starting from day 1, which was optimized. The study did not measure any biomarkers indicating the active components in the herbal formal probably responsible for its efficacy.

12.4 Mechanistic Considerations

12.4.1 Modulation of Phase I and II Enzyme Expression and Activity

Metabolism has been regarded as one of the most important and complex processes in the body, leading to the excretion of most drugs, including anticancer drugs (Lin and Lu 1997). Most anticancer drugs undergo Phase I and/or II metabolism, yielding inactive or active metabolites (Tables 12.1 and 12.2) (Rooseboom et al. 2004). Phase I reactions are mainly oxidative or reductive reactions catalyzed by CYPs, flavin-containing monooxygenases, epoxide hydrolase, carboxylesterase and amidase, peroxidase, alcohol/aldehyde dehydrogenease, monoamine oxidase, or α-nicotinamide adenine dinucleotide phosphate (NADPH) quinone reductase. Phase I reactions usually make a drug more susceptible to Phase II reactions which are conjugative reactions, such as glucuronidation catalyzed by various UGTs, generally producing molecules more amenable to biliary or renal excretion. As such, the disposition and clearance of anticancer drugs may be altered when the enzymes that metabolize them are modulated by coadministered drugs or herbal medicines (Tables 12.1 and 12.2).

Table 12.1 Human CYP enzymes that metabolize anticancer drugs

Drugs	Mechanism of action	CYPs involved	References
5,6-Dimethylxanthenone 4-acetic acid	Antiangiogenic agent and cytokine inducer	CYP1A2	Zhou et al. (2000)
Aminoflavone (NSC686288, Phase I)	Inducer of DNA single-strand breaks	CYP1A2, 1A1, 2C9, 2C19, 2D6, and 3A4	Kuffel et al. (2002); Chen et al. (2006)
Bortezomib	26S proteasome inhibitor	CYP3A4, 2C19, 1A2, 2D6, and 2C9	Pekol et al. (2005); Uttamsingh et al. (2005)
Cyclophosphamide	Alkylating agent	CYP2A6, 2B6, 2C8, 2C9, 3A4, 3A5, and 3A7	Zhang et al. 2005a, b; 2006a)
Dacarbazine	DNA-interacting agent	CYP1A1, 1A2, and 2E1	Reid et al. (1999); Long and Dolan (2001)
Docetaxel	Antimicrotubule agent	CYP3A4, and 3A5	Marre et al. (1996); Royer et al. (1996)
Doxorubicin	Anthracycline antibiotic (DNA intercalator)	CYP2D6	Le Guellec et al. (1993)
Ellipticine	DNA intercalator	CYP1A1, 1A2 and 3A4	Aimova et al. (2007); Stiborova et al. (2008)
Erlotinib	Epidermal growth factor receptor tyrosine kinase inhibitor	CYP3A4, 3A5, 1A1, 1A2, 2C8, and 1B1	Li et al. (2007); Ling et al. (2006)
Etoposide	Topoisomerase II inhibitor	CYP3A4, 3A5, 1A2, and 2E1	Relling et al. (1994); Kawashiro et al. (1998); Zhuo et al. (2004); Zheng et al. (2006)
Gefitinib	Epidermal growth factor receptor kinase inhibitor	CYP3A4, 3A5, 1A1, and 2D6	McKillop et al. (2005); Li et al. (2007)
Ifosfamide	Alkylating agent	CYP2A6, 2B6, 2C8, 2C9, 3A4, and 3A5	Granvil et al. (1999); Roy et al. (1999)
Imatinib	Bcr-Abl and c-kit tyrosine kinase inhibitor	CYP3A4, 3A5, 1A2, 2D6, and 2C9	van Erp et al. (2007)
Indisulam	Carbonic anhydrase inhibitor	CYP2C9, and 2C19	Zandvliet et al. (2007)

Table 12.1 (continued)

Drugs	Mechanism of action	CYPs involved	References
Irinotecan	Topoisomerase I inhibitor	CYP3A4, and 3A5	Rivory et al. (1996b, 1997), Haaz et al. (1998); Santos et al. (2000)
Laromustine (Cloretazine)	Novel sulfonylhydrazine alkylating agent	CYP2B6, 3A4, and 3A5	Nassar et al. (2009)
Methoxymorpholinyl doxorubicin	Prodrug of doxorubicin	CYP3A4, 3A5, and 3A7	Lu and Waxman (2005)
Mofarotene (Ro 40-8757)	Arotinoid	CYP3A4 and 1A2	Valles et al. (1995)
Nemorubicin	DNA intercalator	CYP3A4	Quintieri et al. (2005)
Paclitaxel	Antimicrotubule agent	CYP2C8 and 3A4	Desai et al. (1998)
Sorafenib	Multikinase inhibitor	CYP3A4	Keating and Santoro (2009)
Tamoxifen	Selective estrogen receptor modulator	CYP2D6, 3A4, 2B6, 2C9, 1A1, 1B1, 2C19, and 3A5	Jacolot et al. (1991); Dehal and Kupfer (1997); Crewe et al. (2002); Stearns et al. (2003); Beverage et al. (2007)
Tegafur	Antimetabolite (prodrug of 5-fluorouracil)	CYP2A6, 1A2, and 2C8	Ikeda et al. (2000); Komatsu et al. (2000)
Teniposide	Topoisomerase II inhibitor	CYP3A4 and 2C19	Relling et al. (1994)
TG100855	Novel Src kinase inhibitor	CYP3A4	Kousba et al. (2007)
Thalidomide	Antiangiogenic and immunomodulating agent	CYP2C9, 2C19, 1A1, and 1A2	Miyata et al. (2003)
Tipifarnib	Farnesyltransferase inhibitor	CYP3A4 and 3A5	Sparreboom et al. (2004b)
Trabectedin	DNA-binding agent	CYP3A4, 3A5, 2C8, 2C9, 2D6, 2E1, and 1A2	Reid et al. (2002); Brandon et al. (2006); Vermeir et al. (2009)
TSU-68	Novel inhibitor of angiogenic receptor tyrosine kinases	CYP1A1, 1A2, 2C8, 2D6, and 3A4	Kitamura et al. (2008)
Valspodar (PSC 833)	MDR reversing agent	CYP3A4 and 3A5	Fischer et al. (1998)

Table 12.1 (continued)

Drugs	Mechanism of action	CYPs involved	References
Vinblastine	Antimitotic drug	CYP3A4 and 2D6	Zhou-Pan et al. (1993); Yao et al. (2000)
Vincristine	Antimitotic drug	CYP3A4 and 3A5	Yao et al. (2000); Dennison et al. (2006)
Vindesine	Antimitotic drug	CYP3A4	Zhou et al. (1993)
Vinorelbine (nor-5'-anhydrovinblastine)	Antimitotic agent	CYP3A4	Kajita et al. (2000)

Enzyme induction is considered the major mechanism for the altered plasma levels of SN-38 following irinotecan dosing (Mathijssen et al. 2002) and imatinib (Frye et al. 2004; Smith 2004). Hypericin induces CYP1A2 (Nebel et al. 1999) and hyperforin induces CYP2B6 and 3A4 (Kerb et al. 1996; Moore et al. 2000; Madabushi et al. 2006; Whitten et al. 2006). St John's wort is an inducer of CYP3A4 as indicated by increased urinary 6β-hydroxycortisol/cortisol ratio (Roby et al. 2000) and midazolam clearance in healthy humans (Dresser et al. 2003). Clinical studies using a probe drug cocktail indicated that long-term (2 weeks) administration of St John's wort in humans significantly induced intestinal and hepatic CYP3A4, but did not alter the CYP2C9, 1A2, or 2D6 activities when probe substrates were used (Roby et al. 2000; Wang et al. 2001). The induction of hepatic and intestinal CYP3A4 and other CYPs by St John's wort may partly explain its ability to increase the clearance of a series of coadministered drugs such as indinavir and cyclosporine that are substrates of CYP3A4 (Zhou and Lai 2008).

12.4.2 Modulation of Drug Transporter Expression and Activity

A number of anticancer drugs and their metabolites have been identified as the substrates of P-gp, BCRP, MRP1-MRP9, and/or other transporters (Table 12.3). P-gp/MDR1 is expressed in the apical membrane of many secretory cell types such as kidney, liver, intestine, adrenal gland and the blood-brain barrier where the normal function involves the excretion of drugs and their metabolites (Thiebaut et al. 1987; Dean et al. 2001). Thus, P-gp/MDR1 plays a critical role in drug disposition. Anticancer drugs that are typical substrates of P-gp include actinomycin D, daunorubicin, docetaxel, doxorubicin (adriamycin), docetaxel, etoposide, imatinib, irinotecan, mitomycin C, mitoxantrone, paclitaxel, teniposide, topotecan, vincristine, vinblastine, gimatecan and trabectedin (Jonker et al. 2000; Nakatomi et al. 2001; Chen et al. 2003b; Doyle and Ross 2003; Haimeur et al. 2004; Sarkadi et al. 2004, 2006; Mao and Unadkat 2005; Tian et al. 2006; Wakabayashi et al.

Table 12.2 Human UGTs that conjugate anticancer drugs

Drugs	Mechanism of action	UGTs involved	References
5,6-Dimethylxanthenone 4-acetic acid	Antiangiogenic agent and cytokine inducer	UGT2B7 and 1A2	Miners et al. (1997)
Epirubicin	Anthracycline antibiotic (DNA intercalator)	UGT2B7	Innocenti et al. (2001)
Etoposide	Topoisomerase II inhibitor	UGT1A1, 1A3 and 1A8	Watanabe et al. (2003); Wen et al. (2007)
Flavopiridol (HMR 1275, L86-8275)	Cyclin-dependent kinase inhibitor	UGT1A4 and 1A9	Ramirez et al. (2002); Villeneuve et al. (2003)
Irinotecan (SN-38 as substrate)	Topoisomerase I inhibitor	UGT1A1, 1A7, 1A9 and 1A10	Hanioka et al. (2001); Mathijssen et al. (2001); Oguri et al. (2004); Nagar and Blanchard (2006)
Raloxifene	Selective estrogen receptor modulator	UGT1A10	Jeong et al. (2005)
Seliciclib (*R*-roscovitine)	Cyclin-dependent kinase inhibitor	UGT1A3, 1A9 and 2B7	McClue and Stuart (2008)
Tamoxifen	Selective estrogen receptor modulator	UGT1A4, 1A8, 1A10 and 2B7	Kaku et al. (2004); Ogura et al. (2006); Sun et al. (2006); Sun et al. (2007); Blevins-Primeau et al. (2009)
Tipifarnib	Farnesyltransferase inhibitor	UGT1A1	Sparreboom et al. (2004b)
Topotecan	Topoisomerase I inhibitor	UGTs	Rosing et al. (1998)

2006; Marchetti et al. 2007; Sharom 2008; Noguchi et al. 2009). In addition, mitoxantrone, irinotecan, SN-38, topotecan, 9-aminocamptothecin, daunorubicin, doxorubicin, epirubicin, flavopiridol, MTX and gimatecan, but not *vinca* alkaloids and taxanes, are substrates of BCRP (Jedlitschky et al. 1996; Priebe et al. 1998; Sakamoto et al. 1999) (Table 12.3).

Table 12.3 Anticancer drugs (and their metabolites) as substrates of various drug transporters

Transporter	Symbols	Anticancer drugs as substrates	References
P-gp	ABCB1/MDR1	Actinomycin D, daunorubicin, docetaxel, doxorubicin (adriamycin), docetaxel, etoposide, imatinib, irinotecan, mitomycin C, mitoxantrone, paclitaxel, teniposide, topotecan, vincristine, vinblastine, gimatecan, imatinib & trabectedin	Wils et al. (1994); Alvarez et al. (1995); Seelig and Landwojtowicz (2000); Ambudkar et al. (2003); Hamada et al. (2003); Marzolini et al. (2004); Beumer et al. (2007); Marchetti et al. (2007); Zhou et al. (2007a), (Zhou 2008), Hu et al. (2008); Aller et al. (2009)
BCRP	ABCG2/MXR	Mitoxantrone, irinotecan, SN-38, topotecan, 9-aminocamptothecin, daunorubicin, doxorubicin, epirubicin, flavopiridol, MTX, imatinib & gimatecan (*vinca* alkaloids and taxanes are not substrates)	Jonker et al. (2000); Nakatomi et al. (2001); Chen et al. (2003b); Doyle and Ross (2003); Haimeur et al. (2004); Sarkadi et al. (2004); Mao and Unadkat (2005); Nakanishi et al. (2006); Sarkadi et al. (2006); Tian et al. (2006); Wakabayashi et al. (2006); Marchetti et al. (2007); Hu et al. (2008); Sharom (2008); Noguchi et al. (2009)
MRP1	ABCC1	Doxorubicin, vincristine, etoposide, MTX, camptothecin, CPT-11, SN-38, cyclophosphamide, thiotepa GSH conjugate, cyclophosphamide GSH conjugate, chlorambucil GSH conjugate, melphalan GSH conjugate, flutamide and hydroxyflutamide	Zaman et al. 1993; 1994), Cole et al. (1994); Slapak et al. (1994); Jedlitschky et al. (1996); Priebe et al. (1998); Morrow et al. 1998; 2006), Sakamoto et al. (1999); Hooijberg et al. (2003)

Table 12.3 (continued)

Transporter	Symbols	Anticancer drugs as substrates	References
MRP2	ABCC2	Cisplatin, etoposide, *vinca* alkaloids, anthracyclines and camptothecins (irinotecan, SN-38), MTX, 7-OH-MTX and matecan	Koike et al. (1997); Cui et al. (1999); Hooijberg et al. (1999); Marchetti et al. (2007); Vlaming et al. (2008)
MRP3	ABCC3	Etoposide, teniposide, vincristine, MTX and 7-OH-MTX (but doxorubicin and paclitaxel are not substrates)	Kool et al. (1999); Zeng et al. (1999); Vlaming et al. (2008); Zehnpfennig et al. (2009)
MRP4	ABCC4	MTX, 6-thioguanine, 6-mercaptopurine, topotecan, SN-38, irinotecan, imatinib and leucovorin (but vincristine, etoposide and daunorubicin are not substrates)	Kool et al. (1999); Chen et al. 2001; 2002), Lee et al. (2000); Leggas et al. (2004); Tian et al. (2005); Hu et al. (2008)
MRP5	ABCC5	6-Mercaptopurine and 6-thioguanine (but vincristine, etoposide, MTX and daunorubicin are not substrates)	McAleer et al. (1999); Wijnholds et al. (2000)
MRP6	ABCC6	Etoposide, teniposide, doxorubicin, cisplatin, daunorubicin and dactinomycin (but vincristine and vinblastine are not substrates)	Belinsky et al. (2002)
MRP7	ABCC10	Docetaxel, paclitaxel, vincristine and vinblastine (but MTX is not a substrate)	Chen et al. (2003a); Hopper-Borge et al. (2004)
MRP8	ABCC11	5-FU, MTX and 6-thioguanine	Guo et al. (2003)
MRP9	ABCC12	Does not transport the typical substrates such as drug conjugates and other organic anions transported by other MRP members	Ono et al. (2007)
OAT-1	SLC22A6/PAHT/NKT	MTX	Takeda et al. (2002); Nozaki et al. (2007)
OAT-2	SLC22A7/NLT	MTX	Burckhardt and Burckhardt (2003)
OAT-3	SLC22A8	MTX, topotecan	Cha et al. (2001); Takeda et al. (2002)
OAT-4	SLC22A11	MTX	Takeda et al. (2002)

Table 12.3 (continued)

Transporter	Symbols	Anticancer drugs as substrates	References
OATP1A2	SLCO1A2/ OATP-A/OATP1	Imatinib and MTX	Badagnani et al. (2006); Hu et al. (2008)
OATP1B1	SLCO1B1/ OATP-C	SN-38 and MTX (but CPT-11, paclitaxel and deocetaxel are not substrates)	Nozawa et al. (2005); Smith et al. (2005); Konig et al. (2006); van de Steeg et al. (2009)
OATP1B3	SLCO1B3/ OATP-8	Paclitaxel and docetaxel (but SN-38 is not a substrate)	Nozawa et al. (2005); Smith et al. (2005)
OATP2B1	SLCO2B1/ OATP-B	SN-38 is not a substrate	Nozawa et al. 2004; 2005)
OATP4C1	SLCO4C1/ OATP-H	MTX	Mikkaichi et al. (2004)
ABCA2	ABC2	Estramustine	Laing et al. (1998)
BSEP	ABCB11	Paclitaxel and vinblastine	Childs et al. (1998)
OCT1	SLC22A1	Oxaliplatin, cisplatin, imatinib and *cis*-diammine (pyri-dine)chloroplatinum(II) (but carboplatin and nedaplatin are not substrates)	Yonezawa et al. (2006); Zhang et al. (2006b); Lovejoy et al. (2008)
OCT2	SLC22A2	Oxaliplatin, cisplatin and *cis*-diammine(pyridine) chloroplatinum(II) (but carboplatin and nedaplatin are not substrates)	Yonezawa et al. (2006); Zhang et al. (2006b); Lovejoy et al. (2008)
OCT3	SLC22A3	Oxaliplatin (but carboplatin and nedaplatin are not substrates)	Yonezawa et al. (2006)
OCTN1	SLC22A4/ CT1/SCD	MTX, mitoxantrone and doxorubicin (but cisplatin and oxaliplatin are not substrtes)	Okabe et al. (2008); Yonezawa et al. (2006)
OCTN2	SLC22A5	Cisplatin and oxaliplatin are not substrates	Yonezawa et al. (2006)
OCTN3	SLC22A21	-	Okabe et al. (2008)
ENT1	SLC29A1	6-Mercaptopurine, 6-thioguanine and 5-FU	Lu et al. (2002); Huang et al. (2004)
ENT2	SLC29A2	6-Mercaptopurine, 6-thioguanine and 5-FU	Nagai et al. (2007)
ENT3	SLC29A3	6-Mercaptopurine, 6-thioguanine and 5-FU	Lu et al. (2002)
ENT4	SLC29A4	6-Mercaptopurine, 6-thioguanine and 5-FU	Lu et al. (2002)

Table 12.3 (continued)

Transporter	Symbols	Anticancer drugs as substrates	References
CNT1	SLC28A1	6-Mercaptopurine, 6-thioguanine and 5-FU	Lu et al. (2002)
CNT2	SLC28A2	6-Mercaptopurine, 6-thioguanine and 5-FU	Lu et al. (2002)
CNT3	SLC28A3	6-Mercaptopurine, 6-thioguanine and 5-FU	Lu et al. (2002)
MATE1	FLJ10847	Cisplatin and oxaliplatin (but carboplatin and nedaplatin are not substrates)	Yonezawa et al. (2006)
MATE2	MATE2-K/FLJ31196	Oxaliplatin (but carboplatin and nedaplatin are not substrates)	Yonezawa et al. (2006)
$ATB^{0,+}$	SLC6A14	1-Methyltryptophan	Karunakaran et al. (2008)
RLIP-76	RalBP1	Doxorubicin, daunomycin and vinblastine	Awasthi et al. (1994)

BCRP, breast cancer resistance protein; CNT, concentrative nucleoside transporter; ENT, equilibrative nucleoside transporter; 5-FU, 5-fluorouracil; MTX, methotrexate; MATE, multidrug and toxin extrusion; OAT, organic anion transporter; OATP, organic anion transporting polypeptide; OCT, organic cation transporter; OCTN, novel organic cation/carnitine transporter; RLIP76, 76 kDa Ral-binding GTPase activating protein (RalBP1); SLC, solute carrier.

The MRP/ABCC family contains nine members (MRP1-9) with sizes from 1,325 to 1,545 amino acids (http://www.med.rug.nl/mdl/tab3.htm). Cells that highly express MRP1 confer resistance to a variety of natural product anticancer drugs such as *vinca* alkaloids, anthracyclines and epipodophyllotoxins. MRP1-transfected cells also exhibit decreased drug accumulation and increased drug efflux. MRP1/ABCC1 is capable of transporting the glucuronide conjugate of etoposide and a GSH conjugate of doxorubicin (Koike et al. 1997; Cui et al. 1999; Kawabe et al. 1999). Like MRP1, MRP2 transfected cells are resistant to *vinca* alkaloids (e.g. vincristine), anthracyclines, camptothecins (e.g. CPT-11 and SN-38) and MTX. MRP2 is distinct from MRP1 with the ability to confer resistance to cisplatin (Kool et al. 1999; Zeng et al. 1999). MRP3 confers resistance to a much narrower spectrum of anticancer drugs compared to MRP1 and MRP2, and the drugs are limited to vincristine, MTX, epipodophyllotins (Chen et al. 2001). MRP4 can transport 6-mercaptopurine, and 6-thioguanine (McAleer et al. 1999; Jedlitschky et al. 2000). MRP5 does not interact with typical substrates of MRP1, MRP2 or MRP3, such as vincristine, etoposide or daunorubicin (Oguri et al. 2007). In comparison with MRP1-3, MRP5 has its particular drug resistance selectivity and confers no resistance to natural anticancer compounds or MTX.

The magnitude of the drug interactions (e.g. digoxin) by St John's wort observed in clinical reports is often greater than that predicted by in vitro data (Durr et al. 2000; Perloff et al. 2001; Hennessy et al. 2002), suggesting that induction of

CYP3A4 is unlikely to explain completely some interactions and a second interaction mechanism may exist. St John's wort has been shown to induce intestinal P-gp in vitro and in vivo (Perloff et al. 2001). Treatment of LS-180 intestinal carcinoma cells with St John's wort or hypericin at 3–300 μM caused 4-to 7-fold increase in the expression of P-gp (Durr et al. 2000). The administration of St John's wort extract to rats for 14 days resulted in a 3.8-fold increase of intestinal P-gp expression (Durr et al. 2000). Oral administration of St John's wort for 14 days in healthy volunteers resulted in a 1.4-fold increase in P-gp expression (Dresser et al. 2003; Xie et al. 2005). The probe substrates of P-gp, fexofenadine and cyclosporine were found to have increased clearance in healthy subjects treated with long-term St John's wort (Hennessy et al. 2002). Moreover, chronic treatment with St John's wort (16 days) caused a 4.2-fold increase in P-gp levels in the peripheral blood lymphocytes of healthy volunteers (Durr et al. 2000).

St John's wort appears to have contrary modulating effect on intestinal P-gp and CYP3A compared to grapefruit juice. Grapefruit juice augmented the oral bioavailability of dihydropyridines, terfenadine, saquinavir, cyclosporine, midazolam, triazolam and verapamil (Hunter and Hirst 1997; Zhang and Benet 2001), which was thought to be due to the inhibition of intestinal CYP3A4 and P-gp (Kliewer et al. 1998; Lehmann et al. 1998).

12.4.3 Role of Pregnane X receptor in Herb–Anticancer Drug Interactions

Human pregnane X receptor (PXR/NR1I2) encoded by the nuclear receptor subfamily 1 gene is a member of the orphan nuclear receptor family (Gibson et al. 2002; Kast et al. 2002; Goodwin et al. 2002; Handschin and Meyer 2003; Burk et al. 2004; Wang et al. 2004; Zhou et al. 2004; Ferguson et al. 2005; Itoh et al. 2006). PXR is a master transcriptional regulator of many important genes involved in the detoxification and transport of a number of xenobiotics, including those encoding CYPs including CYP3A4, CYP3A5, CYP2B6, CYP2C19 and CYP2C8 and various drug transporters (e.g. P-gp, and MRP2/ABCC2), and bile acid homeostasis (Orans et al. 2005; Sinz et al. 2006). A wide variety of structurally divergent endobiotics and xenobiotics have been identified as ligands of PXR, including rifampicin, bile acids and their precursors, nifedipine, nicotine, clotrimazole, hyperforin and dexamethasone (Moore et al. 2000). Hyperforin is a more potent activator of PXR ($K_i = 27$ nM) than the known PXR inducer rifampin. The binding of intracellular hyperforin to PXR generates a functional complex which consequently binds to the pregnane response element of *CYP3A4*, *CYP2B6* and *MDR1* genes (Fig. 12.8). The binding will activate and initiate the expression of the target genes. The clinical exposure to hyperforin associated with the ingestion of many available formulations of St John's wort (e.g. plasma concentrations of approximately 200–380 nmol/L) is sufficient to produce activation of PXR and, consequently, induction of CYP3A4 and P-gp. Thus

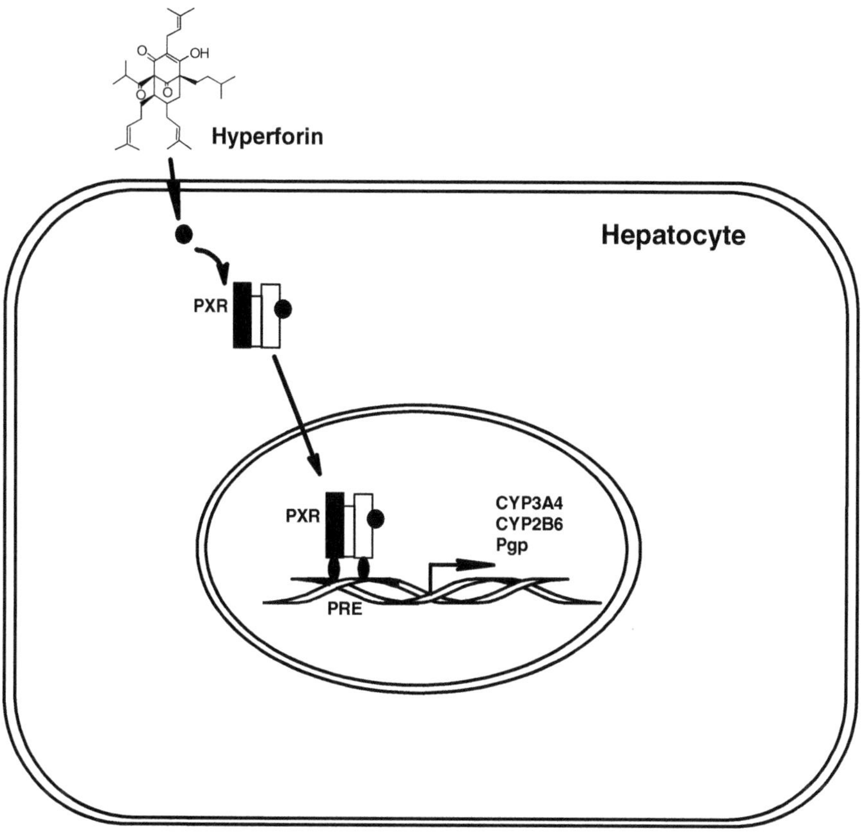

Fig. 12.8 Molecular pathways for the induction of pregnane X receptor (PXR) by hyperforin in human hepatocytes. The binding of intracellular hyperforin to the orphan nuclear receptor, PXR, generates a functional complex which consequently binds to the pregnane response element (PRE) of *CYP3A4*, *CYP2B6* and *MDR1* genes. The binding will activate and initiate the expression of these genes

the potential for clinically significant drug interactions between St John's wort with many CYP3A4 and/or P-gp substrates (e.g., antineoplastic agents) is highly likely (Fig. 12.8).

12.5 Clinical Considerations

Interactions of anticancer drugs with herbal/dietary supplements are difficult to anticipate and predict because of the general lack of information characterizing the pharmacologic actions of these substances. The dramatic rise in the use of herbal remedies means that many more patients on conventional medicines are being exposed to herbal medicines. Thus, timely identification of the herbs involved and victim anticancer drugs is important to remind both physicians and patients of the possible safety concerns arising from combined use of herbs with any anticancer drugs (Zhou et al. 2007b). Unfortunately, in many cases the patients think that herbal remedies are natural products and thus are safe. They are not willing or do not think it is necessary to mention the types and doses of herbal remedies being used to clinicians, so there is little knowledge of who are taking these products and for what indications.

Many individuals regard herbal remedies as natural and therefore safe. However, there is a lack of general advice available to patients who wish to use these products. Patients who notice that their conventional medicine is not working as well as it used to, may seek advice on possible alternatives to this medication, while they continue to concomitantly use herbal remedies, not considering it as a possible culprit or mentioning the use of herbal remedies to their physician. Continued education of consumers and healthcare professionals about the potential for herb–anticancer drug interactions is required to ensure further interactions do not occur. It is therefore essential that patients are asked about the use of over-the-counter medicines, when they receive chemotherapy or present with an adverse reaction. It is also necessary to report all suspected adverse reactions and interactions associated with herbal medicines in order for information about their safety to be established.

Because herbal supplements are becoming increasingly popular, physicians should ask questions about the use of herbal medicines as part of the medication history. Even though herbal products are available without a prescription, medical guidance is necessary because of the adverse effects of these products and the potential for drug interactions. Consequently, physicians need to stay abreast of trends in herbal supplement use, with the realization that for most supplements the adverse effects and potential for anticancer drug interactions are not well characterized.

12.6 Conclusions and Future Perspectives

Caution should be taken when anticancer drugs are used in combination with herbal medicines, particularly for cytotoxic anticancer drugs with narrow therapeutic indices. Monitoring plasma concentrations of concurrently administered anticancer drugs and observing for possible signs of clinical toxicity are necessary when herbal remedies is used concurrently. This will allow early identification of potential drug interactions and severe toxicities.

Cancer patients who take herbal medicine may not wish to discuss their herbal medicine use with their physicians due to various beliefs such as herbal medicines are naturally safe. In addition, patients can access herbal medicine such as St John's wort without the need of prescriptions. This creates a situation that even though the knowledge concerning a herbal medicine interaction with anticancer drugs is available, doctors would not be able to exercise their clinical judgment to make necessary adjustment in their prescribing practice and thus to avoid concurrent medication of such herbs and with a wide range of drugs that may be interacting with this herb.

To date, there are only limited data on herb–anticancer drug interactions in clinical settings. However, currently available data have strongly suggested that caution must be taken when herbal medicines are used concurrently with anticancer drugs. The use of herbal medicines often enlarges the variability in the pharmacokinetics and pharmacodynamics of anticancer drugs. Further clinical studies are warranted to explore the impact of herbal medicines on the clearance, efficacy and toxicity of clinically important anticancer drugs.

References

Aimova D, Svobodova L, Kotrbova V et al. The anticancer drug ellipticine is a potent inducer of rat cytochromes P450 1A1 and 1A2, thereby modulating its own metabolism. Drug Metab Dispos. 2007;35:1926–34.

Albanell J, Rojo F, Averbuch S et al. Pharmacodynamic studies of the epidermal growth factor receptor inhibitor ZD1839 in skin from cancer patients: histopathologic and molecular consequences of receptor inhibition. J Clin Oncol. 2002;20:110–24.

Albanell J, Rojo F, Baselga J. Pharmacodynamic studies with the epidermal growth factor receptor tyrosine kinase inhibitor ZD1839. Semin Oncol. 2001;28:56–66.

Aller SG, Yu J, Ward A et al. Structure of P-glycoprotein reveals a molecular basis for poly-specific drug binding. Science. 2009;323:1718–22.

Alvarez M, Paull K, Monks A et al. Generation of a drug resistance profile by quantitation of mdr-1/P-glycoprotein in the cell lines of the National Cancer Institute Anticancer Drug Screen. J Clin Invest. 1995;95:2205–14.

Ambudkar SV, Kimchi-Sarfaty C, Sauna ZE et al. P-glycoprotein: from genomics to mechanism. Oncogene. 2003;22:7468–85.

Arbuck SG, Douglass HO, Crom WR et al. Etoposide pharmacokinetics in patients with normal and abnormal organ function. J Clin Oncol. 1986;4:1690–5.

Awasthi S, Singhal SS, Srivastava SK et al. Adenosine triphosphate-dependent transport of doxorubicin, daunomycin, and vinblastine in human tissues by a mechanism distinct from the P-glycoprotein. J Clin Invest. 1994;93:958–65.

Badagnani I, Castro RA, Taylor TR et al. Interaction of methotrexate with organic-anion transporting polypeptide 1A2 and its genetic variants. J Pharmacol Exp Ther. 2006;318:521–9.

Bailey DG, Dresser GR, Kreeft JH et al. Grapefruit–felodipine interaction: effect of unprocessed fruit and probable active ingredients. Clin Pharmacol Ther. 2000;68:468–77.

Bailey DG, Malcolm J, Arnold O et al. Grapefruit juice–drug interactions. Br J Clin Pharmacol. 1998;46:101–10.

Bailey DG, Spence JD, Munoz C et al. Interaction of citrus juices with felodipine and nifedipine. Lancet. 1991;337:268–9.

Bauer S, Stormer E, Johne A et al. Alterations in cyclosporin A pharmacokinetics and metabolism during treatment with St John's wort in renal transplant patients. Br J Clin Pharmacol. 2003;55:203–11.

Baumgart A, Schmidt M, Schmitz HJ et al. Natural furocoumarins as inducers and inhibitors of cytochrome P450 1A1 in rat hepatocytes. Biochem Pharmacol. 2005;69:657–67.

Becquemont L, Verstuyft C, Kerb R et al. Effect of grapefruit juice on digoxin pharmacokinetics in humans. Clin Pharmacol Ther. 2001;70:311–6.

Beer TM, El-Geneidi M, Eilers KM. Docetaxel (taxotere) in the treatment of prostate cancer. Expert Rev Anticancer Ther. 2003;3:261–8.

Belinsky MG, Chen ZS, Shchaveleva I et al. Characterization of the drug resistance and transport properties of multidrug resistance protein 6 (MRP6, ABCC6). Cancer Res. 2002;62: 6172–7.

Bencharit S, Morton CL, Howard-Williams EL et al. Structural insights into CPT-11 activation by mammalian carboxylesterases. Nat Struct Biol. 2002;9:337–42.

Beumer JH, Buckle T, Ouwehand M et al. Trabectedin (ET-743, Yondelis) is a substrate for P-glycoprotein, but only high expression of P-glycoprotein confers the multidrug resistance phenotype. Invest New Drugs. 2007;25:1–7.

Beverage JN, Sissung TM, Sion AM et al. *CYP2D6* polymorphisms and the impact on tamoxifen therapy. J Pharm Sci. 2007;96:2224–31.

Bisogno G, Cowie F, Boddy A et al. High-dose cyclosporin with etoposide – toxicity and pharmacokinetic interaction in children with solid tumours. Br J Cancer. 1998;77:2304–9.

Blagden SP, Kaye SB. Docetaxel in the management of ovarian cancer. Expert Rev Anticancer Ther. 2005;5:203–14.

Blevins-Primeau AS, Sun D, Chen G et al. Functional significance of UDP-glucuronosyltransferase variants in the metabolism of active tamoxifen metabolites. Cancer Res. 2009;69:1892–900.

Block KI, Gyllenhaal C, Mead MN. Safety and efficacy of herbal sedatives in cancer care. Integr Cancer Ther. 2004;3:128–48.

Bolton AE, Peng B, Hubert M et al. Effect of rifampicin on the pharmacokinetics of imatinib mesylate (Gleevec, STI571) in healthy subjects. Cancer Chemother Pharmacol. 2004;53:102–6.

Brandon EF, Sparidans RW, Guijt KJ et al. In vitro characterization of the human biotransformation and CYP reaction phenotype of ET-743 (Yondelis, Trabectidin), a novel marine anti-cancer drug. Invest New Drugs. 2006;24:3–14.

Bressler R. Grapefruit juice and drug interactions. Exploring mechanisms of this interaction and potential toxicity for certain drugs. Geriatrics. 2006;61:12–8.

Bruno R, Sanderink GJ. Pharmacokinetics and metabolism of Taxotere (docetaxel). Cancer Surv. 1993;17:305–13.

Bumpus NN, Sridar C, Kent UM et al. The naturally occurring cytochrome P450 (P450) 2B6 K262R mutant of P450 2B6 exhibits alterations in substrate metabolism and inactivation. Drug Metab Dispos. 2005;33:795–802.

Burckhardt BC, Burckhardt G. Transport of organic anions across the basolateral membrane of proximal tubule cells. Rev Physiol Biochem Pharmacol. 2003;146:95–158.

Burk O, Koch I, Raucy J et al. The induction of cytochrome P450 3A5 (CYP3A5) in the human liver and intestine is mediated by the xenobiotic sensors pregnane X receptor (PXR) and constitutively activated receptor (CAR. J Biol Chem. 2004;279:38379–85.

Canal P, Gay C, Dezeuze A et al. Pharmacokinetics and pharmacodynamics of irinotecan during a Phase II clinical trial in colorectal cancer. Pharmacology and Molecular Mechanisms Group of the European Organization for Research and Treatment of Cancer. J Clin Oncol. 1996;14:2688–95.

Cappuzzo F, Gregorc V, Rossi E et al. Gefitinib in pretreated non-small-cell lung cancer (NSCLC): analysis of efficacy and correlation with HER2 and epidermal growth factor receptor expression in locally advanced or metastatic NSCLC. J Clin Oncol. 2003;21:2658–63.

Cha SH, Sekine T, Fukushima JI et al. Identification and characterization of human organic anion transporter 3 expressing predominantly in the kidney. Mol Pharmacol. 2001;59:1277–86.

Chabner BA, Roberts TG, Jr.. Timeline: chemotherapy and the war on cancer. Nat Rev Cancer. 2005;5:65–72.

Chen C, Meng L, Ma X et al. Urinary metabolite profiling reveals CYP1A2-mediated metabolism of NSC686288 (aminoflavone). J Pharmacol Exp Ther. 2006;318:1330–42.

Chen ZS, Hopper-Borge E, Belinsky MG et al. Characterization of the transport properties of human multidrug resistance protein 7 (MRP7, ABCC10). Mol Pharmacol. 2003a;63:351–8.

Chen ZS, Lee K, Kruh GD. Transport of cyclic nucleotides and estradiol 17-β-D-glucuronide by multidrug resistance protein 4. Resistance to 6-mercaptopurine and 6-thioguanine. J Biol Chem. 2001;276:33747–54.

Chen ZS, Lee K, Walther S et al. Analysis of methotrexate and folate transport by multidrug resistance protein 4 (ABCC4): MRP4 is a component of the methotrexate efflux system. Cancer Res. 2002;62:3144–50.

Chen ZS, Robey RW, Belinsky MG et al. Transport of methotrexate, methotrexate polyglutamates, and 17β-estradiol 17-(β-D-glucuronide) by ABCG2: effects of acquired mutations at R482 on methotrexate transport. Cancer Res. 2003b;63:4048–54.
Childs S, Yeh RL, Hui D et al. Taxol resistance mediated by transfection of the liver-specific sister gene of P-glycoprotein. Cancer Res. 1998;58:4160–7.
Chu XY, Kato Y, Niinuma K et al. Multispecific organic anion transporter is responsible for the biliary excretion of the camptothecin derivative irinotecan and its metabolites in rats. J Pharmacol Exp Ther. 1997a;281:304–14.
Chu XY, Kato Y, Sugiyama Y. Multiplicity of biliary excretion mechanisms for irinotecan, CPT-11, and its metabolites in rats. Cancer Res. 1997b;57:1934–8.
Chu XY, Kato Y, Ueda K et al. Biliary excretion mechanism of CPT-11 and its metabolites in humans: involvement of primary active transporters. Cancer Res. 1998;58:5137–43.
Chu XY, Suzuki H, Ueda K et al. Active efflux of CPT-11 and its metabolites in human KB-derived cell lines. J Pharmacol Exp Ther. 1999;288:735–41.
Clark PI, Slevin ML. The clinical pharmacology of etoposide and teniposide. Clin Pharmacokinet. 1987;12:223–52.
Cohen MH, Johnson JR, Chen YF et al. FDA drug approval summary: erlotinib (Tarceva) tablets. Oncologist. 2005a;10:461–6.
Cohen MH, Johnson JR, Pazdur R. U.S. Food and Drug Administration Drug Approval Summary: conversion of imatinib mesylate (STI571; Gleevec) tablets from accelerated approval to full approval. Clin Cancer Res. 2005b;11:12–9.
Cohen MH, Williams G, Johnson JR et al. Approval summary for imatinib mesylate capsules in the treatment of chronic myelogenous leukemia. Clin Cancer Res. 2002;8:935–42.
Cohen MH, Williams GA, Sridhara R et al. FDA drug approval summary: gefitinib (ZD1839) (Iressa) tablets. Oncologist. 2003;8:303–6.
Cole SP, Sparks KE, Fraser K et al. Pharmacological characterization of multidrug resistant MRP-transfected human tumor cells. Cancer Res. 1994;54:5902–10.
Corona G, Aita P, Sorio R et al. Pharmacokinetic interaction between etoposide and tamoxifen in patients with hepatocellular carcinoma. Anticancer Drugs. 1999;10:815–9.
Cortes JE, Pazdur R. Docetaxel. J Clin Oncol. 1995;13:2643–55.
Cotter TG. Apoptosis and cancer: the genesis of a research field. Nat Rev Cancer. 2009;9:501–7.
Cox MC, Low J, Lee J et al. Influence of garlic (*Allium sativum*) on the pharmacokinetics of docetaxel. Clin Cancer Res. 2006;12:4636–40.
Crewe HK, Notley LM, Wunsch RM et al. Metabolism of tamoxifen by recombinant human cytochrome P450 enzymes: formation of the 4-hydroxy, 4'-hydroxy and *N*-desmethyl metabolites and isomerization of *trans*-4-hydroxytamoxifen. Drug Metab Dispos. 2002;30: 869–74.
Crown J. Docetaxel: overview of an active drug for breast cancer. Oncologist. 2001;6 Suppl 3:1–4.
Cui Y, Konig J, Buchholz JK et al. Drug resistance and ATP-dependent conjugate transport mediated by the apical multidrug resistance protein, MRP2, permanently expressed in human and canine cells. Mol Pharmacol. 1999;55:929–37.
Das SK, Vasudevan DM. Protective effects of silymarin, a milk thistle (*Silybium marianum*) derivative on ethanol-induced oxidative stress in liver. Indian J Biochem Biophys. 2006;43:306–11.
Dausch JG, Nixon DW. Garlic: a review of its relationship to malignant disease. Prev Med. 1990;19:346–61.
Dean M, Rzhetsky A, Allikmets R. The human ATP-binding cassette (ABC) transporter superfamily. Genome Res. 2001;11:1156–66.
Dehal SS, Kupfer D. CYP2D6 catalyzes tamoxifen 4-hydroxylation in human liver. Cancer Res. 1997;57:3402–6.
Dennison JB, Kulanthaivel P, Barbuch RJ et al. Selective metabolism of vincristine in vitro by CYP3A5. Drug Metab Dispos. 2006;34:1317–27.
Desai PB, Duan JZ, Zhu YW et al. Human liver microsomal metabolism of paclitaxel and drug interactions. Eur J Drug Metab Pharmacokinet. 1998;23:417–24.

Di Carlo G, Borrelli F, Ernst E et al. St John's wort: Prozac from the plant kingdom. Trends Pharmacol Sci. 2001;22:292–7.
Dodds HM, Haaz MC, Riou JF et al. Identification of a new metabolite of CPT-11 (irinotecan): pharmacological properties and activation to SN-38. J Pharmacol Exp Ther. 1998;286:578–83.
Dowell J, Minna JD, Kirkpatrick P. Erlotinib hydrochloride. Nat Rev Drug Discov. 2005;4:13–4.
Doyle LA, Ross DD. Multidrug resistance mediated by the breast cancer resistance protein BCRP (ABCG2). Oncogene. 2003;22:7340–58.
Dresser GK, Schwarz UI, Wilkinson GR et al. Coordinate induction of both cytochrome P4503A and MDR1 by St John's wort in healthy subjects. Clin Pharmacol Ther. 2003;73:41–50.
Ducharme MP, Warbasse LH, Edwards DJ. Disposition of intravenous and oral cyclosporine after administration with grapefruit juice. Clin Pharmacol Ther. 1995;57:485–91.
Durr D, Stieger B, Kullak-Ublick GA et al. St John's wort induces intestinal P-glycoprotein/MDR1 and intestinal and hepatic CYP3A4. Clin Pharmacol Ther. 2000;68:598–604.
Dutreix C, Peng B, Mehring G et al. Pharmacokinetic interaction between ketoconazole and imatinib mesylate (Glivec) in healthy subjects. Cancer Chemother Pharmacol. 2004;54:290–4.
D'Incalci M, Rossi C, Zucchetti M et al. Pharmacokinetics of etoposide in patients with abnormal renal and hepatic function. Cancer Res. 1986;46:2566–71.
Engels FK, Loos WJ, Mathot RA et al. Influence of ketoconazole on the fecal and urinary disposition of docetaxel. Cancer Chemother Pharmacol. 2007;60:569–79.
Ernst E, Cassileth BR. The prevalence of complementary/alternative medicine in cancer: a systematic review. Cancer. 1998;83:777–82.
Ferguson SS, Chen Y, LeCluyse EL et al. Human CYP2C8 is transcriptionally regulated by the nuclear receptors constitutive androstane receptor, pregnane X receptor, glucocorticoid receptor, and hepatic nuclear factor 4α. Mol Pharmacol. 2005;68:747–57.
Fischer V, Rodriguez-Gascon A, Heitz F et al. The multidrug resistance modulator valspodar (PSC 833) is metabolized by human cytochrome P450 3A. Implications for drug–drug interactions and pharmacological activity of the main metabolite. Drug Metab Dispos. 1998;26:802–11.
Foster BC, Foster MS, Vandenhoek S et al. An *in vitro* evaluation of human cytochrome P450 3A4 and P-glycoprotein inhibition by garlic. J Pharm Sci. 2001;4:176–84.
Frohna P, Lu J, Eppler S et al. Evaluation of the absolute oral bioavailability and bioequivalence of erlotinib, an inhibitor of the epidermal growth factor receptor tyrosine kinase, in a randomized, crossover study in healthy subjects. J Clin Pharmacol. 2006;46:282–90.
Frye RF, Fitzgerald SM, Lagattuta TF et al. Effect of St John's wort on imatinib mesylate pharmacokinetics. Clin Pharmacol Ther. 2004;76:323–9.
Fugh-Berman A. Herb–drug interactions. Lancet. 2000;355:134–8.
Fuhr U, Anders EM, Mahr G et al. Inhibitory potency of quinolone antibacterial agents against cytochrome P450IA2 activity *in vivo* and *in vitro*. Antimicrob Agents Chemother. 1992;36:942–8.
Fulton B, Spencer CM. Docetaxel. A review of its pharmacodynamic and pharmacokinetic properties and therapeutic efficacy in the management of metastatic breast cancer. Drugs. 1996;51:1075–92.
Gardner ER, Burger H, van Schaik RH et al. Association of enzyme and transporter genotypes with the pharmacokinetics of imatinib. Clin Pharmacol Ther. 2006;80:192–201.
Gatenby RA. A change of strategy in the war on cancer. Nature. 2009;459:508–9.
Gatzemeier U, Pluzanska A, Szczesna A et al. Phase III study of erlotinib in combination with cisplatin and gemcitabine in advanced non-small-cell lung cancer: the Tarceva Lung Cancer Investigation Trial. J Clin Oncol. 2007;25:1545–52.
Gibson GG, Plant NJ, Swales KE et al. Receptor-dependent transcriptional activation of cytochrome P4503A genes: induction mechanisms, species differences and interindividual variation in man. Xenobiotica. 2002;32:165–206.
Goodwin B, Moore LB, Stoltz CM et al. Regulation of the human *CYP2B6* gene by the nuclear pregnane X receptor. Mol Pharmacol. 2001;60:427–31.
Goodwin B, Redinbo MR, Kliewer SA. Regulation of *CYP3A* gene transcription by the pregnane X receptor. Annu Rev Pharmacol Toxicol. 2002;42:1–23.

Goryachkina K, Burbello A, Boldueva S et al. CYP2D6 is a major determinant of metoprolol disposition and effects in hospitalized Russian patients treated for acute myocardial infarction. Eur J Clin Pharmacol. 2008;64:1163–73.

Granfors MT, Backman JT, Neuvonen M et al. Ciprofloxacin greatly increases concentrations and hypotensive effect of tizanidine by inhibiting its cytochrome P450 1A2-mediated presystemic metabolism. Clin Pharmacol Ther. 2004;76:598–606.

Granvil CP, Madan A, Sharkawi M et al. Role of CYP2B6 and CYP3A4 in the *in vitro* *N*-dechloroethylation of (*R*)- and (*S*)-ifosfamide in human liver microsomes. Drug Metab Dispos. 1999;27:533–41.

Grenader T, Gipps M, Shavit L et al. Significant drug interaction: phenytoin toxicity due to erlotinib. Lung Cancer. 2007;57:404–6.

Gridelli C, Bareschino MA, Schettino C et al. Erlotinib in non-small cell lung cancer treatment: current status and future development. Oncologist. 2007;12:840–9.

Gridelli C, Butts C, Ciardiello F et al. An international, multicenter, randomized phase III study of first-line erlotinib followed by second-line cisplatin/gemcitabine versus first-line cisplatin/gemcitabine followed by second-line erlotinib in advanced non-small-cell lung cancer: treatment rationale and protocol dynamics of the TORCH trial. Clin Lung Cancer. 2008;9:235–8.

Gschwind HP, Pfaar U, Waldmeier F et al. Metabolism and disposition of imatinib mesylate in healthy volunteers. Drug Metab Dispos. 2005;33:1503–12.

Guo Y, Kotova E, Chen ZS et al. MRP8, ATP-binding cassette C11 (ABCC11), is a cyclic nucleotide efflux pump and a resistance factor for fluoropyrimidines 2',3'-dideoxycytidine and 9'-(2'-phosphonylmethoxyethyl)adenine. J Biol Chem. 2003;278:29509–14.

Gupta E, Lestingi TM, Mick R et al. Metabolic fate of irinotecan in humans: correlation of glucuronidation with diarrhea. Cancer Res. 1994;54:3723–5.

Gupta E, Mick R, Ramirez J et al. Pharmacokinetic and pharmacodynamic evaluation of the topoisomerase inhibitor irinotecan in cancer patients. J Clin Oncol. 1997;15:1502–10.

Gurley BJ, Gardner SF, Hubbard MA et al. In vivo assessment of botanical supplementation on human cytochrome P450 phenotypes: *Citrus aurantium*, *Echinacea purpurea*, milk thistle, and saw palmetto. Clin Pharmacol Ther. 2004;76:428–40.

Haaz MC, Rivory L, Riche C et al. Metabolism of irinotecan (CPT-11) by human hepatic microsomes: participation of cytochrome P-450 3A and drug interactions. Cancer Res. 1998;58:468–72.

Haimeur A, Conseil G, Deeley RG et al. The MRP-related and BCRP/ABCG2 multidrug resistance proteins: biology, substrate specificity and regulation. Curr Drug Metab. 2004;5:21–53.

Hamada A, Miyano H, Watanabe H et al. Interaction of imatinib mesilate with human P-glycoprotein. J Pharmacol Exp Ther. 2003;307:824–8.

Hande KR. Etoposide: four decades of development of a topoisomerase II inhibitor. Eur J Cancer. 1998;34:1514–21.

Handschin C, Meyer UA. Induction of drug metabolism: the role of nuclear receptors. Pharmacol Rev. 2003;55:649–73.

Hanioka N, Ozawa S, Jinno H et al. Human liver UDP-glucuronosyltransferase isoforms involved in the glucuronidation of 7-ethyl-10-hydroxycamptothecin. Xenobiotica. 2001;31:687–99.

Harmsen S, Meijerman I, Beijnen JH et al. Nuclear receptor mediated induction of cytochrome P450 3A4 by anticancer drugs: a key role for the pregnane X receptor. Cancer Chemother Pharmacol. 2009;64:35–43.

Harris JC, Cottrell SL, Plummer S et al. Antimicrobial properties of *Allium sativum* (garlic). Appl Microbiol Biotechnol. 2001;57:282–6.

He K, Iyer KR, Hayes RN et al. Inactivation of cytochrome P450 3A4 by bergamottin, a component of grapefruit juice. Chem Res Toxicol. 1998;11:252–9.

Hennessy M, Kelleher D, Spiers JP et al. St John's Wort increases expression of P-glycoprotein: implications for drug interactions. Br J Clin Pharmacol. 2002;53:75–82.

Herbst RS, Johnson DH, Mininberg E et al. Phase I/II trial evaluating the anti-vascular endothelial growth factor monoclonal antibody bevacizumab in combination with the HER-1/epidermal

growth factor receptor tyrosine kinase inhibitor erlotinib for patients with recurrent non-small-cell lung cancer. J Clin Oncol. 2005;23:2544–55.
Herbst RS, Kies MS. Gefitinib: current and future status in cancer therapy. Clin Adv Hematol Oncol. 2003;1:466–72.
Hooijberg JH, Broxterman HJ, Kool M et al. Antifolate resistance mediated by the multidrug resistance proteins MRP1 and MRP2. Cancer Res. 1999;59:2532–5.
Hooijberg JH, Peters GJ, Assaraf YG et al. The role of multidrug resistance proteins MRP1, MRP2 and MRP3 in cellular folate homeostasis. Biochem Pharmacol. 2003;65:765–71.
Hopper-Borge E, Chen ZS, Shchaveleva I et al. Analysis of the drug resistance profile of multidrug resistance protein 7 (ABCC10): resistance to docetaxel. Cancer Res. 2004;64:4927–30.
Hu S, Franke RM, Filipski KK et al. Interaction of imatinib with human organic ion carriers. Clin Cancer Res. 2008;14:3141–8.
Hu Z, Yang X, Ho PC et al. St. John's wort modulates the toxicities and pharmacokinetics of CPT-11 (irinotecan) in rats. Pharm Res. 2005a;22:902–14.
Hu Z, Yang X, Ho PC et al. Herb–drug interactions: a literature review. Drugs. 2005b;65:1239–82.
Hu ZP, Yang XX, Chan SY et al. St. John's wort attenuates irinotecan-induced diarrhea via down-regulation of intestinal pro-inflammatory cytokines and inhibition of intestinal epithelial apoptosis. Toxicol Appl Pharmacol. 2006;216:225–37.
Hu ZP, Yang XX, Chen X et al. A mechanistic study on altered pharmacokinetics of irinotecan by St. John's wort. Curr Drug Metab. 2007;8:157–71.
Huang Y, Anderle P, Bussey KJ et al. Membrane transporters and channels: role of the transportome in cancer chemosensitivity and chemoresistance. Cancer Res. 2004;64:4294–301.
Huisman MT, Chhatta AA, van Tellingen O et al. MRP2 (ABCC2) transports taxanes and confers paclitaxel resistance and both processes are stimulated by probenecid. Int J Cancer. 2005;116:824–9.
Hukkanen J, Jacob P, 3rd, Benowitz NL. Effect of grapefruit juice on cytochrome P450 2A6 and nicotine renal clearance. Clin Pharmacol Ther. 2006;80:522–30.
Humerickhouse R, Lohrbach K, Li L et al. Characterization of CPT-11 hydrolysis by human liver carboxylesterase isoforms hCE-1 and hCE-2. Cancer Res. 2000;60:1189–92.
Hunter J, Hirst BH. Intestinal secretion of drugs - The role of P-glycoprotein and related drug efflux systems in limiting oral drug absorption. Adv Drug Deliver Rev. 1997;25:129–57.
Ikeda K, Yoshisue K, Matsushima E et al. Bioactivation of tegafur to 5-fluorouracil is catalyzed by cytochrome P450 2A6 in human liver microsomes *in vitro*. Clin Cancer Res. 2000;6:4409–15.
Innocenti F, Iyer L, Ramirez J et al. Epirubicin glucuronidation is catalyzed by human UDP-glucuronosyltransferase 2B7. Drug Metab Dispos. 2001;29:686–92.
Itoh M, Nakajima M, Higashi E et al. Induction of human CYP2A6 is mediated by the pregnane X receptor with peroxisome proliferator-activated receptor-γ coactivator 1a. J Pharmacol Exp Ther. 2006;319:693–702.
Izzo AA. Herb–drug interactions: an overview of the clinical evidence. Fundam Clin Pharmacol. 2005;19:1–16.
Jacolot F, Simon I, Dreano Y et al. Identification of the cytochrome P450 3A family as the enzymes involved in the *N*-demethylation of tamoxifen in human liver microsomes. Biochem Pharmacol. 1991;41:1911–9.
Jedlitschky G, Burchell B, Keppler D. The multidrug resistance protein 5 functions as an ATP-dependent export pump for cyclic nucleotides. J Biol Chem. 2000;275:30069–74.
Jedlitschky G, Leier I, Buchholz U et al. Transport of glutathione, glucuronate, and sulfate conjugates by the *MRP* gene-encoded conjugate export pump. Cancer Res. 1996;56:988–94.
Jeong EJ, Liu Y, Lin H et al. Species- and disposition model-dependent metabolism of raloxifene in gut and liver: role of UGT1A10. Drug Metab Dispos. 2005;33:785–94.
Johnson JA, Burlew BS. Metoprolol metabolism *via* cytochrome P4502D6 in ethnic populations. Drug Metab Dispos. 1996;24:350–5.
Johnson JR, Bross P, Cohen M et al. Approval summary: imatinib mesylate capsules for treatment of adult patients with newly diagnosed philadelphia chromosome-positive chronic myelogenous leukemia in chronic phase. Clin Cancer Res. 2003;9:1972–9.

Johnson JR, Cohen M, Sridhara R et al. Approval summary for erlotinib for treatment of patients with locally advanced or metastatic non-small cell lung cancer after failure of at least one prior chemotherapy regimen. Clin Cancer Res. 2005;11:6414–21.

Jonker JW, Smit JW, Brinkhuis RF et al. Role of breast cancer resistance protein in the bioavailability and fetal penetration of topotecan. J Natl Cancer Inst. 2000;92:1651–6.

Kajita J, Kuwabara T, Kobayashi H et al. CYP3A4 is mainly responsible for the metabolism of a new *vinca* alkaloid, vinorelbine, in human liver microsomes. Drug Metab Dispos. 2000;28:1121–7.

Kakar SM, Paine MF, Stewart PW et al. 6'7'-Dihydroxybergamottin contributes to the grapefruit juice effect. Clin Pharmacol Ther. 2004;75:569–79.

Kaku T, Ogura K, Nishiyama T et al. Quaternary ammonium-linked glucuronidation of tamoxifen by human liver microsomes and UDP-glucuronosyltransferase 1A4. Biochem Pharmacol. 2004;67:2093–102.

Kane GC, Lipsky JJ. Drug–grapefruit juice interactions. Mayo Clin Proc. 2000;75:933–42.

Karunakaran S, Umapathy NS, Thangaraju M et al. Interaction of tryptophan derivatives with SLC6A14 ($ATB^{0,+}$) reveals the potential of the transporter as a drug target for cancer chemotherapy. Biochem J. 2008;414:343–55.

Kase Y, Hayakawa T, Aburada M et al. Preventive effects of *Hange-shashin-to* on irinotecan hydrochloride-caused diarrhea and its relevance to the colonic prostaglandin E_2 and water absorption in the rat. Jpn J Pharmacol. 1997a;75:407–13.

Kase Y, Hayakawa T, Togashi Y et al. Relevance of irinotecan hydrochloride-induced diarrhea to the level of prostaglandin E_2 and water absorption of large intestine in rats. Jpn J Pharmacol. 1997b;75:399–405.

Kast HR, Goodwin B, Tarr PT et al. Regulation of multidrug resistance-associated protein 2 (ABCC2) by the nuclear receptors pregnane X receptor, farnesoid X-activated receptor, and constitutive androstane receptor. J Biol Chem. 2002;277:2908–15.

Kawabe T, Chen ZS, Wada M et al. Enhanced transport of anticancer agents and leukotriene C_4 by the human canalicular multispecific organic anion transporter (cMOAT/MRP2). FEBS Lett. 1999;456:327–31.

Kawashiro T, Yamashita K, Zhao XJ et al. A study on the metabolism of etoposide and possible interactions with antitumor or supporting agents by human liver microsomes. J Pharmacol Exp Ther. 1998;286:1294–300.

Keating GM, Santoro A. Sorafenib: a review of its use in advanced hepatocellular carcinoma. Drugs. 2009;69:223–40.

Kehrer DF, Yamamoto W, Verweij J et al. Factors involved in prolongation of the terminal disposition phase of SN-38: clinical and experimental studies. Clin Cancer Res. 2000;6:3451–8.

Kerb R, Brockmoller J, Staffeldt B et al. Single-dose and steady-state pharmacokinetics of hypericin and pseudohypericin. Antimicrob Agents Chemother. 1996;40:2087–93.

Kitamura R, Asanoma H, Nagayama S et al. Identification of human liver cytochrome P450 isoforms involved in autoinduced metabolism of the antiangiogenic agent (*Z*)-5-[(1,2-dihydro-2-oxo-3*H*-indol-3-ylidene)methyl]-2,4-dimethyl-1*H*-pyrrole-3-propanoic acid (TSU-68. Drug Metab Dispos. 2008;36:1003–9.

Kliewer SA, Moore JT, Wade L et al. An orphan nuclear receptor activated by pregnanes defines a novel steroid signaling pathway. Cell. 1998;92:73–82.

Koike K, Kawabe T, Tanaka T et al. A canalicular multispecific organic anion transporter (cMOAT) antisense cDNA enhances drug sensitivity in human hepatic cancer cells. Cancer Res. 1997;57:5475–9.

Komatsu T, Yamazaki H, Shimada N et al. Roles of cytochromes P450 1A2, 2A6, and 2C8 in 5-fluorouracil formation from tegafur, an anticancer prodrug, in human liver microsomes. Drug Metab Dispos. 2000;28:1457–63.

Konig J, Seithel A, Gradhand U et al. Pharmacogenomics of human OATP transporters. Naunyn Schmiedebergs Arch Pharmacol. 2006;372:432–43.

Kool M, van der Linden M, de Haas M et al. MRP3, an organic anion transporter able to transport anti-cancer drugs. Proc Natl Acad Sci U S A. 1999;96:6914–9.

Kousba A, Soll R, Yee S et al. Cyclic conversion of the novel Src kinase inhibitor [7-(2, 6-dichloro-phenyl)-5-methyl-benzo[1,2,4]triazin-3-yl]-[4-(2-pyrrolid in-1-yl-ethoxy)-phenyl]-amine (TG100435) and its *N*-oxide metabolite by flavin-containing monoxygenases and cytochrome P450 reductase. Drug Metab Dispos. 2007;35:2242–51.

Kris MG, Natale RB, Herbst RS et al. Efficacy of gefitinib, an inhibitor of the epidermal growth factor receptor tyrosine kinase, in symptomatic patients with non-small cell lung cancer: a randomized trial. JAMA. 2003;290:2149–58.

Kroll DJ, Shaw HS, Oberlies NH. Milk thistle nomenclature: why it matters in cancer research and pharmacokinetic studies. Integr Cancer Ther. 2007;6:110–9.

Kudoh S, Fujiwara Y, Takada Y et al. Phase II study of irinotecan combined with cisplatin in patients with previously untreated small-cell lung cancer. West Japan Lung Cancer Group. J Clin Oncol. 1998;16:1068–74.

Kuffel MJ, Schroeder JC, Pobst LJ et al. Activation of the antitumor agent aminoflavone (NSC 686288) is mediated by induction of tumor cell cytochrome P450 1A1/1A2. Mol Pharmacol. 2002;62:143–53.

Kyo E, Uda N, Kasuga S et al. Immunomodulatory effects of aged garlic extract. J Nutr. 2001;131:S1075–S79.

Laing NM, Belinsky MG, Kruh GD et al. Amplification of the ATP-binding cassette 2 transporter gene is functionally linked with enhanced efflux of estramustine in ovarian carcinoma cells. Cancer Res. 1998;58:1332–7.

Le Guellec C, Lacarelle B, Catalin J et al. Inhibitory effects of anticancer drugs on dextromethorphan-*O*-demethylase activity in human liver microsomes. Cancer Chemother Pharmacol. 1993;32:491–5.

Lee K, Klein-Szanto AJ, Kruh GD. Analysis of the MRP4 drug resistance profile in transfected NIH3T3 cells. J Natl Cancer Inst. 2000;92:1934–40.

Leggas M, Adachi M, Scheffer GL et al. Mrp4 confers resistance to topotecan and protects the brain from chemotherapy. Mol Cell Biol. 2004;24:7612–21.

Lehmann JM, McKee DD, Watson MA et al. The human orphan nuclear receptor PXR is activated by compounds that regulate *CYP3A4* gene expression and cause drug interactions. J Clin Invest. 1998;102:1016–23.

Li J, Zhao M, He P et al. Differential metabolism of gefitinib and erlotinib by human cytochrome P450 enzymes. Clin Cancer Res. 2007;13:3731–37.

Lim HK, Duczak N, Jr., Brougham L et al. Automated screening with confirmation of mechanism-based inactivation of CYP3A4, CYP2C9, CYP2C19, CYP2D6, and CYP1A2 in pooled human liver microsomes. Drug Metab Dispos. 2005;33:1211–19.

Lin HL, Kent UM, Hollenberg PF. The grapefruit juice effect is not limited to cytochrome P450 (P450) 3A4: evidence for bergamottin-dependent inactivation, heme destruction, and covalent binding to protein in P450 s 2B6 and 3A5. J Pharmacol Exp Ther. 2005;313: 154–64.

Lin JH, Lu AYH. Role of pharmacokinetics and metabolism in drug discovery and development. Pharmacol Rev. 1997;49:403–49.

Linde K, Mulrow CD, Berner M et al. St John's wort for depression. Cochrane Database Syst Rev. 2005;2:CD000448.

Ling J, Johnson KA, Miao Z et al. Metabolism and excretion of erlotinib, a small molecule inhibitor of epidermal growth factor receptor tyrosine kinase, in healthy male volunteers. Drug Metab Dispos. 2006;34:420–6.

Long L, Dolan ME. Role of cytochrome P450 isoenzymes in metabolism of O^6-benzylguanine: implications for dacarbazine activation. Clin Cancer Res. 2001;7:4239–44.

Lovejoy KS, Todd RC, Zhang S et al. *cis*-Diammine(pyridine)chloroplatinum(II), a monofunctional platinum(II) antitumor agent: Uptake, structure, function, and prospects. Proc Natl Acad Sci U S A. 2008;105:8902–7.

Lu H, Waxman DJ. Antitumor activity of methoxymorpholinyl doxorubicin: potentiation by cytochrome P450 3A metabolism. Mol Pharmacol. 2005;67:212–9.

Lu X, Gong S, Monks A et al. Correlation of nucleoside and nucleobase transporter gene expression with antimetabolite drug cytotoxicity. J Exp Ther Oncol. 2002;2:200–12.

Lum BL, Kaubisch S, Yahanda AM et al. Alteration of etoposide pharmacokinetics and pharmacodynamics by cyclosporine in a Phase I trial to modulate multidrug resistance. J Clin Oncol. 1992;10:1635–42.

Lyseng-Williamson KA, Fenton C. Docetaxel: a review of its use in metastatic breast cancer. Drugs. 2005;65:2513–31.

Ma S, Subramanian R, Xu Y et al. Structural characterization of novel adenine dinucleotide phosphate conjugates of imatinib in incubations with rat and human liver microsomes. Drug Metab Dispos. 2008;36:2414–8.

Ma S, Xu Y, Shou M. Characterization of imatinib metabolites in rat and human liver microsomes: differentiation of hydroxylation from *N*-oxidation by liquid chromatography/atmospheric pressure chemical ionization mass spectrometry. Rapid Commun Mass Spectrom. 2009;23: 1446–50.

Madabushi R, Frank B, Drewelow B et al. Hyperforin in St. John's wort drug interactions. Eur J Clin Pharmacol. 2006;62:225–33.

Mai I, Stormer E, Bauer S et al. Impact of St John's wort treatment on the pharmacokinetics of tacrolimus and mycophenolic acid in renal transplant patients. Nephrol Dial Transplant. 2003;18:819–22.

Maliepaard M, van Gastelen MA, Tohgo A et al. Circumvention of breast cancer resistance protein (BCRP)-mediated resistance to camptothecins *in vitro* using non-substrate drugs or the BCRP inhibitor GF120918. Clin Cancer Res. 2001;7:935–41.

Manthey JA, Buslig BS. Distribution of furanocoumarins in grapefruit juice fractions. J Agric Food Chem. 2005;53:5158–63.

Mao Q, Unadkat JD. Role of the breast cancer resistance protein (ABCG2) in drug transport. AAPS J. 2005;7:E118–E33.

Marchetti S, Oostendorp RL, Pluim D et al. *In vitro* transport of gimatecan (7-*t*-butoxyiminomethylcamptothecin) by breast cancer resistance protein, P-glycoprotein, and multidrug resistance protein 2. Mol Cancer Ther. 2007;6:3307–13.

Marre F, Sanderink GJ, de Sousa G et al. Hepatic biotransformation of docetaxel (Taxotere) *in vitro*: involvement of the CYP3A subfamily in humans. Cancer Res. 1996;56:1296–302.

Marzolini C, Paus E, Buclin T et al. Polymorphisms in human MDR1 (P-glycoprotein): recent advances and clinical relevance. Clin Pharmacol Ther. 2004;75:13–33.

Mathijssen RH, Verweij J, de Bruijn P et al. Effects of St. John's wort on irinotecan metabolism. J Natl Cancer Inst. 2002;94:1247–9.

Mathijssen RHJ, van Alphen RJ, Verweij J et al. Clinical pharmacokinetics and metabolism of irinotecan (CPT-11). Clin Cancer Res. 2001;7:2182–94.

McAleer MA, Breen MA, White NL et al. pABC11 (also known as MOAT-C and MRP5), a member of the ABC family of proteins, has anion transporter activity but does not confer multidrug resistance when overexpressed in human embryonic kidney 293 cells. J Biol Chem. 1999;274:23541–8.

McClue SJ, Stuart I. Metabolism of the trisubstituted purine cyclin-dependent kinase inhibitor seliciclib (R-roscovitine) *in vitro* and *in vivo*. Drug Metab Dispos. 2008;36:561–70.

McKillop D, Guy SP, Spence MP et al. Minimal contribution of desmethyl-gefitinib, the major human plasma metabolite of gefitinib, to epidermal growth factor receptor (EGFR)-mediated tumour growth inhibition. Xenobiotica. 2006;36:29–39.

McKillop D, Hutchison M, Partridge EA et al. Metabolic disposition of gefitinib, an epidermal growth factor receptor tyrosine kinase inhibitor, in rat, dog and man. Xenobiotica. 2004a;34:917–34.

McKillop D, McCormick AD, Millar A et al. Cytochrome P450-dependent metabolism of gefitinib. Xenobiotica. 2005;35:39–50.

McKillop D, McCormick AD, Miles GS et al. *In vitro* metabolism of gefitinib in human liver microsomes. Xenobiotica. 2004b;34:983–1000.

McKillop D, Partridge EA, Hutchison M et al. Pharmacokinetics of gefitinib, an epidermal growth factor receptor tyrosine kinase inhibitor, in rat and dog. Xenobiotica. 2004c;34:901–15.
Mikkaichi T, Suzuki T, Onogawa T et al. Isolation and characterization of a digoxin transporter and its rat homologue expressed in the kidney. Proc Natl Acad Sci U S A. 2004;101:3569–74.
Miners JO, Valente L, Lillywhite KJ et al. Preclinical prediction of factors influencing the elimination of 5,6-dimethylxanthenone-4-acetic acid, a new anticancer drug. Cancer Res. 1997;57:284–9.
Miyata M, Tamura E, Motoki K et al. Thalidomide-induced suppression of embryo fibroblast proliferation requires CYP1A1-mediated activation. Drug Metab Dispos. 2003;31:469–75.
Mohri K, Uesawa Y. Effects of furanocoumarin derivatives in grapefruit juice on nifedipine pharmacokinetics in rats. Pharm Res. 2001;18:177–82.
Mok TS, Yeo W, Johnson PJ et al. A double-blind placebo-controlled randomized study of Chinese herbal medicine as complementary therapy for reduction of chemotherapy-induced toxicity. Ann Oncol. 2007;18:768–74.
Moore LB, Goodwin B, Jones SA et al. St. John's wort induces hepatic drug metabolism through activation of the pregnane X receptor. Proc Natl Acad Sci U S A. 2000;97:7500–2.
Moore MJ, Goldstein D, Hamm J et al. Erlotinib plus gemcitabine compared with gemcitabine alone in patients with advanced pancreatic cancer: a phase III trial of the National Cancer Institute of Canada Clinical Trials Group. J Clin Oncol. 2007;25:1960–6.
Mori K, Kondo T, Kamiyama Y et al. Preventive effect of Kampo medicine (*Hangeshashin-to*) against irinotecan-induced diarrhea in advanced non-small-cell lung cancer. Cancer Chemother Pharmacol. 2003;51:403–6.
Morrow CS, Peklak-Scott C, Bishwokarma B et al. Multidrug resistance protein 1 (MRP1, ABCC1) mediates resistance to mitoxantrone via glutathione-dependent drug efflux. Mol Pharmacol. 2006;69:1499–505.
Morrow CS, Smitherman PK, Diah SK et al. Coordinated action of glutathione *S*-transferases (GSTs) and multidrug resistance protein 1 (MRP1) in antineoplastic drug detoxification. Mechanism of GST A1-1- and MRP1-associated resistance to chlorambucil in MCF7 breast carcinoma cells. J Biol Chem. 1998;273:20114–20.
Moyer JD, Barbacci EG, Iwata KK et al. Induction of apoptosis and cell cycle arrest by CP-358,774, an inhibitor of epidermal growth factor receptor tyrosine kinase. Cancer Res. 1997;57:4838–48.
Nagai K, Nagasawa K, Kihara Y et al. Anticancer nucleobase analogues 6-mercaptopurine and 6-thioguanine are novel substrates for equilibrative nucleoside transporter 2. Int J Pharm. 2007;333:56–61.
Nagar S, Blanchard RL. Pharmacogenetics of uridine diphosphoglucuronosyltransferase (UGT) 1A family members and its role in patient response to irinotecan. Drug Metab Rev. 2006;38:393–409.
Nakanishi T, Shiozawa K, Hassel BA et al. Complex interaction of BCRP/ABCG2 and imatinib in BCR-ABL-expressing cells: BCRP-mediated resistance to imatinib is attenuated by imatinib-induced reduction of BCRP expression. Blood. 2006;108:678–84.
Nakatomi K, Yoshikawa M, Oka M et al. Transport of 7-ethyl-10-hydroxycamptothecin (SN-38) by breast cancer resistance protein ABCG2 in human lung cancer cells. Biochem Biophys Res Commun. 2001;288:827–32.
Narita M, Nagai E, Hagiwara H et al. Inhibition of β-glucuronidase by natural glucuronides of kampo medicines using glucuronide of SN-38 (7-ethyl-10-hydroxycamptothecin) as a substrate. Xenobiotica. 1993;23:5–10.
Nassar AF, King I, Paris BL et al. An *in vitro* evaluation of the victim and perpetrator potential of the anti-cancer agent laromustine (VNP40101M), based on reaction phenotyping and inhibition and induction of cytochrome P450 (CYP) enzymes. Drug Metab Dispos. 2009;in press.
Nathan PJ. *Hypericum perforatum* (St John's Wort): a non-selective reuptake inhibitor? A review of the recent advances in its pharmacology. J Psychopharmacol. 2001;15:47–54.

Nebel A, Schneider BJ, Baker RK et al. Potential metabolic interaction between St. John's wort and theophylline. Ann Pharmacother. 1999;33:502.

Noguchi K, Katayama K, Mitsuhashi J et al. Functions of the breast cancer resistance protein (BCRP/ABCG2) in chemotherapy. Adv Drug Deliv Rev. 2009;61:26–33.

Nozaki Y, Kusuhara H, Kondo T et al. Characterization of the uptake of organic anion transporter (OAT) 1 and OAT3 substrates by human kidney slices. J Pharmacol Exp Ther. 2007;321:362–9.

Nozawa T, Imai K, Nezu J et al. Functional characterization of pH-sensitive organic anion transporting polypeptide OATP-B in human. J Pharmacol Exp Ther. 2004;308:438–45.

Nozawa T, Minami H, Sugiura S et al. Role of organic anion transporter OATP1B1 (OATP-C) in hepatic uptake of irinotecan and its active metabolite, 7-ethyl-10-hydroxycamptothecin: *in vitro* evidence and effect of single nucleotide polymorphisms. Drug Metab Dispos. 2005;33: 434–9.

O'Brien SG, Meinhardt P, Bond E et al. Effects of imatinib mesylate (STI571, Glivec) on the pharmacokinetics of simvastatin, a cytochrome P450 3A4 substrate, in patients with chronic myeloid leukaemia. Br J Cancer. 2003;89:1855–9.

Obach RS. Inhibition of human cytochrome P450 enzymes by constituents of St. John's Wort, an herbal preparation used in the treatment of depression. J Pharmacol Exp Ther. 2000;294:88–95.

Ogura K, Ishikawa Y, Kaku T et al. Quaternary ammonium-linked glucuronidation of *trans*-4-hydroxytamoxifen, an active metabolite of tamoxifen, by human liver microsomes and UDP-glucuronosyltransferase 1A4. Biochem Pharmacol. 2006;71:1358–69.

Oguri T, Bessho Y, Achiwa H et al. MRP8/ABCC11 directly confers resistance to 5-fluorouracil. Mol Cancer Ther. 2007;6:122–7.

Oguri T, Takahashi T, Miyazaki M et al. UGT1A10 is responsible for SN-38 glucuronidation and its expression in human lung cancers. Anticancer Res. 2004;24:2893–6.

Okabe M, Szakacs G, Reimers MA et al. Profiling *SLCO* and *SLC22* genes in the NCI-60 cancer cell lines to identify drug uptake transporters. Mol Cancer Ther. 2008;7:3081–91.

Ono N, van der Heijden I, Scheffer GL et al. Multidrug resistance-associated protein 9 (ABCC12) is present in mouse and boar sperm. Biochem J. 2007;406:31–40.

Oostendorp RL, Buckle T, Beijnen JH et al. The effect of P-gp (Mdr1a/1b), BCRP (Bcrp1) and P-gp/BCRP inhibitors on the *in vivo* absorption, distribution, metabolism and excretion of imatinib. Invest New Drugs. 2009;27:31–40.

Orans J, Teotico DG, Redinbo MR. The nuclear xenobiotic receptor pregnane X receptor: recent insights and new challenges. Mol Endocrinol. 2005;19:2891–900.

Ozvegy-Laczka C, Hegedus T, Varady G et al. High–affinity interaction of tyrosine kinase inhibitors with the ABCG2 multidrug transporter. Mol Pharmacol. 2004;65:1485–95.

Pekol T, Daniels JS, Labutti J et al. Human metabolism of the proteasome inhibitor bortezomib: identification of circulating metabolites. Drug Metab Dispos. 2005;33:771–7.

Perloff MD, von Moltke LL, Stormer E et al. Saint John's wort: an *in vitro* analysis of P-glycoprotein induction due to extended exposure. Br J Pharmacol. 2001;134:1601–8.

Pradhan SC, Girish C. Hepatoprotective herbal drug, silymarin from experimental pharmacology to clinical medicine. Indian J Med Res. 2006;124:491–504.

Priebe W, Krawczyk M, Kuo MT et al. Doxorubicin- and daunorubicin-glutathione conjugates, but not unconjugated drugs, competitively inhibit leukotriene C_4 transport mediated by MRP/GS-X pump. Biochem Biophys Res Commun. 1998;247:859–63.

Quintieri L, Geroni C, Fantin M et al. Formation and antitumor activity of PNU-159682, a major metabolite of nemorubicin in human liver microsomes. Clin Cancer Res. 2005;11:1608–17.

Rakhit A, Pantze MP, Fettner S et al. The effects of CYP3A4 inhibition on erlotinib pharmacokinetics: computer-based simulation (SimCYP) predicts *in vivo* metabolic inhibition. Eur J Clin Pharmacol. 2008;64:31–41.

Ramaswamy B, Puhalla S. Docetaxel: a tubulin-stabilizing agent approved for the management of several solid tumors. Drugs Today (Barc). 2006;42:265–79.

Ramirez J, Iyer L, Journault K et al. *In vitro* characterization of hepatic flavopiridol metabolism using human liver microsomes and recombinant UGT enzymes. Pharm Res. 2002;19:588–94.

Rau T, Wuttke H, Michels LM et al. Impact of the *CYP2D6* genotype on the clinical effects of metoprolol: a prospective longitudinal study. Clin Pharmacol Ther. 2009;85:269–72.
Reid JM, Kuffel MJ, Miller JK et al. Metabolic activation of dacarbazine by human cytochromes P450: the role of CYP1A1, CYP1A2, and CYP2E1. Clin Cancer Res. 1999;5:2192–7.
Reid JM, Kuffel MJ, Ruben SL et al. Rat and human liver cytochrome P-450 isoform metabolism of ecteinascidin 743 does not predict gender-dependent toxicity in humans. Clin Cancer Res. 2002;8:2952–62.
Reif S, Nicolson MC, Bisset D et al. Effect of grapefruit juice intake on etoposide bioavailability. Eur J Clin Pharmacol. 2002;58:491–4.
Relling MV, Nemec J, Schuetz EG et al. *O*-demethylation of epipodophyllotoxins is catalyzed by human cytochrome P450 3A4. Mol Pharmacol. 1994;45:352–8.
Rivory LP. Metabolism of CPT-11. Impact on activity. Ann N Y Acad Sci. 2000;922:205–15.
Rivory LP, Bowles MR, Robert J et al. Conversion of irinotecan (CPT-11) to its active metabolite, 7-ethyl-10-hydroxycamptothecin (SN-38), by human liver carboxylesterase. Biochem Pharmacol. 1996a;52:1103–11.
Rivory LP, Haaz MC, Canal P et al. Pharmacokinetic interrelationships of irinotecan (CPT-11) and its three major plasma metabolites in patients enrolled in phase I/II trials. Clin Cancer Res. 1997;3:1261–6.
Rivory LP, Riou JF, Haaz MC et al. Identification and properties of a major plasma metabolite of irinotecan (CPT-11) isolated from the plasma of patients. Cancer Res. 1996b;56:3689–94.
Roby CA, Anderson GD, Kantor E et al. St John's wort: effect on CYP3A4 activity. Clin Pharmacol Ther. 2000;67:451–7.
Rooseboom M, Commandeur JN, Vermeulen NP. Enzyme-catalyzed activation of anticancer prodrugs. Pharmacol Rev. 2004;56:53–102.
Rosing H, van Zomeren DM, Doyle E et al. *O*-glucuronidation, a newly identified metabolic pathway for topotecan and *N*-desmethyl topotecan. Anticancer Drugs. 1998;9:587–92.
Rothenberg ML, Meropol NJ, Poplin EA et al. Mortality associated with irinotecan plus bolus fluorouracil/leucovorin: summary findings of an independent panel. J Clin Oncol. 2001;19:3801–7.
Roy P, Tretyakov O, Wright J et al. Stereoselective metabolism of ifosfamide by human P-450s 3A4 and 2B6. Favorable metabolic properties of *R*-enantiomer. Drug Metab Dispos. 1999;27:1309–18.
Royer I, Monsarrat B, Sonnier M et al. Metabolism of docetaxel by human cytochromes P450: interactions with paclitaxel and other antineoplastic drugs. Cancer Res. 1996;56:58–65.
Saif MW. Erlotinib: the first biologic in the management of pancreatic cancer. Expert Opin Pharmacother. 2008;9:1595–607.
Sakamoto H, Hara H, Hirano K et al. Enhancement of glucuronosyl etoposide transport by glutathione in multidrug resistance-associated protein-overexpressing cells. Cancer Lett. 1999;135:113–9.
Saloustros E, Mavroudis D, Georgoulias V. Paclitaxel and docetaxel in the treatment of breast cancer. Expert Opin Pharmacother. 2008;9:2603–16.
Santos A, Zanetta S, Cresteil T et al. Metabolism of irinotecan (CPT-11) by CYP3A4 and CYP3A5 in humans. Clin Cancer Res. 2000;6:2012–20.
Sarkadi B, Homolya L, Szakacs G et al. Human multidrug resistance ABCB and ABCG transporters: participation in a chemoimmunity defense system. Physiol Rev. 2006;86:1179–236.
Sarkadi B, Ozvegy-Laczka C, Nemet K et al. ABCG2 - a transporter for all seasons. FEBS Lett. 2004;567:116–20.
Schellens JH, Maliepaard M, Scheper RJ et al. Transport of topoisomerase I inhibitors by the breast cancer resistance protein. Potential clinical implications. Ann N Y Acad Sci. 2000;922:188–94.
Seelig A, Landwojtowicz E. Structure-activity relationship of P-glycoprotein substrates and modifiers. Eur J Pharm Sci. 2000;12:31–40.
Sharom FJ. ABC multidrug transporters: structure, function and role in chemoresistance. Pharmacogenomics. 2008;9:105–27.
Shirakawa K, Takara K, Tanigawara Y et al. Interaction of docetaxel ("Taxotere") with human P-glycoprotein. Jpn J Cancer Res. 1999;90:1380–6.

Sigusch H, Henschel L, Kraul H et al. Lack of effect of grapefruit juice on diltiazem bioavailability in normal subjects. Pharmazie. 1994;49:675–9.

Singh UP, Prithiviraj B, Sarma BK et al. Role of garlic (*Allium sativum* L.) in human and plant diseases. Indian J Exp Biol. 2001;39:310–22.

Sinz M, Kim S, Zhu Z et al. Evaluation of 170 xenobiotics as transactivators of human pregnane X receptor (hPXR) and correlation to known CYP3A4 drug interactions. Curr Drug Metab. 2006;7:375–88.

Slapak CA, Fracasso PM, Martell RL et al. Overexpression of the multidrug resistance-associated protein (*MRP*) gene in vincristine but not doxorubicin-selected multidrug-resistant murine erythroleukemia cells. Cancer Res. 1994;54:5607–13.

Smith P. The influence of St. John's wort on the pharmacokinetics and protein binding of imatinib mesylate. Pharmacotherapy. 2004;24:1508–14.

Smith NF, Acharya MR, Desai N et al. Identification of OATP1B3 as a high-affinity hepatocellular transporter of paclitaxel. Cancer Biol Ther. 2005;4:815–8.

Smith NF, Baker SD, Gonzalez FJ et al. Modulation of erlotinib pharmacokinetics in mice by a novel cytochrome P450 3A4 inhibitor, BAS 100. Br J Cancer. 2008;98:1630–2.

Sparreboom A, Cox MC, Acharya MR et al. Herbal remedies in the United States: potential adverse interactions with anticancer agents. J Clin Oncol. 2004a;22:2489–503.

Sparreboom A, Marsh S, Mathijssen RH et al. Pharmacogenetics of tipifarnib (R115777) transport and metabolism in cancer patients. Invest New Drugs. 2004b;22:285–9.

Sridar C, Goosen TC, Kent UM et al. Silybin inactivates cytochromes P450 3A4 and 2C9 and inhibits major hepatic glucuronosyltransferases. Drug Metab Dispos. 2004;32:587–94.

Standish LJ, Greene KB, Bain S et al. Alternative medicine use in HIV-positive men and women: demographics, utilization patterns and health status. AIDS Care. 2001;13:197–208.

Stearns V, Johnson MD, Rae JM et al. Active tamoxifen metabolite plasma concentrations after coadministration of tamoxifen and the selective serotonin reuptake inhibitor paroxetine. J Natl Cancer Inst. 2003;95:1758–64.

Stiborova M, Arlt VM, Henderson CJ et al. Role of hepatic cytochromes P450 in bioactivation of the anticancer drug ellipticine: studies with the hepatic NADPH:cytochrome P450 reductase null mouse. Toxicol Appl Pharmacol. 2008;226:318–27.

Sugiyama Y, Kato Y, Chu X. Multiplicity of biliary excretion mechanisms for the camptothecin derivative irinotecan (CPT-11), its metabolite SN-38, and its glucuronide: role of canalicular multispecific organic anion transporter and P-glycoprotein. Cancer Chemother Pharmacol. 1998;42 Suppl:S44–S49.

Sun D, Chen G, Dellinger RW et al. Characterization of tamoxifen and 4-hydroxytamoxifen glucuronidation by human *UGT1A4* variants. Breast Cancer Res. 2006;8:R50.

Sun D, Sharma AK, Dellinger RW et al. Glucuronidation of active tamoxifen metabolites by the human UDP glucuronosyltransferases. Drug Metab Dispos. 2007;35:2006–14.

Swaisland HC, Ranson M, Smith RP et al. Pharmacokinetic drug interactions of gefitinib with rifampicin, itraconazole and metoprolol. Clin Pharmacokinet. 2005a;44:1067–81.

Swaisland HC, Smith RP, Laight A et al. Single-dose clinical pharmacokinetic studies of gefitinib. Clin Pharmacokinet. 2005b;44:1165–77.

Takasuna K, Hagiwara T, Hirohashi M et al. Involvement of beta-glucuronidase in intestinal microflora in the intestinal toxicity of the antitumor camptothecin derivative irinotecan hydrochloride (CPT-11) in rats. Cancer Res. 1996;56:3752–7.

Takasuna K, Kasai Y, Kitano Y et al. Protective effects of kampo medicines and baicalin against intestinal toxicity of a new anticancer camptothecin derivative, irinotecan hydrochloride (CPT-11), in rats. Jpn J Cancer Res. 1995;86:978–84.

Takeda M, Khamdang S, Narikawa S et al. Characterization of methotrexate transport and its drug interactions with human organic anion transporters. J Pharmacol Exp Ther. 2002;302:666–71.

Tanovic A, Alfaro V. Gefitinib: current status in the treatment of non-small cell lung cancer. Drugs Today (Barc. 2004;40:809–27.

Thiebaut F, Tsuruo T, Hamada H et al. Cellular localization of the multidrug-resistance gene product P-glycoprotein in normal human tissues. PNAS. 1987;84:7735–8.

Thomas HD, Porter DJ, Bartelink I et al. Randomized cross-over clinical trial to study potential pharmacokinetic interactions between cisplatin or carboplatin and etoposide. Br J Clin Pharmacol. 2002;53:83–91.

Tian Q, Zhang J, Chan SY et al. Topotecan is a substrate for multidrug resistance associated protein 4. Curr Drug Metab. 2006;7:105–18.

Tian Q, Zhang J, Tan TM et al. Human multidrug resistance associated protein 4 confers resistance to camptothecins. Pharm Res. 2005;22:1837–53.

Undevia SD, Gomez-Abuin G, Ratain MJ. Pharmacokinetic variability of anticancer agents. Nat Rev Cancer. 2005;5:447–58.

Uttamsingh V, Lu C, Miwa G et al. Relative contributions of the five major human cytochromes P450, 1A2, 2C9, 2C19, 2D6, and 3A4, to the hepatic metabolism of the proteasome inhibitor bortezomib. Drug Metab Dispos. 2005;33:1723–8.

Valles B, Schiller CD, Coassolo P et al. Metabolism of mofarotene in hepatocytes and liver microsomes from different species. Comparison with *in vivo* data and evaluation of the cytochrome P450 isoenzymes involved in human biotransformation. Drug Metab Dispos. 1995;23: 1051–7.

van Cutsem E, Vervenne WL, Bennouna J et al. Phase III trial of bevacizumab in combination with gemcitabine and erlotinib in patients with metastatic pancreatic cancer. J Clin Oncol. 2009;27:2231–7.

van de Steeg E, van der Kruijssen CM, Wagenaar E et al. Methotrexate pharmacokinetics in *trans* genic mice with liver-specific expression of human organic anion-transporting polypeptide 1B1 (SLCO1B1. Drug Metab Dispos. 2009;37:277–81.

van Erp NP, Baker SD, Zhao M et al. Effect of milk thistle (*Silybum marianum*) on the pharmacokinetics of irinotecan. Clin Cancer Res. 2005;11:7800–6.

van Erp NP, Gelderblom H, Karlsson MO et al. Influence of CYP3A4 inhibition on the steady-state pharmacokinetics of imatinib. Clin Cancer Res. 2007;13:7394–400.

van Zuylen L, Verweij J, Nooter K et al. Role of intestinal P-glycoprotein in the plasma and fecal disposition of docetaxel in humans. Clin Cancer Res. 2000;6:2598–603.

Vermeir M, Hemeryck A, Cuyckens F et al. *In vitro* studies on the metabolism of trabectedin (YONDELIS) in monkey and man, including human CYP reaction phenotyping. Biochem Pharmacol. 2009;77:1642–54.

Villeneuve L, Girard H, Fortier LC et al. Novel functional polymorphisms in the UGT1A7 and UGT1A9 glucuronidating enzymes in Caucasian and African-American subjects and their impact on the metabolism of 7-ethyl-10-hydroxycamptothecin and flavopiridol anticancer drugs. J Pharmacol Exp Ther. 2003;307:117–28.

Vincent J, Harris SI, Foulds G et al. Lack of effect of grapefruit juice on the pharmacokinetics and pharmacodynamics of amlodipine. Br J Clin Pharmacol. 2000;50:455–63.

Vlaming ML, Pala Z, van Esch A et al. Impact of Abcc2 (Mrp2) and Abcc3 (Mrp3) on the *in vivo* elimination of methotrexate and its main toxic metabolite 7-hydroxymethotrexate. Clin Cancer Res. 2008;14:8152–60.

Vogel G, Tuchweber B, Trost W et al. Protection by silibinin against *Amanita phalloides* intoxication in beagles. Toxicol Appl Pharmacol. 1984;73:355–62.

Wakabayashi K, Tamura A, Saito H et al. Human ABC transporter ABCG2 in xenobiotic protection and redox biology. Drug Metab Rev. 2006;38:371–91.

Wakeling AE. Inhibitors of growth factor signalling. Endocr Relat Cancer. 2005;12 Suppl 1: S183–S87.

Wang H, Faucette S, Moore R et al. Human constitutive androstane receptor mediates induction of *CYP2B6* gene expression by phenytoin. J Biol Chem. 2004;279:29295–301.

Wang ZQ, Gorski C, Hamman MA et al. The effects of St John's wort (*Hypericum perforatum*) on human cytochrome P450 activity. Clin Pharmacol Ther. 2001;70:317–26.

Wang Y, Zhou L, Dutreix C et al. Effects of imatinib (Glivec) on the pharmacokinetics of metoprolol, a CYP2D6 substrate, in Chinese patients with chronic myelogenous leukaemia. Br J Clin Pharmacol. 2008;65:885–92.

Wangensteen H, Molden E, Christensen H et al. Identification of epoxybergamottin as a CYP3A4 inhibitor in grapefruit peel. Eur J Clin Pharmacol. 2003;58:663–8.
Warshafsky S, Kamer RS, Sivak SL. Effect of garlic on total serum cholesterol. A meta-analysis. Ann Intern Med. 1993;119:599–605.
Watanabe Y, Nakajima M, Ohashi N et al. Glucuronidation of etoposide in human liver microsomes is specifically catalyzed by UDP-glucuronosyltransferase 1A1. Drug Metab Dispos. 2003;31:589–95.
Wen Z, Tallman MN, Ali SY et al. UDP-glucuronosyltransferase 1A1 is the principal enzyme responsible for etoposide glucuronidation in human liver and intestinal microsomes: structural characterization of phenolic and alcoholic glucuronides of etoposide and estimation of enzyme kinetics. Drug Metab Dispos. 2007;35:371–80.
Wentworth JM, Agostini M, Love J et al. St John's wort, a herbal antidepressant, activates the steroid X receptor. J Endocrinol. 2000;166:R11–R16.
Whitten DL, Myers SP, Hawrelak JA et al. The effect of St John's wort extracts on CYP3A: a systematic review of prospective clinical trials. Br J Clin Pharmacol. 2006;62:512–26.
Wijnholds J, Mol CA, van Deemter L et al. Multidrug-resistance protein 5 is a multispecific organic anion transporter able to transport nucleotide analogs. Proc Natl Acad Sci U S A. 2000;97:7476–81.
Wils P, Phung-Ba V, Warnery A et al. Polarized transport of docetaxel and vinblastine mediated by P-glycoprotein in human intestinal epithelial cell monolayers. Biochem Pharmacol. 1994;48:1528–30.
Xie R, Tan LH, Polasek EC et al. CYP3A and P-glycoprotein activity induction with St. John's Wort in healthy volunteers from 6 ethnic populations. J Clin Pharmacol. 2005;45:352–6.
Yague E, Raguz S. Drug resistance in cancer. Br J Cancer. 2005;93:973–6.
Yang CJ, Horton JK, Cowan KH et al. Cross-resistance to camptothecin analogues in a mitoxantrone-resistant human breast carcinoma cell line is not due to DNA topoisomerase I alterations. Cancer Res. 1995;55:4004–9.
Yao D, Ding S, Burchell B et al. Detoxication of *vinca* alkaloids by human P450 CYP3A4-mediated metabolism: implications for the development of drug resistance. J Pharmacol Exp Ther. 2000;294:387–95.
Yee GC, Stanley DL, Pessa JL et al. Effect of grapefruit juice on blood cyclosporin concentration. Lancet. 1995;345:955–6.
Yonezawa A, Masuda S, Yokoo S et al. Cisplatin and oxaliplatin, but not carboplatin and nedaplatin, are substrates for human organic cation transporters (SLC22A1-3) and multidrug and toxin extrusion family. J Pharmacol Exp Ther. 2006;319:879–86.
You B, Tranchand B, Girard P et al. Etoposide pharmacokinetics and survival in patients with small cell lung cancer: a multicentre study. Lung Cancer. 2008;62:261–72.
Zaman GJ, Flens MJ, van Leusden MR et al. The human multidrug resistance-associated protein MRP is a plasma membrane drug-efflux pump. Proc Natl Acad Sci U S A. 1994;91:8822–6.
Zaman GJ, Versantvoort CH, Smit JJ et al. Analysis of the expression of *MRP*, the gene for a new putative transmembrane drug transporter, in human multidrug resistant lung cancer cell lines. Cancer Res. 1993;53:1747–50.
Zandvliet AS, Huitema AD, Copalu W et al. *CYP2C9* and *CYP2C19* polymorphic forms are related to increased indisulam exposure and higher risk of severe hematologic toxicity. Clin Cancer Res. 2007;13:2970–6.
Zehnpfennig B, Urbatsch IL, Galla HJ. Functional reconstitution of human ABCC3 into proteoliposomes reveals a transport mechanism with positive cooperativity. Biochemistry. 2009;48:4423–30.
Zeng H, Bain LJ, Belinsky MG et al. Expression of multidrug resistance protein-3 (multispecific organic anion transporter-D) in human embryonic kidney 293 cells confers resistance to anticancer agents. Cancer Res. 1999;59:5964–7.
Zhang J, Tian Q, Chan SY et al. Insights into oxazaphosphorine resistance and possible approaches to its circumvention. Drug Resist Updat. 2005a;8:271–97.

Zhang J, Tian Q, Yung Chan S et al. Metabolism and transport of oxazaphosphorines and the clinical implications. Drug Metab Rev. 2005b;37:611–703.
Zhang J, Tian Q, Zhou SF. Clinical pharmacology of cyclophosphamide and ifosfamide. Curr Drug Ther. 2006a;1:104–68.
Zhang S, Lovejoy KS, Shima JE et al. Organic cation transporters are determinants of oxaliplatin cytotoxicity. Cancer Res. 2006b;66:8847–57.
Zhang S, Morris ME. Effects of the flavonoids biochanin A, morin, phloretin, and silymarin on P-glycoprotein-mediated transport. J Pharmacol Exp Ther. 2003;304:1258–67.
Zhang YC, Benet LZ. The gut as a barrier to drug absorption - Combined role of cytochrome P450 3A and P-glycoprotein. Clin Pharmacokinet. 2001;40:159–68.
Zheng N, Pang S, Oe T et al. Characterization of an etoposide-glutathione conjugate derived from metabolic activation by human cytochrome P450. Curr Drug Metab. 2006;7:897–911.
Zhou S, Chan E, Li SC et al. Predicting pharmacokinetic herb–drug interactions. Drug Metabol Drug Interact. 2004;20:143–58.
Zhou S, Paxton JW, Tingle MD et al. Identification of the human liver cytochrome P450 isoenzyme responsible for the 6-methylhydroxylation of the novel anticancer drug 5,6-dimethylxanthenone-4-acetic acid. Drug Metab Dispos. 2000;28:1449–56.
Zhou SF. Structure, function and regulation of P-glycoprotein and its clinical relevance in drug disposition. Xenobiotica. 2008;38:802–32.
Zhou SF, Lai X. An update on clinical drug interactions with the herbal antidepressant St. John's wort. Curr Drug Metab. 2008;9:394–409.
Zhou SF, Xue CC, Yu XQ et al. Clinically important drug interactions potentially involving mechanism-based inhibition of cytochrome P450 3A4 and the role of therapeutic drug monitoring. Ther Drug Monit. 2007a;29:687–710.
Zhou SF, Zhou ZW, Li CG et al. Identification of drugs that interact with herbs in drug development. Drug Discov Today. 2007b;12:664–73.
Zhou XJ, Zhou-Pan XR, Gauthier T et al. Human liver microsomal cytochrome P450 3A isozymes mediated vindesine biotransformation. Metabolic drug interactions. Biochem Pharmacol. 1993;45:853–61.
Zhou-Pan XR, Seree E, Zhou XJ et al. Involvement of human liver cytochrome P450 3A in vinblastine metabolism: drug interactions. Cancer Res. 1993;53:5121–6.
Zhuo X, Zheng N, Felix CA et al. Kinetics and regulation of cytochrome P450-mediated etoposide metabolism. Drug Metab Dispos. 2004;32:993–1000.
Zuber R, Modriansky M, Dvorak Z et al. Effect of silybin and its congeners on human liver microsomal cytochrome P450 activities. Phytother Res. 2002;16:632–8.

Chapter 13
Integrating Chinese and Western Medicine in Cancer Treatment

Delia Chiaramonte and Lixing Lao

Abstract Cancer causes significant physical, psychological and spiritual distress in affected patients, and neither traditional Chinese medicine (TCM) nor Western medicine offers a fully effective and comprehensive treatment approach. While Western medicine provides potentially curative modalities such as surgery, radiation and chemotherapy, these therapies are both invasive and dangerous and can lead to significant side effects. Traditional Chinese medicine modalities tend to be gentler and less toxic yet they are less likely to effectively treat advanced cancers or sequelae of obstructive tumours. Both Western medicine and TCM, although diverse in philosophy and methods, have much to offer the cancer patient. Traditional Chinese medicine can be used to maximize the body's ability to fight cancer, to prepare the body for the assaults of allopathic treatments and to treat resulting side effects as they occur. It can enhance recovery time, improve quality of life, and perhaps even improve prognosis and decrease the risk of recurrence. Risks of integrating Chinese medicine with Western medicine include herb–drug interactions, pursuing supportive treatment in lieu of available curative therapies and a possible decrease in effectiveness of chemotherapy or radiation when combined with Chinese herbs. Neither the allopathic approach nor the TCM approach is sufficient to maximally treat patients with cancer. An integrative treatment plan that harnesses the strengths of each is the most prudent path.

13.1 Introduction

Western medicine and Chinese medicine have vastly divergent world-views, descriptive terms and treatment tools. Integration may seem unlikely, yet each has a weakness that is addressed by the other's strength. Surgery, radiation and chemotherapy are powerful yet dangerous, often causing deleterious side effects.

D. Chiaramonte (✉)
Center for Integrative Medicine, School of Medicine, University of Maryland, Baltimore, MD, USA
e-mail: dc@insightmedicalconsultants.com

W.C.S. Cho (ed.), *Supportive Cancer Care with Chinese Medicine*,
DOI 10.1007/978-90-481-3555-4_13, © Springer Science+Business Media B.V. 2010

In comparison, acupuncture and Chinese herbal medicine tend to exert gentle and subtle actions aimed at restoring homeostasis, however they are less effective at treating advanced oncologic disease. Chinese and Western medical therapies differ philosophically and methodologically, yet when used together these unique health systems effectively complement each other's strengths.

Western physicians and traditional Chinese medicine (TCM) practitioners have, until recently, practiced in separate spheres. In the last few decades, however, some aspects of TCM, particularly acupuncture, have begun to find acceptance within the Western medical community. Acceptance is even wider among the lay public. There are many private TCM practitioners in the West who treat patients with cancer and this number is likely to increase as cancer rates continue to climb.

These two diverse healing methods are often used simultaneously, yet they may not be appropriately integrated. Some patients visit TCM practitioners in the midst of their Western cancer treatments without informing their physicians. This is suboptimal and potentially unsafe. Integrating Western medicine and Chinese medicine requires more than simultaneous use of each modality. Rather, effective integration involves careful selection of treatment methods based on their unique strengths and weaknesses.

Although acupuncture has gained moderate acceptance in the West, Chinese herbal medicine is still widely unknown. Western physicians are generally unfamiliar with the potential benefits of Chinese herbs and may be fearful of drug–herb interactions. Many Chinese medicinals possess complex biological activity affecting diverse aspects of carcinogenesis such as cell growth and proliferation, apoptosis, host–tumour interactions, and immune function. In addition, TCM may be helpful for mitigating the toxicity of Western cancer treatments and improving quality of life. Traditional Chinese medicine has been used for diverse purposes such as reducing post-operative ileus, reducing urinary retention after rectal surgery, treating chemotherapy complications and improving radiation enterocolitis (Tan et al. 2008). Yet many Western physicians dismiss the potential benefits of Chinese herbs for the treatment of cancer without realizing that some of the medications in their arsenal are, in fact, derived from botanicals. Examples include Digitalis from *Digitalis purpurea* (foxglove) and Taxol from *Taxus brevifolia* (Pacific yew).

Western medical diagnostics and therapeutics are often, although not exclusively, based on empiric research. Physicians are trained to value evidence-based information over unconfirmed reports and they tend to be suspicious of unfamiliar medical information that is not backed up by methodologically solid research. In contrast, definitive literature on the therapeutic effects of TCM is scant although it has increased significantly in recent years. Much of the research has been performed in China. A significant proportion of the published work in the field of Chinese medicine in China consists of anecdotal reports or uncontrolled series and many TCM therapies have been empirically applied with clinical results simply observed and described. There are few funding sources available in the United States to evaluate Chinese medical therapeutics, the National Institutes of Health being a notable exception, and without adequate high-quality research Western physicians will continue to resist the idea of integrating TCM with Western oncologic therapeutics.

Misconceptions about Chinese medicine are common in the West. Many physicians are not aware, for example, that there are differences between Chinese herbal and Western herbal therapies. Thus, even though acupuncture has gained some acceptance, the Western medical system has not embraced the full Chinese medical tradition and the culture from which it came. Western physicians tend to view acupuncture as a procedure such as nerve block or minor surgery rather than as a component of a rich and well thought out medical system. Western physicians have begun learning and performing acupuncture on their patients, perhaps believing that a qualified acupuncturist need only learn which acupuncture points treat which conditions. This philosophy is actually antithetical to the Chinese medical world-view, which holds that TCM therapeutics must be individualized based on a patient's unique pattern of underlying imbalances. Therefore use of acupuncture in the midst of chemotherapy or radiation does not necessarily represent a true integration of Western and Chinese medicine.

Western physicians describe cancer as the abnormal and uncontrollable proliferation of cells which have the potential to spread to distant sites. The host is essentially irrelevant to the diagnosis. For example, while it is widely accepted that the toxins contained in cigarettes contribute to lung cancer, Western physicians do not acknowledge the contribution of the patient's constitution or internal imbalances to the development of disease. Cancers are classified by measurable factors such as cell type, stage and aggressiveness and treatment decisions are made based on the qualities and pervasiveness of the cancer itself. While the direct cause of most cancers is unknown, Western medicine does recognize several risk factors for the development of a malignancy including genetic predisposition, environmental toxins, viruses, body habitus, lifestyle choices and radiation exposure.

The essential goal of Western medicine is to isolate disease and control it. Western physicians start with a symptom or abnormal screening test and search for a specific associated disease. Similarly, Western oncology seeks to identify specific malignancies and destroy them. The treatments are not dependent on the cause of the disease, only on the disease itself. That is, a lung cancer initiated by smoking is treated identically to one initiated by radon. This focus on the disease itself, rather than the interplay of host and disease, is one of the key differences between Western and Chinese medicine.

Despite continued advances in cancer screening, surgery, adjuvant radiation and systemic chemotherapy, cancer remains a prevalent and difficult challenge in the West. Western treatments tend to be aggressive and intense and can lead to oncologic cures yet even these powerful therapies have significant limitations, especially in advanced disease. Treatment failures are not uncommon, side effects are almost universal and serious complications are frequent.

Traditional Chinese medicine views health and illness through a different lens. In TCM no single element of illness can be understood in isolation, rather each symptom or imbalance is evaluated in relation to the whole. Whereas a Western physician sees a breast cancer essentially as a parasite attacking a generic host, the Chinese physician will evaluate the imbalance in the patient that led to the development of the tumour and try to correct it. In Chinese medicine each patient is viewed as a cosmos in miniature.

The goal of TCM is to restore harmony and balance to the individual. The emphasis is on comprehensive assessment of physiological and psychological imbalances which have compromised the homeostatic reserve. Western medicine may be thought of as a "search and destroy" mission while Chinese medicine more closely resembles the completion of a complicated puzzle. The TCM practitioner gathers information on patient experiences, bodily functions, emotional reactions and physical symptoms to create a pattern of disharmony, which can then be addressed. The result is not identification of a disease, as a Western medical assessment would provide, but rather a unique picture of the person as a whole. While Western medicine tends to divide the body into unique parts, Chinese medicine is more concerned with function. Thus the TCM spleen is not a specific piece of tissue, as it is to the Western physician, but rather an aspect of function related to transformation, transportation, and the functions of thinking and studying.

A patient with an isolated, advanced cancer would likely benefit from tumour removal using Western surgical techniques. Chinese medicine can be used to accelerate recovery, improve immunity and decrease the likelihood of metastasis and recurrence. Some Chinese herbs seem to have anti-cancer effects however Western chemotherapies are more concentrated and often more powerful. Yet Chinese medicine can augment chemotherapy, perhaps increasing its effectiveness, decreasing its side effects and encouraging the body's intrinsic healing. Radiation can damage surrounding normal tissue and cause significant discomfort, which TCM can help to relieve. In addition, TCM can enhance immune function to support the body's own cancer-fighting abilities.

In the West, the relationship between TCM and Western medicine is an uneasy one. Despite an increasing prevalence of alternative medicine courses in medical school curricula, many Western doctors and scientists remain skeptical about the practical value of TCM. It is the rare oncologist who partners with a Chinese medicine practitioner to holistically treat a patient. Rather, it is often left to the patient to patch together an integrated treatment plan. In contrast, many modern TCM practitioners will refer patients to Western physicians if their medical condition is felt to have put the body too far out of balance for traditional methods to remedy.

Combining the benefits of powerful Western treatment methods with gentler, more holistic TCM tools provides a well-rounded treatment approach for patients with active cancers. In addition, those with known risk factors, such as smoking or chronic Hepatitis C virus might benefit from using TCM to help mitigate their cancer risk.

13.2 Western Cancer Fighting Modalities

Western cancer care is singularly focused on eradicating malignancies. Tumours are surgically removed or irradiated and errant cancer cells are attacked with powerful, and often toxic, pharmaceuticals. Little attention is paid to the underlying status of the patient except to assess his or her ability to tolerate oncologic treatments.

13.2.1 Surgery

Surgical procedures are a cornerstone of Western cancer treatment. They are used for diagnosis, staging, primary treatment, debulking, and even prevention in high-risk patients such as those carrying the *BRCA1* gene who may opt for prophylactic mastectomy. Surgeons have several modalities at their disposal including conventional surgery, cryosurgery, electrosurgery and laser surgery. All surgical procedures are, by definition, invasive and carry the risk of unpleasant or dangerous side effects.

Common side effects include pain, bleeding, wound infection, thrombosis and loss or diminution of organ function. Postoperative bowel and bladder dysfunction is common and can lead to prolonged hospital stays.

13.2.2 Chemotherapy

Some chemotherapy agents are administered orally in the patient's home while others require intravenous infusion at a medical facility. The most common side effects of chemotherapy include neutropenia, anemia, thrombocytopenia, nausea, fatigue, diarrhea and hair loss. Impairments in cardiac function as well as nerve and muscle pain can also occur. Impaired immune function predisposes chemotherapy patients to both common and uncommon infectious illnesses. Medications are available to treat deficiencies in white blood cells and red blood cells, but these medications can have side effects of their own. Transfusions of red blood cells or platelets may be used to treat chemotherapy related deficiencies. Patients with active tissue infections, advanced cardiovascular disease, co-existent immune disorders or advanced age are at particular risk of chemotherapy related complications.

13.2.3 Radiotherapy

High doses of radiation damage cancer cells and impair their growth. However, despite recent advances which have made radiotherapy more accurate, it is impossible to adequately treat the cancer cells without damaging the surrounding normal tissue. Normal cells are better able to repair themselves from radiation damage than cancer cells, however both short term and long term side effects do occur.

Radiotherapy can be used before surgery to shrink a tumour or after surgery to improve outcomes. It can also be used to boost thc cfficacy of chemotherapy and palliate symptoms of advanced cancer.

Short term radiation side effects are variable depending on the site being treated. For example, radiation of the neck can cause impaired saliva production and swallowing dysfunction while radiation to the pelvis can cause dysuria. Regardless of the radiation site, fatigue and dermatitis are common. Longer term side effects, such as secondary cancers and cardiovascular disease, are less common now than in the past as radiation treatments have become more targeted. They may be of particular concern to younger patients receiving curative regimens.

13.3 Traditional Chinese Medicine Cancer Fighting Modalities

Traditional Chinese medicine tools, including acupuncture, Chinese medicinals, qigong and nutrition are useful adjuncts to aggressive Western cancer care.

13.3.1 Acupuncture

Acupuncture can be helpful to support the body's natural healing abilities as well as to treat the side effects of Western cancer treatments. Practitioners of Chinese acupuncture use their knowledge of meridians to achieve free flow of qi, while practitioners of Western medical acupuncture, including physicians, may believe they are stimulating nerves or facilitating the release of endorphins. A Cochrane systematic review of over 3,000 patients in 26 trials found acupuncture to be an effective treatment for chemotherapy-induced nausea and vomiting (Ezza et al. 2006). It has also shown promise in improving psychological well-being in breast cancer patients (Nedstrand et al. 2006), treating cancer pain (Alimi et al. 2003) and improving quality of life in cancer patients (Dang and Yang 1998).

13.3.2 Herbal Therapy

Chinese herbal medicine includes many biologically active agents that can be used to augment Western cancer treatment. Chang (2002) reviewed the nature, extent, bioactivities and applications of polysaccharides in Chinese herbs and found multiple bioactive agents. These agents have varied potential clinical applications for cancer patients such as stimulation of hematopoiesis, antimetastasis, and antiangiogenesis. Some have been developed into pharmaceuticals while the majority remain as nutraceuticals with only preliminary research to support their efficacy.

13.3.3 Qigong

Qigong is a mind-body integrative exercise that aims to improve health and energy levels through regular practice. There is some evidence that qigong can be helpful as an addition to Western cancer treatment, although the studies are of small size and poor quality. A study of 67 patients with breast cancer investigated the effect of qigong on hematologic parameters. Thirty-two patients received 21 days of qigong therapy and the control group of 35 patients had no intervention. All patients received chemotherapy. Hemoglobin, white blood cells and platelets were measured on day 8, 15 and 22. White blood cell levels remained higher in the treatment group, although larger, higher quality studies are needed to confirm this result (Yeh et al. 2006).

Another study evaluated the effect of qigong on quality of life, side effects of Western cancer treatments, and a serum marker of inflammation. Thirty patients with heterogeneous cancers were randomly assigned to two groups: a control group which received usual care and a medical qigong group for 8 weeks in addition to usual care. The patients completed quality of life questionnaires before and after the program and serum C-reactive protein levels were assessed. The intervention group reported significantly improved quality of life scores. In addition, cancer treatment side effects and C-reactive protein levels were lower in the intervention group, although the difference did not reach statistical significance given the small sample size (Oh et al. 2008). Lee et al. (2007) attempted to critically assess the effectiveness of qigong in cancer care by performing a systematic review of the published literature. Only 9 studies met their inclusion criteria and even these studies were of poor quality. All of the included studies assessed qigong as a supportive or palliative modality rather than as a curative one, although two studies suggested effectiveness in prolonging life. The authors concluded that the effectiveness of qigong in cancer care is not yet supported by evidence from rigorous clinical trials, although since it is a pleasant and extremely low risk intervention, it remains appropriate for patients who enjoy it.

13.4 Using Traditional Chinese Medicine to Treat Side Effects of Western Treatments

13.4.1 Surgery

Herbal therapies have been used with some success to improve post-operative recovery after gastrointestinal surgery. One study examined the effect of dai-kenchu-to on gastric motility after gastrectomy for gastric cancer. The patients were randomized to a cross-over study with or without 15 g/day of dai-kenchu-to and questionnaires and emptying tests were used to evaluate gastric function. The treatment group had reduced post-operative symptoms and increased intestinal motility (Endo et al. 2006). Similarly, another study evaluated the effect of dai-kencho-to and keishi-bukuryo-gan on bowel functioning after colorectal surgery. In this study the treatment group of 66 patients took both herbs while the control group took no herbs. The treatment group had a quicker time to flatus, tolerated oral intake sooner and had fewer hospital days than the controls (Suehiro et al. 2005).

Patients commonly experience nausea in the postoperative period, often requiring pharmaceuticals which can lead to further side effects. Stimulation of acupuncture point PC6 can be used to ameliorate this unpleasant surgical side effect. A Cochrane Database systematic review found that PC6 stimulation, via multiple methods, can effectively prevent postoperative nausea and vomiting. Interventions included acupuncture, electro-acupuncture, transcutaneous nerve stimulation, laser stimulation, and acupressure. Forty trials, involving 4,858 patients, were evaluated (Lee and Fan 2009).

13.4.2 Chemotherapy

Traditional Chinese medicine can help mitigate side effects and toxicities in cancer patients who are receiving Western chemotherapy. Haishengsu (isolated from *Tegillarca granosa*) has been tested as an adjunct to conventional chemotherapy in patients with non-small cell lung cancer (Li et al. 2009). This trial was a randomized, double-blind, placebo-controlled trial conducted on 83 patients. Forty-two of the patients received Haishengsu 2.4 mg IV in 250 cc normal saline daily for 15 days. Forty-one patients got 250 cc of normal saline intravenously for 15 days. Each was also treated with 2 cycles of conventional chemotherapy consisting of mitomycin, vindesine, and cisplatin. An improvement in the Karnofsky performance status scores was seen in 66.7% of the Hai Sheng Su group patients and in 17.1% of patients receiving placebo. In addition, the percentage of patients with no or mild gastrointestinal reactions was 83.3% of the Haishengsu group and 39% of placebo group. There was a suggestion of prolongation of life in the treatment group but it did not reach statistical significance.

Another placebo-controlled study evaluated the effect of Chinese herbal therapy on chemotherapy-induced hematological toxicities and nausea. One hundred and twenty early stage breast or colon cancer patients received either Chinese herbal medications in a packet or a placebo packet with non-therapeutic herbs. Both had a similar smell. The intervention had no effect on hematologic toxicities but did significantly decrease nausea (Mok et al. 2007). Fuzheng Yiliu Decoction was found to lower chemotherapy-associated bone marrow toxicity, however since the study was not placebo-controlled confirmation with higher quality study is warranted (Pan et al. 2005).

The Cochrane Database published a systematic review aimed at assessing the effect of herbal medicine plus chemotherapy *versus* chemotherapy alone on quality of life and adverse medication reactions. An extensive literature review was completed including hand searching of relevant Chinese journals. The authors chose randomized trials comparing chemotherapy alone or chemotherapy plus antiemetics with chemotherapy plus Chinese herbs. Four relevant trials were chosen, all of which used a decoction containing *Astragalus membranaceus* (astragalus root) compounds as the intervention. All were of low quality. A significant reduction in nausea and vomiting was found in patients given astragalus root plus chemotherapy as compared to those given chemotherapy alone. A decreased rate of leucopenia was observed in the treatment groups as well as increases in the proportions of T-lymphocyte subsets CD3, CD4 and CD8. The authors concluded that despite the low quality of the studies, the aggregate results suggested that decoctions of astragalus root compounds may stimulate immunocompetent cells and decrease side effects in patients treated with chemotherapy. They noted that no evidence of harm was found but higher quality studies are needed (Taixiang et al. 2005).

13.4.3 Radiation

Panax ginseng (ginseng) has been widely used in TCM as a tonic, immunomodulating agent and antimutagenic, as well as for its antiaging properties. Many of ginseng's effects are attributed to the triterpine glycosides known as ginsenosides (saponins), which are felt to scavenge the free radicals that are responsible for cellular DNA damage. This antioxidative capability may have radioprotective effects. Whole ginseng appears to give better radioprotection than do the isolated ginsenoside fractions (Lee et al. 2005). Radiation mucositis is a common, distressing side effect of radiotherapy, especially to the head and neck. Western treatments, such as oral rinses, are only moderately effective at relieving symptoms. Wu et al. (2007) randomized 60 patients to radiation plus Qingre Liyan Decoction or radiation plus Dobell's Solution, which served as the control. Most patients were treated for 6 weeks. The patients in the intervention group had a statistically significant lower incidence of radiation mucositis as well as increased serum levels of CD4 and CD8. The authors hypothesized that a Decoction of Qingre Liyan may decrease radiation mucositis by enhancing the patient's immunity.

13.5 Improving Prognosis

13.5.1 Increase Potency of Chemotherapy

In addition to helping patients maximize their quality of life and minimize toxic side effects of Western oncology treatments, integrating Chinese and Western medicine may improve survival outcomes. A meta-analysis of 34 studies using astragalus root combined with platinum-based chemotherapy for advanced non-small cell lung cancer showed promising results. Twelve studies (940 patients) showed a reduced risk of death at 12 months and 30 studies (2,472 patients) showed improved tumour response. The authors concluded that astragalus-based Chinese herbal medicine may increase the effectiveness of platinum-based chemotherapy, but they noted that confirmation with rigorously controlled studies is warranted (McCulloch et al. 2006).

13.5.2 Enhance Immune Function

The development of a clinically apparent cancer is due, in part, to the failure of the immune system to adequately recognize and dispose of the initial malignant cells. Thus, cancer can be seen as an immune system failure. The ideal oncologic treatment would not only attack the cancer directly, it would support the immune system's efforts to eliminate any stray malignant cells.

Western cancer treatments focus primarily on damaging the tumour by impacting tumour blood flow, cell division and other vital survival functions. Very little, if any, attention is paid to enhancing immune function. Many traditional Chinese herbs, on the other hand, appear to support immune function. Combining tumour destruction with immune system enhancement epitomizes the integration of Western and Chinese medicine.

Dendritic cells are antigen-presenting cells that play a role in the initiation and regulation of immune responses. Chen et al. (2006) reviewed published studies of TCM's effect on dendritic cells. They found that various Chinese herbal therapies have the capacity to inhibit or promote major functions of the dendritic cells, such as differentiation, maturation, cytokine production, survival, antigen uptake and antigen presentation. Accumulating evidence indicates that many of TCM's clinical effects can be attributed to the up or down regulation of immune responses such as these. Curcumin, the principle component of *Curcuma longa* (common turmeric), has also been shown to affect cytokine production, humoral and cell mediated immunity, and antigen presentation (Gautam et al. 2007).

Ganoderma lucidum (lucid ganoderma) is a medicinal mushroom that is widely used in China for health promotion. A review of the literature performed by Yuen and Gohel (2005) found three trials, two randomized and one non-randomized, showing that lucid ganoderma enhanced cellular immune responses in cancer patients. In one study it also improved quality of life in 65% of patients. A Decoction of Wuye has been shown to improve immune parameters in patients with non-small cell lung cancer. Eighty-two patients who had completed operative treatment and chemotherapy for their lung cancer were randomly assigned to receive Wuye Decoction or no herb. Levels of CD4, CD16, CD19 and CD4/CD8 were measured. Both groups had depressed immune cell volume as would be expected after chemotherapy. However in the group given the Wuye Decoction all of the measured immune parameters increased to near-normal levels. In the control group immune parameters remained low (Zheng et al. 2006).

Astragalus root is a common Chinese herb with well-documented immunomodulating properties. Cho and Leung (2007a, b) isolated a potent bioactive fraction from astragalus root that demonstrated varied immune stimulating actions, both *in vitro* and *in vivo*. Specifically, macrophage volume and phagocytic activity were increased, interleukin-2 expression was enhanced and mouse model tumours were suppressed. A decoction containing astragalus root and *Angelica sinensis* (Chinese angelica root) induced secretion of interleukin-2 (Gao et al. 2006) and astragalus root alone was found to regulate macrophage immune responses (Clement-Kruzel et al. 2008). A meta-analysis designed to evaluate the efficacy of astragalus root combined with chemotherapy in non-small cell lung cancer suggested that the combination may be more efficacious than chemotherapy alone. An extensive literature search revealed 1,305 relevant publications of which 34 studies (2,815 patients) met inclusion criteria. Thirty studies revealed improved tumour response and twelve showed increased survival at 1 year (McCulloch et al. 2006).

13.5.3 Attack Cancer Directly

Many Chinese herbs have multiple actions. *Glycyrrhiza uralensis* (licorice root), one of the oldest and most frequently used botanicals, has several known effects, including inducing apoptosis in cancer cells and protection against carcinogen-induced DNA damage (Wang and Nixon 2001). Another common botanical, *Rheum palumatum* (rhubarb), has several bioactive antineoplastic anthraquinones. The most abundant one, emodin, was found to be capable of inhibiting cellular proliferation, inducing apoptosis and preventing metastasis (Huang et al. 2007).

Mushrooms such as *Coriolus versicolor* (multicolored polypore) have been found to inhibit cancer growth (Chu et al. 2002) as have multiple herbs (Thatte et al. 2000) such as *Artemisia annua* (sweet wormwood herb) (Efferth 2006).

Several studies have investigated the use of TCM for hepatocellular carcinoma. A meta-analysis of 26 studies (2,079 patients) showed a statistically significant increase in survival for those who used TCM plus chemotherapy compared to those who used chemotherapy alone. However the trials were of low quality and confirmation with large, quality studies is needed (Shu et al. 2005). Another meta-analysis reviewed the efficacy and safety of TCM plus transcatheter arterial chemoembolization (TACE) for patients with unresectable hepatocellular carcinoma. An extensive literature review yielded 37 trials with 2,653 patients. The combination improved survival, quality of life, symptoms and tumour response. No serious events were reported (Meng et al. 2008). Another meta-analysis reviewing TACE with or without Chinese herbal therapy for hepatocellular carcinoma arrived at a similar conclusion (Cho and Chen 2009a). These same authors performed a meta-analysis of TCM plus conventional therapy *versus* conventional therapy alone for nasopharyngeal carcinoma. Eighteen controlled trials (1,732 patients) met inclusion criteria and six of them reported improved tumour response in the combination group (Cho and Chen 2009b).

13.6 Improve Quality of Life

Western oncologic treatment modalities may prolong life, but they usually worsen its quality, at least temporarily. The aggressiveness and toxicity of surgery, chemotherapy and radiation leave many patients fatigued, nauseous and debilitated. Chinese herbs such as Fuzheng Yiliu Decoction (Pan et al. 2005) and Shenfu Preparation (Wu et al. 2006) have been shown to improve performance status and quality of life in patients undergoing Western cancer treatments.

Piao et al. (2004) performed a prospective, randomized controlled trial of *Viscum album* (European mistletoe) extract in patients with breast, ovarian and non-small cell lung cancer. Two hundred and twenty four patients were randomized to receive standardized mistletoe extract or lentinan, an anti-tumour polysaccharide from the *Lentinus edodes* (Shiitake mushroom). The lentinan group served as a control. All patients received chemotherapy. Quality of life was significantly improved in patients getting mistletoe as determined by approved quality of life assessments such as the Functional Living Index – Cancer and the Karnofsky Performance Index, in comparison to the control group. In addition, the occurrence of adverse events was lower in the mistletoe group than in the control group, although there were several mild side effects and one serious side effect of angioedema.

Pain is a common side effect of advanced cancer that negatively affects quality of life. Western therapeutics for pain tends to have significant side effects, including somnolence, which may worsen quality of life. Chinese herbal medicine has been used extensively to treat cancer pain and there is some evidence that botanicals can both decrease pain and reduce the side effects of Western analgesics. A large review of 115 articles evaluated multiple Chinese herbal medicine modalities including oral administration, intravenous infusion, inhalation and external application. Forty-one of the studies were randomized and controlled. Both Chinese and English studies were evaluated. The authors assessed that TCM may be effective for cancer pain and may reduce the side effects of Western analgesics. Multiple modalities (topical, oral and IV) can be used. As is often the case, the quality of the studies was variable (Xu et al. 2007).

Acupuncture is another effective tool for increasing quality of life in patients undergoing Western cancer treatments. One small pilot study of acupuncture for the treatment of cancer-related menopausal symptoms in tamoxifen treated patients showed a positive effect. The patients were evaluated using the Greene Menopause Index before treatment began and again at 1, 3 and 6 months. Anxiety, depression and vasomotor symptoms improved but libido did not. However larger, randomized, controlled studies are needed to confirm this preliminary result (Porzio et al. 2002).

13.7 Cancer Prevention

Preventing a cancer is preferable to treating it after it has become established. Western medicine attempts to prevent certain cancers, such as cervical cancer and colon cancer, by identifying pre-cancerous lesions using common screening tests such as PAP smear and colonoscopy. Yet there are many cancers for which effective prevention strategies have yet to be developed.

Traditional Chinese medicine may be a helpful adjunct to Western medicine in the prevention of certain cancers. A double-blind placebo-controlled study was done to evaluate this possibility. Fifty-nine patients with oral leukoplakia were randomly assigned to receive an intervention consisting of a mixed tea product plus a topical treatment developed by the authors or a placebo drink and topical glycerin treatment. After 6 months the size of the lesion decreased in 37.9% of the 29 intervention patients and increased in 3.4%. In the control group only 10% of the lesions decreased in size and 6.7% increased. Pathologic indices also indicated decreased cell proliferation in the intervention group (Li et al. 1999).

13.8 Risks of Integrating Chinese and Western Medicine

Chinese medicine, while generally gentler than Western medicine, does carry some risk. Both acupuncture and Chinese medicinals have caused significant complications, some of which have been fatal.

Some patients might choose Chinese herbal treatments over Western allopathic treatments because they believe that natural therapies are without risk. Despite the general safety of TCM treatments, this assumption is invalid. A new renal disease called Chinese-herb nephropathy has been recognized and side effects have occasionally been severe. Nortier and Vanherweghem (2002) described cases of severe nephrotoxicity in patients who ingested weight loss remedies containing *Aristolochia fangchi* (Guangfangji). They developed significant atrophy of the proximal tubules requiring dialysis or transplant. Just as with Western pharmaceuticals, toxicities resulting from Chinese medicinals may be secondary to inadequate testing, unintentional contamination, inappropriate prescribing or due to the properties of the individual herb or formula.

Acupuncture can, rarely, cause complications such as infection, syncope, local hematoma, and pneumothorax (Lao et al. 2003). Many of the serious complications can be attributed to poor technique or substandard practices, such as using nonsterile acupuncture needles. Since pneumothorax is a recognized complication of acupuncture, attention should be paid to the baseline respiratory status of the patient. Patients with end stage lung cancer and underlying chronic obstructive pulmonary disease (COPD) might not have the pulmonary reserve to tolerate such a complication. Acupuncture violates the integrity of the skin and therefore caution should be used in patients with bleeding diatheses or severely compromised immune systems. Patients with hematologic cancers or those undergoing aggressive chemotherapy may be significantly hemo- or immuno-compromised and thus might be at increased risk of bleeding or infection. Skin that has been radiated may be more sensitive to complications of acupuncture, and if possible, these areas should be avoided. In addition since deep vein thrombosis and pulmonary embolism are more common in cancer patients, practitioners should screen for anticoagulant use prior to starting treatment. Coumadin is generally considered a contraindication to acupuncture. Despite these cautions, acupuncture is considered safe for most patients with cancer. Table 13.1 lists conditions that increase the risk for serious acupuncture complications.

Chinese medicinals have more potential risks than do acupuncture or qigong. Botanicals and other TCM agents may cause direct effects such as fatigue, dizziness and stomach upset, as well as exacerbating presenting symptoms if an inaccurate TCM diagnosis is made. These symptoms may be misinterpreted as pharmaceutical side effects if the patient has recently started a new medication. Chinese medicinals can also interact with Western pharmaceuticals or cause IgE mediated allergic reactions. And they have, on occasion, been adulterated with Western medications, tainted with toxins or heavy metals or been found to have inconsistent levels of the herbs they claim to contain. Some Chinese medicinals, such as arsenic, have intrinsic toxic properties.

Table 13.1 Conditions increasing risk for serious acupuncture complications

Condition	Risk
Severe underlying lung disease such as extensive lung cancer, chronic obstructive pulmonary disease or poorly controlled asthma	Pulmonary compromise in the event of pneumothorax (White 2004)
Peripheral neuropathy such as that caused by some chemotherapy regimens	Burns resulting from moxibustion (MacPherson et al. 2001)
Skin with radiation damage	Risk of poor wound healing (Hill et al. 2004)
Bleeding diathesis due to bone marrow dysfunction	Bleeding (Witt et al. 2009)
Severe immunocompromise	Infection (White 2004)

Equally concerning is the risk that a patient will choose TCM over Western medicine for a serious ailment when an effective Western treatment is available. A patient with early stage breast cancer, for example, would be at great risk if she took an herbal formula rather than pursuing surgical excision of the cancer. It is thus important for Chinese medicine practitioners to be able to recognize life-threatening illnesses for which there are Western cures, and refer to their Western colleagues when appropriate. If a patient has recently had a medical procedure or taken a Western pharmaceutical, the TCM practitioner must be alert for complications. Some complications, such as headache, may be appropriately treated with Chinese medicine, while others, such as wound infection or hives, may require a return visit to the Western physician or discontinuation of the therapy. A patient who presents to an inexperienced TCM practitioner risks having these complications missed.

Perhaps the most controversial issue regarding the use of TCM for cancer patients is the question of whether herbal formulae can be safely used concomitantly with chemotherapy and radiation. The primary concern verbalized by Western doctors is that Chinese herbal medicines may decrease the effectiveness of radiotherapy and Western oncologic medications. Chemotherapy is often presumed to work via the creation of oxygen free radicals which damage cancer cells and impair their reproduction. The use of herbs, many of which have antioxidant properties, may interfere with this action. Patients receiving Western cancer treatment are often instructed to avoid all herbal therapy during chemotherapy and radiation.

Free radicals are molecules with an odd, unpaired electron. These molecules are unstable and quickly react with other molecules in an effort to acquire another electron to regain stability. They accomplish this by stealing an electron from a nearby molecule, thus creating a new free radical which then steals an electron from another nearby molecule, and so on. This chain reaction can lead to tissue damage and dysfunction, age related illnesses and possibly cancer. Antioxidants are able to donate an electron to unstable free radicals without becoming unstable themselves, thus inhibiting free-radical cellular damage and stopping the negative electron-stealing reaction.

Both antioxidants and free radicals are normally present in the body and a careful balance between them is required. Radiotherapy and chemotherapy generate increased free radicals, potentially damaging both normal and malignant tissues. Some cancer patients may already be antioxidant deficient making them more susceptible to the negative effects of free radicals. Thus, the risk-benefit equation is as follows: does the oncologist want the patient to be antioxidant deficient in order to increase the free radical damage to both the cancer and healthy tissues? Or is it preferable to have the tissue support of antioxidants while the patient undergoes free radical-inducing radiation and chemotherapy? Definitive answers to these questions are lacking.

Oncologists are primarily interested in maximizing tissue damage in an effort to eradicate the malignancy under treatment. There is some evidence to support this position. A recent review published in the Journal of the National Cancer Institute assesses the conflicting evidence regarding antioxidant use with chemotherapy and radiation (Lawenda et al. 2008). The authors acknowledge the controversy and mention several randomized clinical trials that have demonstrated that taking antioxidants concurrent with radiation or chemotherapy may reduce treatment-related side effects. They note that some data indicate that antioxidants may protect normal tissues from chemotherapy or radiation induced damage without decreasing tumour control. Yet after their review of the evidence, the authors conclude that the use of supplemental antioxidants during chemotherapy and radiation should be discouraged because of the possibility of tumour protection and reduced survival.

The controversy remains, however, because there is published evidence that chemotherapy may not produce its effect via oxidation and that antioxidants may actually improve treatment outcomes (Block et al. 2007). In this chapter, randomized, controlled clinical trials that reported survival and/or tumour response were reviewed. Of the 845 trials considered, 19 met the inclusion criteria. Multiple antioxidant supplements (not TCM herbs) were evaluated and the subjects of most studies had advanced or relapsed disease. None of the trials reported evidence of significant decreases in efficacy from antioxidant supplementation during chemotherapy. In fact, many of the studies showed either increased survival times, increased tumour response or both. However the authors noted that lack of statistical power was a consistent limitation. A review of the literature completed by Weijl et al. (1997) suggests that chemotherapy-induced oxidation is the cause of chemotherapy side effects and toxicity, but may not be related to the drugs' ability to control cancer. Ralph Moss, a well-respected authority on alternative treatments for cancer, has reviewed and summarized hundreds of studies assessing antioxidant use in cancer treatment and interpreted the literature as a whole to be in support of its use (Moss 2000).

The research needed to definitively evaluate the safety of antioxidant herbal therapy during chemotherapy has not yet been completed. Large, randomized, double-blind, placebo-controlled trials are needed. Until such data is available, Western physicians and Chinese practitioners will likely remain on opposite sides of this controversial issue and patients attempting to integrate the two modalities into their cancer care will need to participate fully in their treatment decisions. Patients who wish to use TCM as part of their cancer care but are concerned about the risks of using supplemental antioxidants during chemotherapy may choose a modified treatment plan (Table 13.2).

Table 13.2 Cautious use of traditional Chinese medicine with chemotherapy and radiation

Phase of treatment	Traditional Chinese medicine modalities
Pre-chemotherapy	• Chinese medicinals to address constitutional imbalances and antioxidant deficiency • Qigong and acupuncture as indicated for stress reduction and constitutional imbalances
During chemotherapy and radiation	• Avoid Chinese medicinals with antioxidant properties due to risk of decreasing effectiveness of chemotherapy and radiotherapy (Lawenda et al. 2008) • No need to restrict nutritional antioxidants or qigong • Acupuncture for chemotherapy-induced nausea and vomiting (Ezza et al. 2006), cancer pain (Alimi et al. 2003) and improved psychological well-being (Nedstrand et al. 2006)
Between chemotherapy and radiation	• Consider short course of Chinese medicinals to modify toxicity of Western therapeutics and stabilize free radicals • Continue qigong and acupuncture as indicated
Post-chemotherapy and radiation	• Restart Chinese medicinals • Continue qigong and acupuncture to treat cancer pain, treatment related side effects and improve psychological well-being

13.9 Integration Is the Way of the Future

Despite wider acceptance of Chinese medicine into Western medical spheres, a lack of true integration remains. Patients may visit both Western physicians and Chinese medicine practitioners for the same illness, often not discussing either practitioner's suggestions with the other. This is not integration. Simultaneous, yet non-integrated use of both modalities is inefficient and potentially dangerous. Herbs and pharmaceuticals may interact with each other and herb side effects may be inaccurately attributed to medications, leading to inaccurate diagnoses. True integration requires a collaborative approach whereby Western and Chinese practitioners agree on a coordinated treatment plan that is accepted by, and fully explained to, the patient. This ideal scenario faces some challenges.

Problems include a lack of consensus on treatment regimens, both Western medicine and TCM, and questions about the reliability, validity and applicability of published TCM studies. Much of the published work in TCM is in the form of anecdotal reports or uncontrolled series and many TCM therapies have been empirically applied to patients based on knowledge taken from ancient Chinese texts. Definitive research that meets Western standards is scant and therefore these important and helpful modalities have not been fully integrated into the mainstream medical community. In addition, the emphasis that Chinese medicine places on energy flow and the terms used to describe unfamiliar concepts, such as qi, are challenging for some Western physicians to understand. The inability to objectively measure qi adds to the difficulty.

Lack of adequate insurance coverage hinders many patients' access to TCM. Some insurance companies cover acupuncture but may not cover CPT codes for integrative care. Medicare and Medicaid do not cover TCM services at all.

However, despite the reluctance of some Western physicians to embrace Chinese medicine, TCM is making inroads into Western culture. A number of Chinese herbs such as ginseng, astragalus root and Chinese angelica root have become well known to the lay public and even to some conventional physicians. Many large health centers now offer some form of TCM to their patients, including acupuncture for chemotherapy-induced nausea or qigong for stress reduction. Chinese medicine practitioners are now often invited to join the faculty or staff of integrative medical centers.

Despite this increasing popularity of TCM in Western culture, most medical students know very little about the coordinated Chinese medical system. They may have a lecture on the value of acupuncture for pain control, yet they are unlikely to learn many of the terms or diagnostic modalities of Chinese medicine. The difference between Chinese and Western herbal therapies is likely to elude them, making it difficult to accept integration of these therapies into their treatment plans once they go into practice.

In recent years, more research has been done on the benefits of integrating Western and Chinese treatments for cancer, although not all studies have shown positive effects (Zhou et al. 2008). Reports of negative studies or adverse effects of TCM are often highlighted in the Western media, adding to the suspicion some physicians feel about the benefits of TCM. A product called PC-Spes, available in the US from 1997 to 2002, was beginning to gain acceptance from Western physicians before it was withdrawn from the market. PC-Spes was a patented mixture of 8 Chinese herbs thought to be useful in prostate cancer. It was found to be contaminated with prescription drugs such as DES, indomethacin and warfarin and was thus withdrawn from the market. This unfortunate event negatively affected the reputation of Chinese herbal therapy in the Western medical community. If TCM is to be effectively integrated into the Western medical consciousness, manufacturers must commit themselves to rigorous product purity.

Encouraging TCM and Western practitioners to work together is an important and achievable goal, but it is not the only way to integrate Chinese and Western modalities. Wong et al. (2003) designed an interesting study that integrated both methodologies into one treatment modality. They used a transcutaneous nerve stimulation method to mimic the action of acupuncture needles for radiation-induced xerostomia. The stimulation was applied over pre-selected acupuncture points, according to TCM principles. Xerostomia was assessed by questionnaire and direct measurement of saliva in response to citric acid. Forty-six patients were treated and significant improvement in xerostomia was shown over 3 and 6 months. There were no complications. The lack of a control group is a significant weakness of the study, thus validation of the efficacy of this intervention is needed.

Literature reviews have been published that attempt to evaluate the efficacy of Chinese medicinal herbs in the adjunctive treatment of cancer. One such review, published in 2007 in the Cochrane Database, evaluated the safety and efficacy of Chinese herbs in alleviating chemotherapy-related side effects in breast cancer patients. The authors performed an extensive review of the literature and found 7 randomized controlled trials involving 542 breast cancer patients (Zhang et al. 2007). All studies were conducted and published in China. Each study evaluated Chinese herbs plus chemotherapy *versus* chemotherapy alone, however no more than 2 studies used the same intervention. The studies were assessed by the authors to be of low quality. This review did not show a consistent therapeutic effect, however that is not surprising since the studies did not use consistent herbal therapies. It is hard to imagine a Western literature review that would attempt to evaluate the effects of diverse and unrelated pharmaceuticals.

Chinese and Western researchers must work together to identify the most promising herbal formulae and then rigorously test them with large, well-designed studies. Attempting to evaluate TCM as a whole is unproductive. Just as Western medicines should not be accepted or rejected en masse, we must uncover which of TCM's tools are most beneficial to cancer patients and then learn to effectively integrate them into Western cancer treatment.

An important partnership is evolving between Western and Chinese medicine in cancer care. Western physicians surgically remove malignancies and aggressively attack tumours with powerful procedures and pharmaceuticals. They may save lives, but often leave their patients fatigued and depleted. Chinese medicine practitioners, although unable to cure advanced cancers, attempt to correct imbalances that predispose patients to cancer, stimulate the immune system and ameliorate the side effects of radiation, chemotherapy and surgery.

Western physicians and TCM practitioners each have a valuable place at the table.

References

Alimi D, Rubino C, Pichard-Léandri E et al. Analgesic effect of auricular acupuncture for cancer pain: a randomized, blinded, controlled trial. J Clin Oncol. 2003;21:4120–6.

Block KJ, Koch AC, Mead MN et al. Impact of antioxidant supplementation on chemotherapeutic efficacy: a systematic review of the evidence from randomized controlled trials. Cancer Treat Rev. 2007;33:407–18.

Chang R. Bioactive polysaccharides from traditional Chinese medicine herbs as anticancer adjuvants. J Altern Complement Med. 2002;8:559–65.

Chen X, Yang L, Howard OM et al. Dendritic cells as a pharmacological target of traditional Chinese medicine. Cell Mol Immunol. 2006;3:401–10.

Cho WC, Chen HY. Transcatheter arterial chemoembolization combined with or without Chinese herbal therapy for hepatocellular carcinoma: meta-analysis. Expert Opin Investig Drugs. 2009a;18:617–635.

Cho WC, Chen HY. Clinical efficacy of traditional Chinese medicine as a concomitant therapy for nasopharyngeal carcinoma: a systematic review and meta-analysis. Cancer Invest. 2009b;27:334–44.

Cho WC, Leung KN. *In vitro* and *in vivo* anti-tumor effects of *Astragalus membranaceus*. Cancer Lett. 2007a;252:43–54.

Cho WC, Leung KN. *In vitro* and *in vivo* immunomodulating and immunorestorative effects of *Astragalus membranaceus*. J Ethnopharmacol. 2007b;113:132–41.

Chu KK, Ho SS, Chow AH. Coriolus versicolor: a medicinal mushroom with promising immunotherapeutic values. J Clin Pharmacol. 2002;42:976–84.

Clement-Kruzel S, Hwang SA, Kruzel MC et al. Immune modulation of macrophage pro-inflammatory response by goldenseal and Astragalus extracts. J Med Food. 2008;11:493–8.

Dang W, Yang J. Clinical study on acupuncture treatment of stomach carcinoma pain. J Tradit Chin Med. 1998;18:31–8.

Efferth T. Molecular pharmacology and pharmacogenomics of artemisinin and its derivatives in cancer cells. Curr Drug Targets. 2006;7:407–21.

Endo S, Nishida T, Nishikawa K et al. Dai-kenchu-to, a Chinese herbal medicine, improves stasis of patients with total gastrectomy and jejunal pouch interposition. Am J Usrg. 2006;192:9–13.

Ezza J, Streitberger K, Schneider A. Cochrane systematic reviews examine P6 acupuncture-point stimulation for nausea and vomiting. J Altern Complement Med. 2006;12:489–95.

Gao QT, Cheung JK, Li J et al. A Chinese herbal decoction, Danggui Buxue Tang, prepared from *Radix Astragali* and *Radix Angelicae Sinensis* stimulates the immune responses. Planta Med. 2006;72:1227–31.

Gautam SC, Gao X, Dulchavsky S. Immunomodulation by curcumin. Adv Exp Med Biol. 2007;595:321–41.

Hill A, Hanson M, Bogle MA et al. Severe radiation dermatitis is related to Staphylococcus aureus. Am J Clin Oncol. 2004;27:361–3.

Huang O, Lu G, Shen HM et al. Anti-cancer properties of anthraquinones from rhubarb. Med Res Rev. 2007;27:609–30.

Lao L, Hamilton G, Fu J et al. Is acupuncture safe? A systematic review of case reports. Altern Ther. 2003;9:72–83.

Lawenda BD, Kelly KM, Ladas EJ et al. Should supplemental antioxidant administration be avoided during chemotherapy and radiation therapy? J Natl Cancer Inst. 2008;100:773–83.

Lee A, Fan LT. Stimulation of the wrist acupuncture point P6 for preventing postoperative nausea and vomiting. Cochrane Database Syst Rev. 2009;2:CD003281.

Lee MS, Chen KW, Sancier KM et al. Qigong for cancer treatment: a systematic review of controlled clinical trials. Acta Oncol. 2007;46:717–22.

Lee TK, Johnke RM, Allison RR et al. Radioprotective potential of ginseng. Mutagenesis. 2005;20:237–43.

Li GY, Yu XM, Shang HW et al. Haishengsu as an adjunct therapy to conventional chemotherapy in patients with non-small cell lung cancer: a pilot randomized and placebo-controlled clinical trial. Complement Ther Med. 2009;17:51–5.

Li N, Sun Z, Han C et al. The chemopreventive effects of tea on human oral precancerous mucosa lesions. Proc Soc Exp Biol Med. 1999;220:218–24.

MacPherson H, Thomas K, Walters S et al. A prospective survey of adverse events and treatment reactions following 34,000 consultations with professional acupuncturists. Acupunct Med. 2001;19:93–102.

McCulloch M, See C, Shu XJ et al. Astragalus-based Chinese herbs and platinum-based chemotherapy for advanced non-small-cell lung cancer: meta-analysis of randomized trials. J Clin Oncol. 2006;24:419–30.

Meng MB, Cul YL, Guan YS et al. Traditional Chinese medicine plus transcatheter arterial chemoembolization for unresectable hepatocellular carcinoma. J Altern Complement Med. 2008;14:1027–42.

Mok TS, Yeo W, Johnson PJ et al. A double-blind placebo-controlled randomized study of Chinese herbal medicine as complementary therapy for reduction of chemotherapy-induced toxicity. Ann Oncol. 2007;18:768–74.

Moss RW. Antioxidants against cancer. New York: Equinox Press; 2000.

Nedstrand E, Wyon Y, Hammar M et al. Psychological well-being improves in women with breast cancer after treatment with applied relaxation or electro-acupuncture for vasomotor symptom. J Psychosom Obstet Gynaecol. 2006;27:193–9.

Nortier JL, Vanherweghem JL. Renal interstitial fibrosis and urothelial carcinoma associated with the use of a Chinese herb (*Aristolochia fangchi*). Toxicology. 2002;181–2:577–80.

Oh B, Butow P, Mullan B et al. Medical qigong for cancer patients: pilot study of impact on quality of life, side effects of treatment and inflammation. Am J Chin Med. 2008;36:459–72.

Pan B, Cheng T, Nan KJ et al. Effect of Fuzheng Yiliu Decoction combined with chemotherapy on patients with intermediate and late stage gastrointestinal cancer. World J Gastroenterol. 2005;11:439–42.

Piao BK, Wang YX, Xie GR et al. Impact of complementary mistletoe extract treatment on quality of life in breast, ovarian and non-small cell lung cancer patients. A prospective randomized controlled clinical trial. Anticancer Res. 2004;24:303–9.

Porzio G, Trapasso T, Martelli S et al. Acupuncture in the treatment of menopause-related symptoms in women taking tamoxifen. Tumori. 2002;88:128–30.

Shu X, McCulloch M, Xiao H et al. Chinese herbal medicine and chemotherapy in the treatment of hepatocellular carcinoma: a meta-analysis of randomized controlled trials. Integr Cancer Ther. 2005;4:219–29.

Suehiro T, Matsumata T, Shikada Y et al. The effect of the herbal medicines dai-kenchu-to and keishi-bukuryo-gan on bowel movements after colorectal surgery. Hepatogastroenterology. 2005;52:97–100.

Taixiang W, Munro AJ, Guanlian L. Chinese medical herbs for chemotherapy side effects in colorectal cancer patients. Cochrane Database Syst Rev. 2005;1:CD004540.

Tan KY, Liu CB, Chen AH et al. The role of traditional Chinese medicine in colorectal cancer treatment. Tech Coloproctol. 2008;12:1–6.

Thatte U, Bagadey S, Dahanukar S. Modulation of programmed cell death by medicinal plants. Cell Mol Biol. 2000;46:199–214.

Wang ZY, Nixon DW. Licorice and cancer. Nutr Cancer. 2001;39:1–11.

Weijl NI, Cleton J, Osanto S. Free radicals and antioxidants in chemotherapy-induced toxicity. Cancer Treat Rev. 1997;23:209–40.

White A. A cumulative review of the range and incidence of significant adverse events associated with acupuncture. Acupuncture Med. 2004;22:122–33.

Witt CM, Pach D, Brinkhaus B et al. Safety of acupuncture; results of a prospective observational study with 229,230 patients and introduction of a medical information and consent form. Forsch Komplementmed. 2009;16:91–7.

Wong RK, Jones GW, Sagar SM et al. A Phase I–II study in the use of acupuncture-like transcutaneous nerve stimulation in the treatment of radiation-induced xerostomia in head-and-neck cancer patients treated with radical radiotherapy. Int J Radiat Oncol Biol Phys. 2003;57:472–80.

Wu MH, Yuan B, Liu OF et al. Study of Qingre Liyan Decoction in treating and preventing acute radioactive oral mucositis. Chin J Integr Med. 2007;13:280–4.

Wu WY, Long SQ, Shang HB et al. Improvement of quality of life with Shenfu injection in non small cell lung cancer patients treated with gemcitabine plus cisplatin regimen. Chin J Integr Med. 2006;12:50–4.

Xu L, Lao LX, Ge A et al. Chinese herbal medicine for cancer pain. Integr Cancer Ther. 2007;6:208–34.

Yeh ML, Lee TI, Chen HH et al. The influences of Chan-Chuang qi-gong therapy on complete blood cell counts in breast cancer patients treated with chemotherapy. Cancer Nurs. 2006;29:149–55.

Yuen JW, Gohel MD. Anticancer effects of *Ganoderma lucidum*: a review of scientific evidence. Nutr Cancer. 2005;53:11–17.

Zhang M, Liu X, Li J et al. Chinese medicinal herbs to treat the side-effects of chemotherapy in breast cancer patients. Cochrane Database Syst Rev. 2007;2:CD004921.

Zheng SL, Yang OS, Ma XH. Effect of Wuye Decoction on lymphocyte phenotype in patients with non-small cell lung cancer. Chin J Integr Med. 2006;12:118–21.

Zhou Y, Li N, Zhuang W et al. Green tea and gastric cancer risk: meta-analysis of epidemiologic studies. Asia Pac J Clin Nutr. 2008;17:159–65.

Chapter 14
Traditional Chinese Medicine in the Prevention and Treatment of Cancer Disease: A Review of the Evidence

Jianping Liu, Xun Li, Huijuan Cao, and Torkel Snellingen

Abstract During the past decades, studies have suggested that traditional Chinese medicine (TCM) may be effective for the prevention of cancer and cancer-related health problems. For primary prevention one systematic review demonstrated a potential benefit of green tea consumption for cancer prevention especially for gastrointestinal cancers. A meta-analysis involving 4,654 patients with high-grade esophageal epithelial cells hyperplasia found herbal medicines more effective than placebo in preventing esophageal cancer. Another review evaluated herbal medicine for gastric cancer prevention in people with precancerous lesions and showed beneficial effect of Chinese medicine from 3 randomized trials. For secondary and tertiary prevention 21 and 28 randomized trials were identified respectively with the majority of the trials reported positive findings in the alleviation of symptoms of the side effects of treatment, recurrence of disease and metastasis from primary tumour. Although there were beneficial effects from Chinese medicine for prevention of cancer or cancer-related complications, we found significant heterogeneity in the meta-analyses and there were severe limitations due to poor methodological quality of the included studies. Few observational studies were found. Future studies of TCM for the prevention and treatment of cancer need to be more rigorous in study design using existing guidelines such as the CONSORT Statement. More studies should be designed as observational cohort studies to better reflect the nature of TCM treatment modalities.

14.1 Introduction

More than 2 million new cancer cases were diagnosed in 1997. One in every four deaths in the United States – approximately 550,000 individuals per year – is the result of cancer (National Cancer Institute Cancer Prevention Program Review

J. Liu (✉)
Centre for Evidence Based Chinese Medicine, Beijing University of Chinese Medicine, Beijing, China
e-mail: jpliutcm@yahoo.co.uk

W.C.S. Cho (ed.), *Supportive Cancer Care with Chinese Medicine*,
DOI 10.1007/978-90-481-3555-4_14,

Group 1997). World Health Organization (WHO) has reported that cancer killed 7.6 million people in 2005, yet 40% of all cancer deaths can be prevented (WHO 2007).

WHO has urged the member states in the 58th World Health Assembly to give priority also to research on cancer prevention, early detection and management strategies, including, where appropriate, traditional medicines and therapies, including for palliative care (WHO 2005).

Prevention of cancer disease is divided into three categories, namely primary, secondary and tertiary prevention (Haas et al. 2001). Primary prevention consists of health promotion activities which focus on protecting against the occurrence of cancer. Secondary prevention refers to health behaviors that promote early detection, early treatment, and prevention of cancer in high risk populations such as people with pre-cancerous conditions. Tertiary prevention seeks to minimize disability, protect cancer patients against suffering from complications, and help patients to live well (Linda 2009).

Allopathic medical practitioners provide advice and various interventions that are believed to be based on sound laboratory and clinical research. On the other hand, complementary and alternative medicine (CAM) is believed to lack scientific evidence for their claimed effectiveness. However, CAM practices are becoming more widely employed.

As one of the mainstream of CAM therapies, traditional Chinese medicine (TCM) is a 3,000-year-old holistic system of medicine, including medicinal herbs, acupuncture, food therapy, massage and therapeutic exercise for both prevention and treatment of diseases (Fulder 1996). Emphasizing the holistic harmonization of human body and strengthening the body itself in order to fight against the "evil", TCM regards the capability of treating diseases before they happen as of the highest value. Based on the theory of TCM, Chinese medicine practice addresses ZhiWeiBing, meaning treating pre-disease conditions and preventing the deterioration of existing diseases through balancing yin and yang and promoting self-healing ability of human body.

14.2 Chinese Medicine Used for Prevention of Cancer

Chinese medicine practitioners use herbal decoction, Chinese patent medicine, acupuncture, therapeutic exercise and other treatment modalities according to the theory of syndrome differentiation to prevent cancer at the primary, secondary and tertiary levels.

For primary prevention of cancer disease, TCM practitioners include consultation on lifestyle, diet, and physical exercises. For secondary prevention, TCM interventions target persons with precancerous lesions having high risk of developing cancer.

For tertiary prevention, different TCM therapies can be applied to improve survival and quality of life by treating the side effects of chemo/radiotherapy-related symptoms in cancer patients such as pain, nausea and vomiting. TCM is also used to prevent the recurrence of metastasis of cancers.

14.3 Information Resources of the Evidence Summary

We searched the current literature about cancer prophylaxis related to TCM, using the searching words as precancerous (Aiqian), prevention/prophylaxis (Yufang), herbal medicine (Zhongyao), Chinese medicine (Zhongyi), Chinese medicine (Zhongyiyao), herbal medicine (Zhongcaoyao), medicinal herb (Caoyao), needle/acupuncture (Zhen), moxibustion (Jiu) in searching PubMed, the Cochrane Library (Issue 1, 2009), EMBASE, CINAHL, China National Knowledge Information (CNKI), Chinese Biological Medicine (CBM), Chinese Scientific Journal Database (VIP) and WanFang Database, the authors totally retrieved 514 Chinese publications and 302 publications in other languages.

14.4 Selection Criteria

Excluding the duplication of the publications, we included papers according to the following criteria: Study design should include (1) systematic review or meta-analysis related to TCM for cancer prevention; (2) randomized clinical trial (RCT). We excluded non-randomized clinical trial (CCT), or observational studies such as case-control study.

Participants included healthy people for the primary prophylaxis, people with precancerous conditions confirmed by histopathological examination for the secondary prophylaxis, and cancer patients received chemo/radiotherapy or/and surgery for tertiary prophylaxis of adverse effects, complications, or relapse or metastasis.

Interventions include all kinds of TCM therapies defined as herbal decoction, Chinese patent medicine, herbal extracts, acupuncture and moxibustion; control may include no intervention, placebo, or any non-TCM interventions; We included studies reporting outcome such as survival and quality of life indicators, any biochemical indicators that can predict prognosis of cancer, or complications of cancer such as recurrence rate, metastasis, or prevention of adverse effects of chemo/radiotherapy or operation.

14.5 Summary of Evidence

14.5.1 Primary Prophylaxis

There was one systematic review demonstrating a potential benefit of green tea consumption on cancer prevention especially gastrointestinal cancers (Liu et al. 2008).

The studies included were clinical trials and observational studies and excluded were in vitro and animal studies. Forty-one epidemiological studies, 3 randomized trials, and 1 meta-analysis were identified that investigated green tea in prevention of cancer. There was lack of randomized trials following up the participants till incidence of cancer. The findings were not consistent across all studies although some studies showed that green tea had benefit in reducing the risk of gastrointestinal cancers when comparing among green tea-drinkers to non-drinkers, or highly consuming drinkers to low consuming drinkers. Thirty-three out of 48 studies showed significant benefits. The positive findings were mainly from women who were drinking green tea in large amount. However, the author also mentioned that the benefit claim needed to be confirmed in large and long term cohort studies and clinical trials. Potential known or unknown factors and heterogeneity in green tea such as quality of product, frequency, quantity and duration of drinking, diet, environment and populations may influence the positive findings or interpret inconsistent results among studies. Drinking green tea appeared safe at regular, habitual and moderate use.

No clinical trial or epidemiological study related to other TCM for primary prophylaxis was found.

14.5.2 Secondary Prophylaxis

A meta-analysis published in 1998 included 6 randomized trials that included 4,654 patients with high-grade esophageal epithelial cell hyperplasia (Chen et al. 1998). The study found Chinese patent medicines more effective than placebo in preventing esophageal cancer. This was the earliest meta-analysis we could find published in Chinese about TCM for secondary prevention in a high risk population. It demonstrated that use of Chinese patent medicines reduced the canceration rate (i.e. absolute risk reduction, ARR, 6.13%, 95% CI 4.56–7.69) as compared with placebo in people with the precancerous lesions which were believed to be the predecessor of esophageal cancer. However, in the included 6 RCTs, 3 were conducted in the same area in China, and 2 studies were published by the same authors (Hou et al. 1992a, b, 1996), and have not been confirmed by other researchers. Therefore, publication bias may not be excluded.

Another meta-analysis of 3 randomized trials (153 receiving Chinese medicine and 137 control) evaluated herbal medicine for prevention of gastric cancer in people with precancerous lesions and found Chinese medicine more effective than control intervention (folic acid and sivyer in 1 trial, and Vitacoenzyme tablets in another 2 trials) (Liu and Zhang 2005). However, the author stated that the three included trials were of low methodological quality, so that the conclusion should be taken with caution.

A systematic review demonstrated a significant decrease of 8-hydroxydeoxyguanosine by green tea polyphenols intake compared with placebo in 124 individuals with sero-positive HBsAg and aflatoxin-albumin adducts (Chen et al. 1998). Green tea catechins could significantly reduce the incidence of prostate cancer in a group of 60 volunteers with high-grade prostate intraepithelial neoplasia compared with placebo.

In total, 21 randomized clinical trials included secondary prophylaxis of cancer (Table 14.1). They all tested TCM interventions for precancerous lesions, including chronic atrophic gastritis (CAG) with intestinal metaphases (IM) and atypical hyperplasia (ATP), cirrhosis, or esophageal epitheliosis. Among the trials, 8 trials applied herbal decoction, 12 applied Chinese patent medicines, 1 on Kampo medicine (originated from Chinese herbal medicine Xiaochaihu Decoction). The treatment duration varied from 5 days to 5 years (average 13.2 ±1 9.5 months), with 4 trials unspecified. The preventive effect was highly significant according to the trial reports. In majority of the trials, usual care was tested as comparator, defined as routine procedures that were used to manage health-related problems, yet having not been proved to be effective for prevention of cancer in rigorous studies.

Table 14.1 Summary of Chinese herbal interventions for secondary prophylaxis for cancer in RCTs

Study	Participants, T/C	Intervention (duration)	Control	Main finding (*P*-value)
Wei et al. (1998)	CAG with IM/ATP, 31/29	Weiansu capsule (3–6 months)	Usual care	Histo/pathological changes (IM, ATP) ($P < 0.05$)
Kan et al. (1999)	CAG with IM/ATP, 49/34	Yangyin Rongwei decoction (3 months)	Usual care	Histo/pathological changes (IM, ATP) ($P < 0.05$)
Yao et al. (1999)	CAG with IM/ATP, 50/50	Weisuokang (3 months)	Usual care	Histo/pathological changes (IM, ATP) ($P < 0.05$)
Liu et al. (2000)	CAG with IM/ATP, 84/36	Weiyanqing (2 months)	Usual care	Histo/pathological changes (IM, ATP) ($P < 0.001$)
Tian and Xu (2000)	CAG with IM/ATP, 75/30	Modified Shenyi decoction (2 months)	Usual care	Histo/pathological changes (IM, ATP) ($P < 0.05$)
Chen et al. (2002)	CAG with IM/ATP 30/30	Weier Fang	Usual care	Histo/pathological changes (IM, ATP) ($P < 0.05$)
Li (2004)	CAG with IM/ATP, 61/36	Qilian Shupi powder (3 months)	Usual care	Histo/pathological changes (IM, ATP) ($P < 0.05$)
Mo et al. (2005)	CAG with IM/ATP, 62/62	Yiqi Yangyin Huayu decoction (3 months)	Usual care	Histo/pathological changes (IM, ATP) ($P < 0.05$)
Zhang et al. (2007)	CAG with IM/ATP, 30/30	Self-prescribed herbal decoction (2 months)	Usual care	Histo/pathological changes (IM, ATP) ($P < 0.05$)

Table 14.1 (continued)

Study	Participants, T/C	Intervention (duration)	Control	Main finding (*P*-value)
Yu et al. (2008)	CAG with IM/ATP, 120/86	Xialian Yiying decoction (3 months)	Usual care	Histo/pathological changes (IM, ATP) ($P < 0.05$)
Wang et al. (2006)	Gastric ulcer with IM/ATP, 52/50	Jiedu Huoxue decoction (3 months)	Usual care	Histo/pathological changes (IM, ATP) ($P < 0.05$)
Chen et al. (2008)	Gastric ulcer with IM/ATP, 58/57	Jiedu Huoxue powder (3 months)	Usual care	Histo/pathological changes (IM, ATP) ($P < 0.05$)
Lin et al. (1990)	Esophageal epitheliosis, 568/566	Kangai II pill	Placebo	Incidence of cancer ($P < 0.05$)
Zhang et al. (1990)	Esophageal epitheliosis, 822/826	Kangai II pill	Placebo	Incidence of cancer ($P < 0.01$)
Hou et al. (1992a)	Esophageal epitheliosis, 234/44	Compound Dangshen pill (2 years)	Placebo	Incidence of cancer ($P < 0.05$)
Hou et al. (1992b)	Esophageal epitheliosis, 400/237	Compound Cangdou pill (2 years)	Placebo	Incidence of cancer ($P < 0.05$)
Hou et al. (1996)	Esophageal epitheliosis, 396/223	Compound Cangdou pill (5 years)	Placebo	Incidence of cancer ($P < 0.05$)
He et al. (1998)	Esophageal epitheliosis, 214/128	Liuwei Dihuang pill (2 years)	Not stated	Incidence of cancer ($P < 0.05$)
Lin et al. (1998)	Esophageal epitheliosis, 2168/4583	Zengsheng pill	Placebo	Incidence of cancer ($P < 0.05$)
Oka et al. (1995)	Cirrhosis, 260	Sho-saiko-to (TJ-9) + usual care (5 years)	Usual care	Incidence of cancer and survival rate ($P < 0.05$)
Luo et al. (2005)	Gular precancerous lesion, 17/16	Self-prescribed herbal decoction (5–20 days)	Usual care	Incidence of cancer ($P < 0.05$) Reduction of recurrence rate ($P > 0.05$)

CAG: chronic atrophic gastritis; IM: intestinal metaplasia; ATP: atypical hyperplasia

Among the trials, over half (12 of 21 trials) used histopathological changes (surrogate outcome) as the outcome measures instead of confirmed end-point such as incidence of cancer. We don't have solid evidence that pathological diagnosis is a reliable indicator to predict cancer. Therefore, further evidence from long-term follow up studies is needed to confirm the positive conclusions.

No cohort study on secondary prophylaxis of cancer in relation to TCM was identified.

14.5.3 Tertiary Prophylaxis

Nineteen trials investigated TCM interventions for the control of treatment related side effects such as nausea and vomiting related to chemo/radiotherapy (Table 14.2). Thirteen trials studied the recurrence of diseases and cancer metastasis (Table 14.3).

Table 14.2 Summary of Chinese herbal interventions for prevention for complication of chemo/radiotherapy in RCTs

Study	Participants, T/C	Intervention	Control	Main finding (*P*-value)
Deng and Zhou (2002)	Nasopharyngeal carcinoma, 50/50	Jinyinhua Decoction	No treatment	Grade of radioactivity stomatitis ($P < 0.05$)
Lin (2003)	Nasopharyngeal carcinoma, 50/50	Biyanling Pill and radiotherapy	Radiotherapy and usual care	Incidence rate of radioactivity stomatitis ($P < 0.05$)
Zhao et al. (2003)	Nasopharyngeal carcinoma, 21/20	Yangyin Shengjin Tea and radiotherapy	Radiotherapy	Radiotherapy reaction on oral mucous membrane ($P < 0.05$)
Su and Han (2004)	Nasopharyngeal carcinoma, 41/41	Yangyin Shengjin Tea and radiotherapy	Radiotherapy and usual care	Radiotherapy reaction on oral mucous membrane ($P < 0.01$)
Wang (2008)	Nasopharyngeal carcinoma, 13/13	Yiqi Shengjin Jiedu Decoction and radiotherapy	Radiotherapy	Radiotherapy reaction on oral mucous membrane ($P < 0.05$)
Zhou et al. (2005)	Nasopharyngeal carcinoma, 20/20	Self-prescribed herbal decoction and radiotherapy	Radiotherapy	Incidence rate of oral ulcer ($P < 0.01$)
Zou et al. (2005)	Nasopharyngeal carcinoma, 55/54	Self-prescribed herbal decoction and radiotherapy	Radiotherapy/ usual care	Incidence rate of radioactivity stomatitis ($P < 0.05$)
Liang et al. (2006)	Pectoral tumour, 70/78	Kangxian Decoction and radiotherapy	Radiotherapy and placebo	Incidence rate of radioactivity pneumonia/pulmonary fibrosis ($P < 0.01$)
Fei et al. (2008)	Pectoral cancer, 69/76	Huaxian Decoction and radiotherapy	Radiotherapy	Incidence rate of radioactivity pneumonia/pulmonary fibrosis ($P < 0.001$)

Table 14.2 (continued)

Study	Participants, T/C	Intervention	Control	Main finding (P-value)
Mori et al. (1998)	Non-resectable and untreated non-small cell lung cancer, 18/23	Hangeshashin-to (TJ-14)	No treatment	Improvement in the grade of diarrhea ($P = 0.044$), incidence of diarrhea grade 3 and above ($p = 0.018$), frequency of diarrhea and duration of diarrhea ($p>0.05$)
Cao et al. (2006)	Advanced non-small cell lung cancer, 25/20	Shenmai Injection and chemotherapy	Chemotherapy	Karnofsky scoring and body weight ($P < 0.05$), reduction of decrease of leukocyte and hemoglobin ($P < 0.05$), improvement of thrombocytopenia, reduction of occurrence of nausea/vomiting, alleviating injury of liver and kidney function (only lower value in treatment group with $P > 0.05$)
Liu et al. (2005)	Liver cancer, 33/33	Fuzheng Yiai Decoction and chemotherapy	Chemotherapy	Incidence rate of nausea/vomiting ($P < 0.05$)
Zhang et al. (2006)	Acute leukemia, 17/14	Self-prescribed herbal decoction	Usual care	Incidence rate of complication ($P < 0.05$)
Lu (1998)	Trophobiastic disease, 96/32	Self-prescribed herbal decoction and chemotherapy	Chemotherapy	Chemo reaction of gastrointestinal tract and incidence rate of complication ($P < 0.05$)
Bao et al. (2008)	Colon cancer, 50/47	Self-prescribed herbal decoction and chemotherapy	Chemotherapy/ usual care	Incidence rate/grade of dental ulcer ($P < 0.05$)

Table 14.2 (continued)

Study	Participants, T/C	Intervention	Control	Main finding (*P*-value)
Mok et al. (2007)	Breast or colon cancer, 60/60	Self-prescribed herbal tea	Placebo	Incidence of grade 3/4 anemia, leukopenia, neutropenia and thrombocytopenia ($P = 0.27, 0.37, 0.63$ and 0.13, respectively); incidence of grade 2 nausea ($P = 0.04$)
Liu (2009)	Gastric/colon/rectal cancer, 34/34	Huoxue Tongluo Decoction and usual care	Usual care	Incidence rate of reaction of neurotoxicity ($P < 0.01$)
Yuan and Jiang (2007)	Cancer (totally 4 types of cancer, all revived chemotherapy), 30/30	Xuanfu Daizhe Decoction and chemotherapy and usual care	Chemotherapy/ usual care	Incidence rate of nausea/vomiting ($P < 0.05$)
Chen and Zheng (2005)	Cancer (totally 5 types of cancer, all received surgery), 33/33	Self-prescribed herbal decoction and Chinese patent medicine and chemotherapy	Chemotherapy/ usual care	Incidence rate of dental ulcer ($P < 0.01$)

Table 14.2 summarized 19 RCTs testing Chinese patent medicine (3 trials), herbal decoction (15 trials) and 1 Kampo-medicine (originated from Chinese herbal medicine Banxia Xiexin Decoction) in relieving post-chemo/radiotherapy nausea and vomiting (4 trials) and cancer-related complications (17 trials). The conditions were related to chemo/radiotherapy, including neurotoxicity, oral mucous ulcers, nausea/vomiting, radiotherapy related pneumonia or pulmonary fibrosis, stomatitis. All the trials reported positive findings favoring herbal medicines in prevention of chemo/radiotherapy related conditions.

Thirteen RCTs studied Chinese herbal interventions for prevention of cancer recurrence or metastasis after surgery or chemo/radiotherapy (Table 14.3), and the tested herbal interventions included Chinese patent medicine (3 trials), herbal extract (1 trial) and herbal decoctions (9 trials). Majority of the trials reported increased survival by preventing the recurrence of cancer or tumour metastasis. The treatment duration varied from 7 days to 1 year (mean 7.0 ± 8.2 months). One RCT found no significant effect on cancer recurrence rate between herbal decoction and chemotherapy (Han 2005).

Oral mucositis caused by chemo/radiotherapy (including bone marrow transplant) for cancer can lower the quality of life in patients, causing discomfort, pain,

Table 14.3 Summary of Chinese herbal interventions for prevention of cancer recurrent or metastasis after surgery in RCTs

Study	Participants, T/C	Intervention (duration)	Control	Main finding (*P*-value)
Chen et al. (1996)	Bladder cancer 58/45	Compound Ezhuye (>2 months)	Usual care	Reduction of recurrence rate ($P < 0.05$)
Guan et al. (2006)	Bladder cancer, 48/48	Donglingcao Decoction (2 years)	Usual care	Reduction of recurrence rate ($P < 0.05$)
Chang (2007)	Bladder cancer, 82/72	Donglingcao Decoction (12–18 months)	Usual care	Reduction of recurrence rate ($P < 0.05$)
Li et al. (2004)	Gastric cancer(postoperative), 45/43	Jianpi Xiaoliu Decoction and chemotherapy (3 months)	Chemotherapy	1/2/3 years survival rate and recurrence/metastasis rate ($P < 0.05$)
Yang et al. (2003)	Progressive staged gastric cancer 59/58/31[a]	Weichangan/ Weichangan and chemotherapy (> = 6 months)	Chemotherapy	1/2/3 years survival rate and metastasis rate, quality of life, tumour-bearing survival time (apart from 2/3 years metastasis rate, the rest showed significant result with $P < 0.05$)
Xiang et al. (2002)	Breast cancer, 50/50	Juzao Pill and chemotherapy	Chemotherapy	5 years survival rate and recurrence/metastasis rate ($P < 0.05$)
Ma et al. (2005)	Colon cancer (postoperative), 28/25	Herbal decoction and chemotherapy (3 months)	Chemotherapy	1/2/3 years survival rate and recurrence/metastasis rate ($P < 0.05$)
Zhu et al. (2006)	Poorly differentiated adenocarcinoma on antrum of stomach with cancerous ascites, 40/40	Fuzheng Kang'ai Powder and chemotherapy	Chemotherapy	Median survival time and 1 year survival rate ($P < 0.05$)
Han (2005)	Cancer (including 5 different types of cancer, all received surgery), 52/47	Self-prescribed herbal decoction	Chemotherapy	Reduction of recurrence rate ($P > 0.05$)
Feng et al. (2005)	Primary liver carcinoma, 20/20/20/20[b]	Ginsenosides (7 days)	Dexamethasone, placebo	Prevention of postembolization syndrome after TACE

Table 14.3 (continued)

Study	Participants, T/C	Intervention (duration)	Control	Main finding (*P*-value)
Chang et al. (1999)	Nasopharyngeal carcinoma, 60/46	Shengjinye and radiotherapy	Radiotherapy	1/2 years survival rate and recurrence/metastasis rate ($P < 0.05$)
He (2007)	Esophageal cancer, 137/130	Shunshi decoction and radiotherapy	Radiotherapy	Incidence of radioactivity esophagitis ($P < 0.05$)
Rao et al. (2002)	Multiple adenomatous polyposis coli, 110/100	Self-prescribed herbal decoction and usual care (3 months)	Usual care	Reduction of recurrence rate ($P < 0.05$)

[a]This trial has three-arm trial with the third group as control.
[b]This trial has four arms, 3 of which were treatment groups while 1 was control group applying placebo.
TACE: transcatheter arterial chemoembolization

difficulties in eating, and prolonged stay in hospital. One Cochrane review that included 2 randomized trials evaluated the effectiveness of prophylactic agents for oral mucositis in cancer patients receiving chemo/radial therapy (Worthington et al. 2007). In patients with head and neck cancer and other solid cancers, Chinese herbal medicine was found to be more effective than Dobell's Solution. Chinese medicine showed a benefit for increased levels of mucositis severity in patients with head and neck cancer and other solid cancers with RR of 0.44 (95% CI 0.20–0.96), 0.44 (95% CI 0.33–0.59) and 0.16 (95% CI 0.07–0.35), respectively. The strength of the evidence (33% of trials were deemed at low risk of bias, 32% at medium risk of bias and 36% high risk of bias) and implications for practice include consideration that benefits may be specific for certain cancer types and treatment. There was a need for trials that included sufficient numbers of participants to enable subgroup analyses by type of disease and chemotherapeutic agents.

One Cochrane review studied the use of stimulating acupuncture points for alleviation of chemotherapy treatment related nausea and vomiting (Ezzo et al. 2006). Acupuncture points could be stimulated by electroacupuncture, manual acupuncture, acupressure (finger pressing on acupuncture points) or electrical stimulation on the skin surface such as wristwatch-like devices. Data from 11 trials involving 1,247 patients were pooled. Overall, acupuncture-point stimulation of all methods combined reduced the incidence of acute vomiting (RR = 0.82; 95% CI 0.69 to 0.99; $P = 0.04$), but not acute or delayed nausea severity compared to control. Modality, stimulation with needles reduced the severity of acute vomiting (RR = 0.74; 95% CI 0.58–0.94; $P = 0.01$), but did not reduce the severity of acute nausea. Electroacupuncture reduced the proportion of acute vomiting in patients (RR = 0.76; 95% CI 0.60–0.97; $P = 0.02$), while manual acupuncture did not. Exact symptoms for acupuncture treatment were not reported. Acupressure reduced mean acute nausea severity (SMD = –0.19; 95% CI –0.37 to –0.01; $P = 0.04$) but not acute vomiting or delayed symptoms. Noninvasive electrostimulation showed no benefit for any outcome. All trials used concomitant pharmacologic antiemetics, and all, except electroacupuncture trials, used state-of-the-art antiemetics. The author concluded that the review suggested a possible biologic effect of acupuncture-point stimulation on the severity and frequency of nausea as side effects of chemotherapy treatment. Electroacupuncture demonstrated benefit for chemotherapy-induced acute vomiting, but studies combining electroacupuncture with state-of-the-art antiemetics and in patients with refractory symptoms were needed to determine clinical relevance. Self-administered acupressure appeared to have a protective effect against acute nausea though studies did not involve placebo control. Noninvasive electrostimulation appears unlikely to have clinically relevant impact when patients were given state-of-the-art pharmacologic antiemetic therapy.

To sum up, electroacupuncture reduced first-day vomiting, but manual acupuncture did not. Acupressure reduced first-day nausea, but was not effective on later days. Acupressure showed no benefit for vomiting. Electrical stimulation on the skin showed no benefit. All trials also gave antiemetics, but the drugs used in the electroacupuncture trials were not the most modern drugs, so it was not known whether electroacupuncture adds anything to modern drugs. Trials of electroacupuncture with modern drugs are needed.

We have identified 2 more RCTs evaluating acupuncture or auricular therapy for the prophylaxis of chemotherapy-induced nausea/vomiting, which showed significant positive results. One RCT with 60 cancer participants compared auricular acupuncture plus acupuncture and chemotherapy with chemotherapy and usual care, and the results showed a reduction of incidence rate of nausea and vomiting ($P < 0.05$) (Cao and Cao 2007). Another RCT with 43 cancer participants comparing auricular acupuncture plus chemotherapy and usual care with chemotherapy and usual care also demonstrated beneficial effect on reducing the severity of nausea and vomiting ($P < 0.05$) (Fu 2007).

One RCT evaluating the effectiveness of using acupressure in Pericardium 6 (Neiguan) acu-point in managing chemotherapy-induced nausea and vomiting in 36 patients with breast cancer (17 in treatment and 19 in control) found that the treatment could significantly reduce nausea and retching experience, occurrence and distress ($P < 0.05$), and it showed a close to significance ($P = 0.06$) in vomiting experience (Molassiotis et al. 2007).

One randomized multicenter crossover pilot trial in Germany found in 23 children receiving highly emetogenic chemotherapy for treatment of solid malignant tumours and together with standard antiemetic medication that acupuncture seemed to be effective in preventing nausea and vomiting as it showed significant reduction in number of episodes of vomiting ($P = 0.001$) and episodes of vomiting ($P = 0.01$) compared with the control which did not receive acupuncture (Gottschling et al. 2008).

One randomized crossover trial in USA (Jones et al. 2008) determining the feasibility and effectiveness of acupressure in preventing chemotherapy-associated nausea in children receiving standard antiemetics at the same time found no significantly more effectiveness of the treatment than placebo among 21 patients.

One randomized cross-over pilot study (Melchart et al. 2006) investigating whether a combination of acupuncture and acupressure was effective for reducing chemotherapy-induced nausea and vomiting in 28 patients receiving moderately of highly emetogenic chemotherapy and conventional standard antiemesis found no difference between the treatment at PC6 Point and at the sham point for the nausea score, but the level of nausea was very low in both phases, 6.2 (standard deviation 9.0) for treatment at PC6 and 6.3 (9.1) for treatment at the sham point (mean difference –0.1, 95% CI –3.9 to 3.7; $P = 0.96$). Seventeen of 21 participants completing the study would desire acupuncture and acupressure for future chemotherapy cycles, but there was no clear preference for either point.

14.6 Conclusion

We totally included 5 systematic reviews/meta-analysis and 61 clinical trials. Of the total number of trials (61), 85.2% were published in Chinese. The majority of these were of poor quality. In majority of studies, outcome measures were poorly defined, and there were significant differences in the sample size of study groups and follow up.

More rigorously designed and conducted studies are needed to establish a stronger evidence base for TCM interventions at different levels of cancer prevention. Observational studies should be promoted as these will have the capability to better reflect the whole TCM system theory on syndrome differentiation, which is the basis for the TCM treatment modalities.

With the knowledge of the need for improvement of the quality of studies addressing benefits of TCM in prevention of cancer disease current existing guidelines – the Consolidated Standards of Reporting Trials (CONSORT) statement should be promoted and actively used in the planning and implementation of clinical trials (Altman 1996; Rennie 1996; Altman et al. 2001; Moher et al. 2001). CONSORT statement has been translated into several languages to facilitate awareness and dissemination. More recently, an elaborated CONSORT Statement (CONSORT Statement for Herbal Medicine) was published in the aim of leading and encouraging more complete and accurate reporting of herbal trials (Gagnier et al. 2006). For acupuncture, or acupoint stimulations, the Standards for reporting interventions in controlled trials of acupuncture (STRICTA) recommendations have been available since 2001 (Macpherson et al. 2001). For the meta-analysis of observational studies, Meta-analysis Of Observational Studies in Epidemiology (MOOSE) can be followed (Stroup et al. 2000).

References

Altman DG. Better reporting of randomized controlled trials: the CONSORT statement. BMJ. 1996;313:570–1.

Altman DG, Schulz KF, Moher D, et al. CONSORT GROUP (Consolidated Standards of Reporting Trials). The revised CONSORT statement for reporting randomized trials: explanation and elaboration. Ann Intern Med. 2001;134:663–94.

Bao NX, Zeng GZ, Zhou LW, et al. Preventive effect of self-made gargle solution on chemotherapy-induced oral ulcer in patient with colorectal carcinoma. J Nurs Sci. 2008;23:44–5.

Cao CC, Cao XJ. Effect of acupuncture therapy and auricular points compression on nausea and vomiting caused by chemotherapy. J Nurs Sci. 2007;22:29–30.

Cao Y, Li P, Tan KJ. Clinical observation on Shenmai injection in preventing and treating adverse reaction of chemotherapy on advanced non-small cell lung cancer. Zhongguo Zhong Xi Yi Jie He Za Zhi. 2006;26:550–2.

Chang J. Thermotherapy with rabdosia rubesens in preventing recurrence of tumor of bladder. J Med Forum. 2007;28:103.

Chang ZL, Lin XM, Wang XL, et al. Effect of combination of traditional Chinese medicine and radiotherapy on nasopharyngeal carcinoma. J Oncol. 1999;5:230–1.

Chen CY, Zheng YZ. Clinical study on prevention of oral ulcers caused by chemotherapy with combined therapy of centrum and specific Chinese herbs that invigorate the function of the spleen and regulate the flow of qi. Chin J Clin Nutr. 2005;13:398–400.

Chen GH, Liu HJ, Li HH, et al. Clinical observation on therapeutic effect of Jiedu Huoxue decoction on gastric ulcer complicated with gastric precancerous lesion. J Sichuan Tradit Chin Med. 2008;26:51–2.

Chen JZ, Ji WS, Pei JY, et al. Observation of therapeutic effect of compound Ezhu decoction in preventing postoperative superficial bladder tumor recurrence. Shandong Med J. 1996;36:55.

Chen WL, Pan YB, Cai G. 30 cases of clinical study of modified Weierfang Decoction on gastric precancerous lesions. J Tradit Chin Med. 2002;43:275–6.

Chen ZF, Hou J, Zhang JH. Meta-analysis of the studies on Chinese herbal medicine for esophageal epitheliosis. Pract J Integr Chin Mod Med. 1998;11:746.

Deng ZX, Zhou FL. Evaluation on the effects of Jinyin flower liquor for mouthwash in the prevention of pharyngo – oral complication of NPC patents treated with radiotherapy. Guangxi Med J. 2002;24:1744–5.

Ezzo JM, Richardson MA, Vickers A, et al. Acupuncture-point stimulation for chemotherapy-induced nausea or vomiting. Cochrane Database Syst Rev. 2006;2:CD002285.

Fei Y, Kong QZ, Zhang LJ. Clinical research for radiation pulmonary injuries caused by radiotherapy for chest tumors with melt fibrosis traditional Chinese medicine. Liao Ning J Traditional Chin Med. 2008;35:225–6.

Feng YL, Ling CQ, Zhu DZ, et al. Ginsenosides combined with dexamethasone in preventing and treating postembolization syndrome following transcatheter arterial chemoembolization: a randomized, controlled and double-blinded prospective trial. Zhong Xi Yi Jie He Xue Bao. 2005;3:99–102.

Fu Y. Effectiveness observation on auricular acupuncture for nausea and vomiting induced by chemotherapy. Pract Diagn Ther Integr Tradit Chin West Med. 2007;7:49–50.

Fulder S. The handbook of alternative and complementary medicine. Oxford: Oxford University Press. 1996

Gagnier JJ, Boon H, Rochon P, et al. CONSORT Group. Reporting randomized, controlled trials of herbal interventions: an elaborated CONSORT statement. Ann Intern Med. 2006;144:364–7.

Gottschling S, Reindl TK, Meyer S, et al. Acupuncture to alleviate chemotherapy-induced nausea and vomiting in pediatric oncology – A randomized multicenter crossover pilot trial. Klinische Padiatrie. 2008;220:365–70.

Guan JY, Zhao GX, Zhang WX, et al. The anticancer recurrence effects of rabdosia rubescens (hemls) hara on the hyperthermia therapy of bladder cancer. Central Plains Med J. 2006;33: 24–5.

Haas SA, Hackbarth DR, Black JM, et al. Medical-surgical nursing: Clinical management for positive outcomes, 6th edn. Philadelphia: WB Saunders; 2001: 84–7.
Han KX. Clinical study of therapeutic effect of self-refit Kangai Yihao decoction in preventing tumor recurrence or metastasis after surgery. Chin Med Hyg. 2005;6:34–5.
He FX. Clinical study on the prevention and cure effect of Shunshi decoction. China Med Her. 2007;4:36–8.
He XX, Yan SC, Wang ED, et al. The result analysis of cytology diagnosis when Liuwei Dihuang pill is used to treat the precancerous lesion in oesophagus and gastric cardia. Hebei Med. 1998;4:1–3.
Hou J, Yan FR, Li SS, et al. A clinical research on precancerous lesion of esophagus treated with compound Dang Shen pill. China J Tradit Chin Med Pharm. 1992a;7:11–2.
Hou J, Yan FR, Li SS, et al. Clinical study of compound Cang Dou pill on esophageal precancerous lesion. Chin J Integr Med. 1992b;12:604–6.
Hou J, Chen ZF, Li SS, et al. Clinical study on treatment of esophageal precancerous lesion with Cang Dou pill. Chin J Clin Oncol. 1996;24:117–20.
Jones E, Isom S, Kemper K.J. Acupressure for chemotherapy-associated nausea and vomiting in children. J Soc Integr Oncol. 2008;6:141–5.
Kan SY, Chen RF, You ZS, et al. 49 cases clinical study of therapeutic effect of Yangyin Rongwei Decoction on chronic atrophic gastritis complicated with precancerous lesions. J Tradit Chin Med. 1999;40:601–2.
Li M. The clinical and experimental studies of QLSP Granule in treating precancerous lesions of chronic atrophic gastritis (CAG). Shandong, China: Dissertation for Master Degree of Shandong University of Traditional Chinese Medicine; 2004.
Li YM, Yue FH, Tan XY, et al. Clinical observation of Jianpi Huatan Decoction in preventing post-operative gastric tumor recurrence and metastasis. Chin Arch Tradit Chin Med. 2004;22:1337, 57.
Liang PY, Li Q, Chen XX, et al. Clinical research for radiation pulmonary injuries caused by radiotherapy for chest tumors with ant-fibrosis traditional Chinese medicine. Cancer Res Clin. 2006;18:608–9.
Lin GH. Effectiveness observation on Bi Yan Ling pill for treatment and prevention of radioactive oropharyngeal reaction. Henan J Oncol. 2003;16:385.
Lin PZ, Zhang JS, Rong ZP, et al. Therapeutic block of medicine in treating esophageal precancerous lesion: triennial and lustrum effect for therapeutic block of Kang Ai Yi Tablet, Viaminati and Riboflavin. Acta Acad Med Sin. 1990;12:235–45.
Lin PZ, Chen ZF, Hou J, et al. Chemoprophylaxis of esophageal cancer. Acta Acad Med Sin. 1998;20:413–8.
Linda H Yoder. Let's talk 'cancer prevention'. MedSurg Nursing. In: Fulder S (Ed). The handbook of alternative and complementary medicine. Oxford: Oxford University Press; 1996. http://findarticles.com/p/articles/mi_m0FSS/is_3_14/ai_n17209497/. Accessed 24 May 2009.
Liu J, Xing J, Fei Y. Green tea (*Camellia sinensis*) and cancer prevention: a systematic review of randomized trials and epidemiological studies. Chin Med. 2008;3:12.
Liu JL, Wang XH, Guo XG, et al. Chemotherapy combined with Fuzheng Yi'ai Decoction for advanced liver cancer in 33 cases. Tradit Chin Med Res. 2005;34:6.
Liu SQ. Care observation of Huoxue Tongluo Decoction for prevention of neurotoxicity reaction induced by oxaliplatin chemotherapy. Beijing J Tradit Chin Med. 2009;28:45–6.
Liu YS, Wei YZ, Tang YQ. Clinical observation of therapeutic effect of Weiyan Qing Tablet on gastric precancerous lesions. J Liaoning Coll Tradit Chin Med. 2000;2:197–8.
Liu ZW, Zhang XX. Meta-analysis of effectiveness of Chinese medicine for gastric precancerous lesion. Mod J Integr Tradit Chin West Med. 2005;14:2818–20.
Lu XH. Chinese medicine for the prevention and treatment of gastrointestinal reaction by chemotherapy. Res Pract Chin Med. 1998;12:62.

Luo KQ, Zhang XB, Wang NY, et al. A comparative study on the therapeutic effects of laryngomicrosurgery and integrative medicine therapy on precancerous lesions in the larynx. Chin Otorhinolaryngol J Integr Med. 2005;13:262–4.

Ma J, Wang GH, Cai DF, et al. Clinical observation of Jianpi Xiaoliu Decoction in preventing postoperative colorectal carcinoma recurrence and metastasis. Shanghai J Tradit Chin Med. 2005;39:24–5.

MacPherson H, White A, Cummings M, et al. Towards better standards of reporting controlled trials of acupuncture: the STRICTA statement. Complement Ther Med. 2001;9:246–249.

Melchart D, Ihbe-Heffinger A, Leps B, et al. Acupuncture and acupressure for the prevention of chemotherapy-induced nausea – A randomised cross-over pilot study. Support Care Cancer. 2006;14:878–82.

Mo TS. Clinical observation of Yiqi Yangyin Huayu decoction on chronic atrophic gastritis complicated with precancerous lesion. J Emerg Tradit Chin Med. 2005;14:523–4.

Moher D, Schulz KF, Altman DG, et al. The CONSORT statement: revised recommendations for improving the quality of reports of parallel-group randomized trials. J Am Podiatr Med Assoc. 2001;91:437–42.

Mok TS, Yeo W, Johnson PJ, et al. A double-blind placebo-controlled randomized study of Chinese herbal medicine as complementary therapy for reduction of chemotherapy-induced toxicity. Ann Oncol. 2007;18:768–74.

Molassiotis A, Helin AM, Dabbour R, et al. The effects of P6 acupressure in the prophylaxis of chemotherapy-related nausea and vomiting in breast cancer patients. Complement Ther Med. 2007;15:3–12.

Mori K, Hirose T, Machida S, et al. Kampo medicines for the prevention of irinotecan-induced diarrhea in advanced non-small cell lung cancer. Gan To Kagaku Ryoho. 1998;25:1159–63.

National Cancer Institute Cancer Prevention Program Review Group. Report of the National Cancer Institute Cancer Prevention Program Review Group. http://deainfo.nci.nih.gov/ADVISORY/bsa/bsa_program/bsacaprevnt.htm#1. Accessed 16 June 2009.

Oka H, Yamamoto S, Kuroki T, et al. Prospective study of chemoprevention of hepatocellular carcinoma with Sho-saiko-to (TJ-9). Cancer. 1995;76:743–9.

Rao ZF, Chen B, Liu WQ. Using herbal medicine to treat 110 patients with multiple adenomatous polyp of colon to prevent the recurrence. J Tradit Chin Med. 2002;43:131.

Rennie D. How to report randomized controlled trials: the CONSORT statement. JAMA. 1996;276:649.

Stroup DF, Berlin JA, Morton SC, et al. Meta-analysis of observational studies in epidemiology: a proposal for reporting. Meta-analysis Of Observational Studies in Epidemiology (MOOSE) group. JAMA. 2000;283:2008–12.

Su QZ, Han XY. Prevention from radiation reaction on nasopharyngeal carcinoma (NPC) patients by YangYinShengJin Tea. J Qilu Nurs. 2004;10:163–4.

Tian LX, Xu HD. 45 cases clinical observation of Shenyi Decoction on chronic atrophic gastritis. Hunan Guid J Tradit Chin Med Pharmacol. 2000; 6:21–2.

Wang SS. Observation on tonifying qi, producing fluid and detoxify methods preventing and treating pharynx mucosa injury after radiotherapy nasopharyngeal carcinoma in clinic. Liao Ning J Tradit Chin Med. 2008;35:1176–7.

Wang ZK, Liu QQ, Liu XH, et al. Clinical observation of Jiedu Huoxue Decoction in treating precancerous lesion of gastric cancer with gastric ulcer. Shanghai J Tradit Chin Med. 2006;40:23–4.

Wei BH, Zhang ZH, Yang LC, et al. Clinical and experimental study of Wei An Su in chronic atrophic gastritis. World Chin J Digestol. 1998;6:114–7.

World Health Organization 2005. WHA58.22 Cancer prevention and control, The Fifty-eighth World Health Assembly. http://www.who.int/cancer/media/news/WHA58%2022-en.pdf. Accessed 16 June 2009.

World Health Organization 2007. The World Health Organization's fight against cancer: strategies that prevent, cure and care. http://www.who.int/cancer/publicat/WHOCancerBrochure2007.FINALweb.pdf. Accessed 16 June 2009.

Worthington HV, Clarkson JE, Eden OB. Interventions for preventing oral mucositis for patients with cancer receiving treatment. Cochrane Database Syst Rev. 2007;4: CD000978.
Xiang LP, Ouyang H, Xiao YL. Clinical observation of Ju Zao pill in preventing postoperative mammary cancer recurrence and metastasis. Chin J Clin Pharmacol Ther. 2002;7:63–4.
Yang J.K, Zhen J, Shen KP. Clinical study on post-operative metastasis prevention of progressive stage of gastric cancer by Weichang'an. Zhongguo Zhong Xi Yi Jie He Za Zhi. 2003;3:580–2.
Yao BT, Wang L, Wang HJ, et al. Clinical observation and experimental study of therapeutic effect of Weisuo Kang Granules on chronic atrophic gastritis complicated with precancerous lesions. J Tradit Chin Med. 1999;40:673–6.
Yu DM, Sun CD, Lu WJ, et al. The clinical effect by using Xialian Yiying Soup in CAG of humid heat to hinder type. Chin Arch Tradit Chin Med. 2008;26:2621–2.
Yuan TC, Jiang JB. Effectiveness observation on modified Xuanfu Daizhe decoction combined with Ondansetron for the prevention of nausea and vomiting after chemotherapy. Clin J Tradit Chin Med. 2007;19:4–5.
Zhang H, Tong CZ, Qi Y. Clinical observation of therapeutic effect of modified Si Ni powder on chronic atrophic gastritis. J Hubei Coll Tradit Chin Med. 2007;9:45–6.
Zhang JS, Lin PZ, Rong ZP, et al. Therapeutic block with Kang Ai Yi tablet for esophageal precancerous lesion. J Tradit Chin Med. 1990;31:23–5.
Zhang YY, Lan H, Zhao F, et al. Treatment based on syndrome differentiation on refractory leukemia. Int Med Health Guid News. 2006;12:157–9.
Zhao T, Wei BH, Li X. Observation on preventing and vontrolling mouth mucositis of 41 cases with therapy of nourishing Yin to produce body fluid after radiotherapy of nasopharyngeal cancer. J Beijing Univ Tradit Chin Med (Clin Med). 2003;10:16–7.
Zhou ZX, Zhang ZR, Qian HX, et al. Prevention and treatment with traditional Chinese medicine for dental ulcer caused by radiotherapy and chemotherapy. Henan J Oncol. 2005;339:40.
Zou YH, Liu XM, Tan LR. Clinical study on Chinese herbal medicine for prevention and treatment of 60 cases of acute radiation oropharyngeal inflammation of nasopharyngeal carcinoma. J Tradit Chin Med. 2005;30:520–2.
Zhu JS, Song MQ, Wang L, et al. Immunoregulation and short-term therapeutic effects of superselective intra-arterial chemotherapy combined with traditional Chinese drugs on gastric cancer patients. J Chin Integr Med. 2006;4:478–81.

Index

DOI 10.1007/978-90-481-3555-4,